Treating NVLD in Children

Jessica Broitman · John M. Davis
Editors

Treating NVLD in Children

Professional Collaborations for Positive Outcomes

Springer

Editors
Jessica Broitman
Clinic and Training Center
San Francisco Psychotherapy
Research Group
San Francisco, CA, USA

John M. Davis
California State University, East Bay
Hayward, CA, USA

ISBN 978-1-4614-6178-4 ISBN 978-1-4614-6179-1 (eBook)
DOI 10.1007/978-1-4614-6179-1
Springer New York Heidelberg Dordrecht London

Library of Congress Control Number: 2012955367

Printed on acid-free paper

Springer is part of Springer Science+Business Media (www.springer.com)

To J the start of it all, who still continues to amaze us in every way!

Foreword

Fifteen years ago, my daughter was diagnosed with a nonverbal learning disorder (NVLD) by her fourth grade educational team. At the time, there was scant literature for parents or providers on this complex disorder and I remember the avalanche of questions that began to erupt as our family came to grips with trying to understand this new condition, how to find professionals who understood NVLD, how to provide our daughter with the appropriate treatment, and the implications NVLD had for her growth and development. At the time, I was starting a tenure track, academic position in nursing and decided to study the families of children with NVLD and Asperger Syndrome (Little, 2002, 2003, 2006). Since then, there has been a steady increase in the literature on NVLD and a number of related fields.

Nonverbal Learning Disorder or (NVLD) is a brain-based, neurodevelopmental childhood disorder that expresses itself in several different domains: serious problems in the area of social competencies, academic performance in math, reading comprehension and reasoning, visual–spatial perception, and motor coordination. Part of the challenge in diagnosis is that children with NVLD may exhibit different degrees of severity in each domain, or not exhibit any deficits in some domains. Although classified as a learning disorder, it shares characteristics with autism spectrum disorders such as Asperger's yet receives far less attention, funding, and research focus than autism-related disorders.

Broitman and Davis describe in this comprehensive, and thoughtful, new book a breathtakingly comprehensive history and evolution of our understanding of NVLD, followed by in-depth treatment reviews from those practitioners most likely to be involved in the treatment and care of children and young adults with NVLD.

What is different and welcomed about Broitman and Davis's book is that they frame each chapter by posing the same essential questions regarding the identification and treatment of children with NVLD to each contributor, thereby highlighting the importance of the multidisciplinary team approach in treating children with NVLD, and providing readers with an integrated synthesis and thread to essential questions in the identification and treatment of the various problems children with NVLD face. Psychologists and neuropsychologists, occupational therapists, special education teachers, speech and language therapists, coaches and parents will all benefit from this content. Moreover, the early chapters on interdisciplinary assessment provide new ideas regarding the diagnosing of NVLD moving our thinking from a subtype model to a multidisciplinary conceptualization of the disorder.

Broitman and Davis's careful attention to current evidence-based treatments or lack thereof for this complex disorder from the perspective of the different practitioners is a helpful addition to the current field. A developing child with NVLD is likely to have deficits in a significant number of different domains, all requiring remediation and treatment. This volume pulls together the treatment interventions available from the perspective of the occupational therapist, reading and math educators, speech and language therapist, clinical therapist, vocational counselor, and college guidance specialist thereby addressing the essential treatment needs in individual domains. Each chapter contains a wealth of careful detail to current research and evidence to validate current treatment recommendations.

Different from previous volumes on NVLD, Broitman and Davis include chapters on services for young adults with NVLD who are entering college and the work force and provide the reader with materials that target developmental transitions and possible pitfalls for young adults with NVLD. As the field has grown over the last 15 years, so has the need for attention to the issues facing the young adult with NVLD. Family and first-person accounts also grace the book, adding a textured and grounded perspective to the rigorous chapters on treatment.

Some of the seminal writing on nonverbal learning disorders in the 1980s and 1990s is now dated, and this book honors those early contributions to our understanding while moving forward with detailed descriptions of current diagnostic practices and treatment perspectives. As in much of the past writing on NVLD, Broitman and Davis's volume does not offer new answers to the ongoing controversies concerning diagnostic criteria, etiology, and overlaps with other neurodevelopmental disorders but does highlight how these questions continue to evolve in the field's research. What the book does provide is a thorough, current, and detailed evidence-based review of treatments for NLVD.

- Little, L. & Clark, R. (2006) The wonders and worries of parenting a child with Asperger Syndrome and nonverbal learning disorder: A qualitative study of 103 couples. *Maternal Child Nursing, 31*(1), 13–16.
- Little, L. (2003). Maternal perceptions of the availability, helpfulness and importance of needs for children with Asperger syndrome and nonverbal learning disorders. *Focus on Autism and Other Developmental Disabilities, 18*(4), 257–267.
- Little, L. (2002). Maternal discipline of children with Asperger Syndrome and nonverbal learning disorders. *American Journal of Maternal Child Nursing, 27*(6), 349–354.

- Little, L (2002). Differences in stress and coping of mothers and fathers of children with Asperger's syndrome and nonverbal learning disorders. *Pediatric Nursing*, *28*(6), 565569.
- Little, L. (2002). Middle-class mothers' perceptions of peer and sibling victimization among children with Asperger's syndrome and nonverbal learning disorders. *Issues in Comprehensive Pediatric Nursing, 25,* 43–57.

Biddeford, ME, USA Liza Little, Psy.D., A.P.R.N-B.C.

Acknowledgments

We would to thank Tekoa King and Gibor Basri for their careful reading, editing, and overall support during the process of writing our book. We also thank Wendy Williams for her very detailed edits! All of their thoughtful recommendations and insights proved invaluable. We also acknowledge and appreciate the patience of all our friends and families when we couldn't come out to play.

About the Editors

Jessica Broitman, Ph.D. (Coeditor) is the coauthor of Nonverbal Learning Disabilities in Children: Bridging the Gap Between Science and Practice (2011). She is the President emeritus of the San Francisco Psychotherapy Research Group and Executive Director of its Clinic and Training Center. She frequently lectures on Weiss's Control Mastery Theory worldwide. Currently a psychoanalyst in private practice since 1980, she has worked with families who have learning-disabled children for more than 10 years. She is currently involved in several research projects concerning the treatment and understanding of NVLD and has a special interest in helping professionals and families understand and treat this disorder. She is available for consultations and can be reached at: drjess@comcast.net.

John M. Davis, Ph.D. (Coeditor) is the coauthor of Nonverbal Learning Disabilities in Children: Bridging the Gap Between Science and Practice (2011). He is currently a Professor at California State University, East Bay, and Chair of the Educational Psychology Department, where he teaches and supervises. He received his Ph.D. from the U. C. Berkeley School Psychology program and did clinical postdoctoral studies to become a licensed psychologist. He has a special interest in learning and developmental disorders having been the director of a school and clinic for students with learning disabilities for 13 years, which provided diagnostic and intervention services. His current clinical work is primarily with children and adults with learning disorders. His writing and research interests include articles and book chapters in the areas of mental health consultation, suicide/crisis intervention, and learning disorders. He is available for consultation and evaluations can be reached at: jack.davis@csueastbay.edu.

Contents

Contributors

Catherine M. Brown, Ph.D., is a Licensed Educational Psychologist and coauthor of publications in the area of disabilities, directs Accessibility Services at California State University East Bay (CSUEB). Dr. Brown's research interests include individuals with disabilities, parent involvement, and multicultural issues in education. At CSUEB she developed and coordinated the College Link Program for students on the autism spectrum. This program provides academic, social, and residential "coaching" support on campus to manage students' strengths and challenges. She can be reached at: katie.brown@csueastbay.edu.

Bernadette Evans-Smith, Ph.D., is a clinical psychologist and the Clinical Director at Rush Neurobehavioral Center (RNBC), Rush University Medical Center, in Chicago, IL. She holds an Assistant Professor position in Pediatrics and Behavioral Sciences. In addition, she oversees the intervention studies conducted at RNBC and continues to provide treatment to children, teens, and families. Dr. Evans-Smith has worked at the ground level with the Social–Emotional Learning Framework (SELF) model that drives much of the research at RNBC. Her work experience extends past 27 years as a teacher and psychologist, with an expertise in servicing children with significant neurodevelopmental delays, emotional disturbance, social emotional learning problems (Autistic Spectrum Disorders, Nonverbal Learning Disabilities), chronic illness, anxiety, and attachment and mood disorders. In addition to psychotherapy, Dr. Evans-Smith has taught at universities and presented at national and international conferences regarding social skill development and intervention for children with NLD, Autism, and social emotional learning deficits for approximately the last 11 years. She can be reached at: Bernadette_evans-smith@rush.edu or address: Rush Neurobehavioral Center, 4711 West Golf Road, Suite 1100, Skokie, IL 60076, USA.

Jodene Goldenring Fine, Ph.D., is an Assistant Professor of School Psychology at Michigan State University. She received her Ph.D. in School Psychology at The University of Texas at Austin, and completed a 2-year combined clinical and research postdoctoral fellowship at Michigan State University. Her research activities are focused on neurodevelopmental barriers to learning in children and she has published numerous articles on this topic. She can be reached at: jodene.fine@gmail.com.

Lynn Koch, Ph.D., CRC, is a Professor in the Rehabilitation Education and Research Program at the University of Arkansas. She has authored or coauthored more than 85 publications on the topics of psychosocial and vocational adjustment to emerging disabilities, vocational rehabilitation consumer expectations, employment discrimination and disability, and transition of students with disabilities into postsecondary education and employment. She can be reached at: lckoch@uark.edu or address: Rehabilitation Education and Research Program, University of Arkansas, 106 Graduate Education Building, Fayetteville, AR 72701, USA.

Bridget Leary has a B.A. in psychology and is an afterschool teacher currently working in the field of educational research and applying to graduate programs in the area of School Counseling.

Meryl E. Lipton, M.D., Ph.D. is a Behavioral Pediatric Neurologist and Assistant Professor of Pediatrics at Rush University Medical Center. She is the Founder and Medical Director of the Rush Neurobehavioral Center (RNBC), an intradisciplinary clinic where neuropsychologists, pediatric neurologists, psychologists, speech/language pathologists, and education specialists serve children with a range of social emotional and neurobehavioral challenges. Dr. Lipton specializes in the diagnostic evaluation, neuropharmacology, and treatment and case management of children with brain-based social and academic learning in Chicago and Northern California. A popular speaker, Dr. Lipton regularly presents to a variety of professional organizations, schools and community groups. She can be reached at: Meryl_Lipton@rush.edu or address: 4711 W. Golf Road, Suite 1100, Skokie, IL 60076, USA.

Jennifer Wheeler Maedgen, Ph.D. is a Senior Associate Vice President in the Division of Diversity and Community Engagement and a Clinical Associate Professor in the Department of Educational Psychology at The University of Texas at Austin. She can be reached at: maedgen@austin.utexas.edu.

Marion Marshall, M.S., B.C.E.T., F.A.E.T., is an Associate Professor of Education, Holy Names University and the Coordinator of the Educational Therapy Certificate Program. Previously she was the Clinical Director of the Raskob Learning Institute. Ms. Marshall is an award-winning educator who has taught in public and independent schools and has been an Educational Therapist for the past 20 years. She is a sought-after presenter for regional, statewide and national conferences. Her current interests are linking assessment to remediation, collaborating with allied professionals across disciplines, and mentoring those who are new to the dynamic field of Educational Therapy. She can be reached at: marshall@hnu.edu.

Dianne Matthaei, E.T., is an Educational Therapist in private practice for the last 15 years. Her business, Lighthouse Learning, LLC, provides assessment and instruction for the atypical learner. Currently she also serves as a learning specialist and mathematics teacher for the Annie Wright Upper School, an International Baccalaureate school in Tacoma, Washington. She can be reached at: dmatthaei@harbornet.com or address: PO Box 64543 University Place, WA 98464, USA.

Jane McClure, M.A., is a Licensed Educational Psychologist. The focus of her work has been on college counseling and conducting psycho-educational evaluations. Jane was a partner at McClure, Mallory & Baron for more than 20 years. She frequently conducts workshops and has participated in sessions at the annual conferences for guidance counselors related to counseling college bound students who have learning disabilities and/or Attention Deficit Hyperactivity Disorder (ADHD). Jane also frequently speaks at schools throughout California on various aspects of the college admission process. She has worked as a consultant for College Board on issues related to services for students with disabilities. Jane works with students from public and independent schools throughout the Bay Area, and beyond. The most important aspect of Jane's work with students, she believes, is to find the best fit between students and the group of colleges to which they apply. She can be reached at: janemcclr@aol.com or address: McClure, Mallory, Baron & Ross, 200 Lombard Street, San Francisco, CA 94111, USA.

Brett Mills is a recent college graduate. He is happy to correspond with anyone and can be reached through the editors.

Rebecca Schatz, M.S., O.T.R/L., is a Pediatric Occupational Therapist. During the past 17 years she has worked both in Israel and Chicago, Illinois. Currently she practices in Chicago (Lincoln Park), where she works exclusively with children who have sensory processing disorders, learning disabilities, and pervasive developmental disorders. Schatz conducts both individual and group therapies for her clients utilizing the environment(s) that is most effective for each child. She frequently conducts in-services focusing on sensory integration and motor skill development for preschool and lower school programs within many of the private schools in the Chicago area. She consults and provides training for elementary school teachers in motor skill development and sensory integration techniques to use in their classrooms and leads parent discussion groups to enable parents to incorporate appropriate therapy ideas at home. She can be reached at: Rebecca.Schatz@comcast.net or address: Rebecca Schatz & Associates, Inc., 2000 N. Racine #3600 Chicago, IL 60614, USA.

Margaret Semrud-Clikeman, Ph.D., is currently a professor of Pediatrics and Division Head of Pediatric Behavioral Neuroscience at the University of Minnesota Medical School. After receiving her doctorate from the University of Georgia in 1990 she completed a postdoctoral fellowship at the Massachusetts General Hospital/Harvard Medical School, studying neuropsychological and brain morphology in children with ADHD. She continues her research interests in the areas of ADHD and educational neuroscience currently working on research in ADHD, and autistic spectrum disorders. Dr. Semrud-Clikeman and her students have developed a social competence intervention that has been successfully piloted. Dr. Semrud-Clikeman has received numerous awards and grants for her work. She has published more than 60 articles, 75 chapters, and 6 books as well as has made over 200 presentations at national and international conferences. She can be reached at: semru002@umn.edu or address: Department of Pediatrics, University of Minnesota Medical School, MMC, 486 Mayo, 8486A, 420 Delaware St. SE, Minneapolis, MN 55455, USA.

Joanne Volden, Ph.D., S-LP (C), R. S-LP is the Associate Dean of Graduate Studies and Research, Faculty of Rehabilitation Medicine, University of Alberta, and a Professor, Speech-Language Pathology. Her research interests include Pragmatic Communication Impairments and Social Cognition, Autism Spectrum Disorder, Nonverbal Learning Disability, Social Communication Disorder, and she has published widely on these topics. She can be reached at: joanne.volden@ualberta.ca or address: Joanne Volden, Ph.D., Associate Dean, Graduate Studies and Research, Professor, Speech Pathology and Audiology, Faculty of Rehabilitation Medicine, University of Alberta, 3-48 Corbett Hall, Edmonton, AL T6G 2G4, USA.

Chapter 1
Introduction

Jessica Broitman and John M. Davis

The Centers for Disease Control and Prevention currently estimates that 8.7% of the school population children from ages 6 to 17 have learning disabilities (Pastor & Reuben, 2008), and this accounts for roughly half of all students currently receiving special educational services. Informal estimates are that 10–15% of these students identified as having a learning disability have a nonverbal learning disorder (NVLD) Rourke, 1985. Over the last 20 years there has been a significant increased interest in the treatment of children with NVLD. The number of publications concerning NVLD has risen from 15 in the years between 1981 and 1990 to 85 in the years 2001–2010 (Semrud-Clikeman, Fine, & Bledsoe, 2008). Unfortunately, efficacious treatments for children with NVLD have not progressed at the same rate, and most interventions that are published are based on anecdotal or clinical experience. It is imperative that practitioners know how to treat students who are at risk for and manifest this disorder.

We believe that it is important to collect such information in one volume so we can more fully understand and determine the efficacy of such treatments and to begin to establish empirical bases for such treatments. The role of the school professional in providing or guiding these services has increased and it is expected that this book will serve as a resource for all psychologists and all other education professionals, both within and outside of educational agencies, and to students training to be clinical or school psychologists, educational therapists, speech and language specialists, occupational therapists, and special education teachers.

J. Broitman, Ph.D. (✉)
San Francisco Psychotherapy Research Group, 9 Funston Street,
San Francisco, CA 94129, USA
e-mail: drjess@comcast.net

J.M. Davis, Ph.D.
California State University, East Bay, 25800 Carlos Bee Blvd,
Hayward, CA 94542-3095, USA
e-mail: jack.davis@csueastbay.edu

J. Broitman and J.M. Davis (eds.), *Treating NVLD in Children: Professional Collaborations for Positive Outcomes*, DOI 10.1007/978-1-4614-6179-1_1,

The purpose of this book will be to provide practitioners with an understanding of the treatment needs of children with NVLD and more importantly knowledge of the roles of the many varied professionals with whom they will be interacting. Unlike other learning disabilities, the number of professionals involved in treatment for students with NVLD for *best practice* is often many and varied. Treatment is further complicated due to the difficulty in accurately diagnosing children with NVLD and the differing labels and names associated with this disorder, for example: developmental coordination disorder, dyspraxia, mathematics disorder, semantic pragmatic disorder, etc. The reader will see that we advocate for a team approach with one member of the team serving as the case manager. Which professional takes the *lead* role is likely to shift over the course of a child with NVLD's lifetime as at different ages the most crucial needs will shift. This publication is intended to be a useful resource that follows up on our first book, NVLD in Children: Bridging the Gap Between Science and Practice (Davis & Broitman, 2011). It will not only inform the reader upon first reading, but will also be a handbook to which the practitioner can turn when considering possible cases of NVLD.

The role of the school psychologist is evolving and knowledge regarding effective practices for understanding and treating the many areas of NVLD is of renewed relevance to school psychology practice (Davis & Broitman, 2006, 2007; Forrest, 2004; Myklebust, 1975; Palombo, 2006; Tanguay, 2002). Books on NVLD developed for classroom teachers and school-based professionals are beginning to emerge (e.g., *Nonverbal Learning Disabilities and Their Clinical Subtypes: A Handbook for Parents and Professionals* (Mamen, 2006) and *Nonverbal Learning Disorders at School* (Tanguay, 2002)). However, there are no previously published books addressing the different professionals who must all be involved in the treatment of a child with NVLD over the course of his or her lifespan. Each chapter of this edited book is written by a different and necessary member of the team. A treatment team for a child with NVLD might include:

- *Professional services*:
  Child psychiatrist or developmental pediatrician
  Pediatric neuropsychologist
  Occupational therapist
  Physical therapist
  Speech and language therapist
  Psychologist for assessment
  Psychotherapist
  Coach
  Social skills specialist

- *Educational intervention and placement*:
  Educational therapist
  Special education teacher
  Math tutor
  Written expression tutor
  Reading comprehension tutor
  Educational consultant

Advocate
Specialized school consultant
College counselor
Vocational and rehabilitation consultant

- *Family members*:
  Child or young adult with NVLD
  Parents

In this volume each practitioner will answer similar crucial questions and issues (as it relates to their field) regarding the treatment of children with NVLD. A selection of the following questions will be considered:

- An overview of how their discipline understands the theory or theories of NVLD.
- What are the instruments of assessment used to assess the area(s) of difficulty treated within their discipline (as clinically appropriate)?
- An overview and example of a treatment plan with a case study illustrating how they might work with a child with NVLD.
- Sample school or parent report for their discipline with recommendations/referrals for other professional services.
- How they monitor treatment effectiveness?
- What, if any, are any evidence base for the treatments offered?
- How the diagnosis was made, i.e., what were the essential symptoms used to establish the diagnosis?
- Do they consider medications and if so why (where clinically relevant)?
- What kind of psycho-education do they provide for the parents of children with NVLD?
- References and resources.

In Chap. 2 the authors will provide an overview of NVLD. We will survey the history, etiology, and symptoms of the disorder. We will offer a developmental picture of how the child with NVLD might appear throughout his/her lifespan. In addition we offer a new four-subtype model for NVLD and list the supporting research.

In Chap. 3 occupational therapist Rebecca Schatz will provide the same overview of assessment in the OT field as well as how the information would go into a report, be presented to parents and educators, and would serve to develop an OT treatment plan. Interventions, especially as pertains to any evidence-based interventions, will be included.

In Chap. 4 speech and language therapist Joanne Volden, PhD, will offer a variation of the clinician's assessment, intervention plan, and interventions available as outlined above.

In Chap. 5 psychologists John M. Davis, PhD, and Jessica Broitman, PhD (coeditors), will address the role of a comprehensive psychoeducational and neuropsychological assessment in the identification of the issues which need to be better understood and addressed.

In Chap. 6 pediatric neurologist Meryl Lipton, MD, will cover the role of a developmental pediatrician in how these professionals may encounter and work with children with NVLD and their parents. Here, the topic of whether any medications may be useful for the client and how the developmental pediatrician goes about thinking about the issues to help make those decisions will be explored.

In Chap. 7 school psychologist Dr. Cathrine Brown and her student Bridget Leary will discuss the role of the coach and what services parents, teachers, and professionals working with the child with NVLD in pre-K-12 may need to consider for future academic and social success. Most K-12 students with NVLD will receive recommendations and mandated accommodations from a school psychologist who completes classroom observations, reviews health and academic history, assesses and diagnoses NVLD, and makes the appropriate recommendations for the related subtypes of NVLD. The psychologist's primary focus is to determine eligibility for special education including waivers for testing, course substitutions, modifications to course content, and para-educator assistance in the classroom as mandated by law. These recommendations may also include transportation, counseling, physical, occupational, and speech therapy. Often, other psychosocial issues and executive functioning issues are associated with students with NVLD. These issues most often include comorbid diagnoses and delayed development of social and independent living skills. Therefore, some parents of children with specific types of NVLD may opt to provide additional non-mandated social supports outside of the school setting such as the use of *coaches* or tutors in order to better prepare children with NVLD for positive psychosocial outcomes in various environments.

In Chap. 8 Marion Marshall, MS, BCET, FAET, will discuss the role of the educational therapist and academic interventions. This chapter will have three main foci. First will be an introduction and overview of what an educational therapist does. Second will be specific recommendations for treatment of reading comprehension disorders. And third will be recommendations for treatment of written expression disorders. The recommendations will be cited as evidence based whenever possible.

In Chap. 9 Dianne Matthaei, ET, will specifically address how to work on math with the children who have NVLD. She will describe how to learn the *vocabulary* of mathematics, the *procedures* of mathematics, and the *major concepts* of mathematics. She will show how, with support, students with NVLD can become competent at mathematics and achieve their learning goals.

In Chap. 10 psychologist and social skills specialist Bernadette Evans, PhD, will discuss what assessments will need to be employed to better understand and plan for social skills interventions for NVLD students. It will not be profession specific, but rather more focused on discussing the variety of treatments needed. In addition she will offer a review of existing treatments from two complementary theoretical perspectives, neurodevelopmental behavioral (Lipton & Evans-Smith, 2006; Lipton & Nowicki, 2009; Siegel, 1999; Stern, 2000) and interpersonal neurobiology (Palombo, Bendicsen, & Koch, 2011; Schore, 2005; Siegel, 1999).

In Chap. 11 licensed educational psychologist Jane McClure, MA/LEP, will talk about the role of a college counselor and the process of helping young adults with

NVLD finding their best fit for college. She will identify the crucial issues to be considered and discuss the application process including considerations regarding disclosure. Dr. McClure will also discuss the role of a counselor in K-12 placement decisions including private school vs. public schools and homeschooling.

In Chap. 12 school psychologist Dr. Cathrine Brown and her student Bridget Leary will address the issues that children with NVLD face as they transition from high school to college. Most students with NVLD will receive recommendations and mandated accommodations from a case counselor such as the disability resource counselor who is designated to review documentation of students with NVLD and other disabilities. The counselor's primary focus is to determine academic accommodations needed to provide the student with equal access to the curriculum as mandated by law, such as extra time on tests, note takers in the classroom, etc. However, they must also be ware of other psychosocial issues associated with students with NVLD. These issues most often include comorbid diagnoses, delayed development of social and independent living skills, and significant deficits in executive functioning. Therefore, some students with specific types of NVLD are using non-mandated supports in college to address these psychosocial issues.

In Chap. 13 psychologist and vocational specialist Lynn C. Koch will review post-high-school nonacademic services, for those students with NVLD who are not college bound. She will provide an overview of the kinds of services a vocational rehabilitation counselor and workforce specialist can provide.

In Chap. 14 neuropsychologist Margaret Semrud-Clikeman, PhD, and Dr. Jennifer Wheeler Maedgen will cover the role of the pediatric neuropsychologist as an advocate in the treatment of NVLD. Pediatric neuropsychologists are often looked upon to provide recommendations to the school system for the clients with whom they work. The purpose of these recommendations is generally to establish academic accommodations and/or special education services within the school setting that are appropriate to the child's disability and functional limitations. However, clinicians often do not have more than a basic understanding of the legislation that determines the provision of these services, which are at times conflicting, often reinterpreted based on relevant court decisions, and dramatically different in purpose and scope between the secondary and postsecondary setting (Gordon, Lewandowski, Murphy, & Dempsey, 2002; Ranseen & Parks, 2005). In addition, the definitions set forth in disability-related legislation are often at odds with standard practices surrounding clinical diagnostic procedures. Clinicians may find themselves confused when their recommendations are not incorporated within the secondary school environment and/or the client is not considered eligible for academic accommodations in college. The purpose of this chapter is to familiarize neuropsychologists with the laws affecting the provision of accommodations in the secondary and postsecondary settings through a discussion of their scope, purposes, and how related legislation has been interpreted by the courts and educational institutions. Issues related to the transition from high school to college and how this affects neuropsychologists who are working with incoming college students will also be reviewed. Finally, practical strategies relating to how clinicians can best work with school personnel and clients in secondary and postsecondary settings will be considered, as well as a discussion of why neuropsychologists, by virtue of their training, may be especially well suited to perform disability- and education-related evaluations.

In Chap. 15 research psychologist Jodene Fine, PhD, will offer an update on what is known about the ongoing research on children, adolescents, and adults with NVLD.

In Chap. 16 Brett Mills will offer his personal account of growing up with NVLD (previously heard from in the afterword of our last book). This chapter will include some of the most important things parents/educators must know about dealing with a child with NVLD from the perspective of a young adult with NVLD and his family.

In Chap. 17 the authors will offer their final thoughts and summarize the main themes of the book.

References

Davis, J., & Broitman, J. (2006). A brief overview of nonverbal learning disorders. *The Educational Therapist, 27*(3), 5–10.

Davis, J., & Broitman, J. (2007). Nonverbal learning disabilities: Models of proposed subtypes, part II. *The Educational Therapist, 27*(4), 5–10.

Davis, J. M. & Broitman, J. (2011). Nonverbal Learning Disability in Children: Bridging the Gap Between Science and Practice. New York: Springer.

Forrest, B. J. (2004). The utility of math difficulties, internalized psychopathology, and visual-spatial deficits to identify children with nonverbal learning disability syndrome: Evidence for a visual spatial disability. *Child Neuropsychology, 10*(2), 129–146.

Gordon, M., Lewandowski, L., Murphy, K., & Dempsey, K. (2002). ADA-based accommodations in higher education: A survey of clinicians about documentation requirements and diagnostic standards. *Journal of Learning Disabilities, 35*(4), 357–363.

Lipton, M. & Evans-Smith, B. (2006, August). "Social Emotional Learning Framework (SELF): Conceptual, Clinical, and Research Aspects." The Summer Institute on Neurodevelopmental Disorders, MIND Institute, University of California, Davis, CA.

Lipton, M., & Nowicki, S. (2009). The social emotional learning framework (SELF): A guide for understanding brain-based social emotional learning impairments. *Journal of Developmental Processes, 4*(2), 99–115.

Mamen, M. (2006). *Nonverbal learning disabilities and their clinical subtypes: A handbook for parents and professionals—new edition*. Ottawa, ON: Centrepointe Professional Services.

Myklebust, H. R. (1975). Nonverbal learning disabilities: Assessment and intervention. In H. R. Myklebust (Ed.), *Progress in learning disabilities* (Vol. III, pp. 85–121). New York, NY: Grune & Stratton.

Palombo, J. (2006). *Nonverbal learning disabilities: A clinical perspective*. New York, NY: WW Norton.

Palombo, J., Bendicsen, H., & Koch, B. (2011). Guide to Psychoanalytic Developmental Theories. USA: Springer.

Pastor, P. N., & Reuben, C. A. (2008). Diagnosed attention deficit hyperactivity disorder and learning disability: United States, 2004–2006. National Center for Health Statistics. *Vital Health Stat, 10*(237), 1–14.

Ranseen, J. D., & Parks, G. S. (2005). Test accommodations for post-secondary students: The quandary resulting from ADA's disability definition. *Psychology, Public Policy, and Law, 11*, 83–108.

Rourke, B. P. (Ed.). (1985). *Neuropsychology of learning disabilities: Essentials of subtype analysis*. New York: Guilford Publications.

Schore, A. (2005). Attachment, affect regulation, and the developing right brain: Linking developmental neuroscience to pediatrics. *Pediatrics in Review, 26*(6), 204–217.

Semrud-Clikeman, M., Fine, J. G., & Bledsoe, J. (2008). *Meta-analysis of empirical literature on NVLD*. Paper presented at the International Neuropsychological Society.

Stern, D. (2000). *The interpersonal world of the infant: A view from psychoanalysis and developmental psychology*. New York: Basic Books.

Tanguay, P. B. (2002). *Nonverbal learning disabilities at school*. London, England: Jessica Kingsley.

Chapter 2
Overview of NVLD

Jessica Broitman and John M. Davis

This chapter provides an overview of the evolution of what we, today, call a nonverbal learning disorder (or nonverbal learning disability) (NVLD). Although there was increased interest in this disorder in the 1980s and 1990s, researchers and practitioners have not even been able to agree whether nonverbal learning disabilities should be abbreviated as NLD (mostly used on the West Coast) or NVLD (preferred by East Coast clinicians), nor have they arrived at an accepted definition for this condition, although Rourke's definition is the most frequently noted (Pelletier, Ahmad, & Rourke, 2001). We will use the abbreviation NVLD for the purposes of this book.

Estimates vary about how prevalent NVLD is, but the most frequently cited estimate is that 10–15% of all learning-disabled students have NVLD (Ozols & Rourke, 1988). It is imperative that practitioners know how to identify and treat students who are at risk for, and manifest, this disorder. Although data has been accumulating since Johnson and Myklebust's (1967) classic work, *Learning Disabilities: Educational Principles and Practices*, nonverbal learning disabilities are still the least known and the least understood learning disorder.

We begin with a review of the clinician's concept of the child with NVLD. Next we present a brief overview of the pioneers' thoughts about this disorder, and then we discuss the most common definition of NVLD, and then the current dominant model of the etiology of NVLD. Unfortunately, as is the case with other learning

J. Broitman, Ph.D. (✉)
San Francisco Psychotherapy Research Group, 9 Funston Street,
San Francisco, CA 94129, USA
e-mail: drjess@comcast.net

J.M. Davis, Ph.D.
California State University, East Bay, 25800 Carlos Bee Blvd,
Hayward, CA 94542-3095, USA
e-mail: jack.davis@csueastbay.edu

J. Broitman and J.M. Davis (eds.), *Treating NVLD in Children: Professional Collaborations for Positive Outcomes*, DOI 10.1007/978-1-4614-6179-1_2,

disabilities (LD) (Duane, 1991) and developmental disorders (DD) (Ozonoff & Rogers, 2003), the exact cause or causes of NVLD are not yet clear. However, the most current model of understanding NVLD which is from a neurological perspective commonly called the *white matter model* will be presented.

Additionally, we describe the symptoms as they manifest at different developmental stages, along with the professionals likely to become involved in each stage whose work is represented in other chapters of this book. Lastly we broaden our understanding of NVLD as a neurobiologically based learning disorder by looking at it through the clinical lens of multiple subtypes. Due to the limitations of space we present only a very brief review of these important topics. For a more comprehensive treatment we direct the reader to *Nonverbal Learning Disabilities in Children: Bridging the Gap Between Science and Practice* (Davis & Broitman, 2011).

Overview of NVLD

In order to help readers develop a *feeling* for this disorder, let us review a clinician's concept of the child with NVLD. Judy Lewis' overview on the website www.NLDline.com, which is based on educator Sue Thompson's (1997) groundbreaking work, *The Source for Nonverbal Learning Disorders*, is a useful reference. Lewis lists early speech and vocabulary development; remarkable rote memory; strong auditory retention; attention to detail, at times good early reading skills; and excellent spelling skills, as among the assets of some children with NVLD.

Five major categories of deficits and dysfunction are identified: motor, visual–spatial, organizational, social, and sensory. Motor deficits include poor coordination, severe balance problems, and difficulties with graphomotor skills. Visual–spatial/organizational deficits reflect a lack of image formation, poor visual recall, faulty spatial perceptions, and difficulties with executive functions. These executive functioning difficulties include decision making, planning, initiative, assigning priority, sequencing, motor control, emotional regulation, problem-solving, impulse control, establishing goals, monitoring results of action, self-correcting, and problems with spatial relations. Social deficits include difficulties comprehending nonverbal communication and adjusting to transitions and novel situations, along with deficits in social judgment and social interaction. The last category refers to sensitivity in any of the sensory modes: visual, auditory, tactile, taste, or olfactory.

Defining NVLD

The definition of NVLD is crucial to how we assess, diagnose, understand, and intervene for effected children. As is similar with dyslexia, NVLD's better known learning disorder cousin, NVLD is not currently in any formal eligibility or diagnostic codes such as the Diagnostic and Statistical Manual of Mental Disorders-IV-TR (American Psychiatric Association, 2000). Some researchers do not view NVLD as a specific learning syndrome and argue against it even being considered as an *official* diagnosis (Pennington, 2009), while others argue that creating a formal diagnostic code will aid in the understanding, research, and treatment of NVLD and for insurance reimbursement for services (Davis & Broitman, 2011; Rourke, 1985). A recently released draft of the DSM-V does not include the diagnosis NVLD.

We assert that NVLD should be a formalized diagnosis, not only to aid research but also to make it easier for parents to be able to receive benefits for intervention for the disorder. In addition, we believe that having a formalized diagnostic category will be a useful heuristic tool for guiding assessment and intervention. But let us begin with a historical perspective for how our understanding of the syndrome of NVLD has progressed over time.

Historical Perspective

Josef Gerstmann, an Austrian-born neurologist who fled Nazi Europe to the United States in the late 1930s, wrote the first published article on symptoms which seemed like what we now call nonverbal learning disorders (Gerstmann, 1940). He conceptualized a syndrome that took his name, the Gerstmann syndrome (Gerstmann, 1940). This syndrome consisted of difficulties in the areas of finger agnosia, right–left orientation, agraphia, and acalculia. From the beginning, these nonverbal processes were linked to problems in math and writing, but for Gerstmann, the primary focus was on sensorimotor or fine motor control and function.

In 1967, Johnson and Myklebust (Johnson & Myklebust, 1967) added to our thinking about NVLD in their book entitled *Learning Disabilities: Educational Principles and Practices*. In this work they described their version of the syndrome of nonverbal learning disorders. Whereas Gerstmann (1940) had noted fine motor difficulties and difficulties with math and writing, Johnson and Myklebust (1967) observed additional difficulties in visual–spatial processing and something they called *social perception*. They suggested that children with these learning disabilities had difficulties in understanding gesture, nonverbal motor learning, body image, spatial orientation, right–left orientation, and social perception. Additionally, these children also demonstrated distractibility, perseveration, and disinhibition. Johnson and Mykelbust's vision generally holds true to current thinking about NVLD. Later work by Landau and colleagues (Landau, Gross-Tsur, Auerback, Van der Meere, & Shalev, 1999) found overlap between learning disabilities and ADHD and executive function issues.

The next major advances in research and thinking about NVLD were made by Byron Rourke and his many colleagues. Rourke is the leading exponent of the dominant model and/or definition of NVLD today. After decades of research and two seminal books, *Neuropsychology of Learning Disabilities: Essentials of Subtype*

Table 2.1 Rourke's diagnostic criteria for NVLD

1. Target test at least 1 standard deviation (SD) below the mean
2. No, or very minimal, simple tactile imperception and suppression versus very poor finger agnosia and/or finger dysgraphesthesia
3. The highest scores on two subtests of the Verbal Scale of the Wechsler Intelligence Scale for Children-III (WISC-III): Vocabulary, Similarities, or Information
4. Two of the subtests from the WISC-III nonverbal subtests of Block Design, Object Assembly, or Coding fall among the lowest scores of the Performance Scale
5. Wide Range Achievement Test-Revised (WRAT-R) standard score for reading is at least 8 points higher than arithmetic
6. Tactual Performance Test, right, left, and both hand times become progressively worse vis-à-vis the norms
7. Normal to superior grip strength versus mildly to moderately impaired Grooved Pegboard
8. WISC-III: VIQ exceeds PIQ by at least 10 points

Analysis (1985) and *Syndrome of Nonverbal Learning Disabilities: Neurodevelopmental Manifestations* (1995), Rourke has left a significant mark on the field both by trying to establish a diagnostic set of criteria for NVLD and offering a theory for the cause of the disorder.

Diagnostic Criteria for NVLD

Rourke's diagnostic criteria have remained fairly stable over time. Most recently, Rourke and his colleagues (Pelletier et al., 2001) have stated that the following criteria have to be met to determine NVLD (Table 2.1):

The following conditions meet Rourke's criteria for a *diagnosis* of NVLD:

- Children presenting with the first six criteria would definitely be diagnosed with NVLD.
- If seven or eight of any of the features are present, it would constitute a positive diagnosis.
- Five or six of any of the criteria suggest probable NVLD.
- Three or four of any of the criteria suggest questionable NVLD.
- One or two of any of the criteria suggest low probability of NVLD.

Those of us who do assessments will find problems with Rourke's algorithm. First, all of the instruments would be considered outdated today. Second, although many newer, better standardized tests are available, none have been utilized to update the definition. This will be addressed in the chapter on assessment. We turn now to the question of the etiology of NVLD.

Etiology of NVLD: White Matter Model

Unfortunately the exact cause or causes of NVLD are not yet clear. We will, however, review the most current model of understanding NVLD which is from a neurological perspective commonly called the *white matter model*. For a more comprehensive review of the current available information from the areas typically addressed when considering the causality of NVLD—genetics, neurobiology, and environment—we refer the reader to Rourke's *Syndrome of Nonverbal Learning Disabilities: Neurodevelopmental Manifestations* (Rourke, 1995) or *Nonverbal Learning Disabilities in Children: Bridging the Gap Between Science and Practice* (Davis & Broitman, 2011).

Initially, authors like Semrud-Clikeman and Hynd (1990), Voeller (1986), and Weintraub and Mesulam (1983) conceptualized these nonverbal difficulties as *right hemisphere learning disorders*, all of which (including Rourke's later work) were based on Goldberg and Costa's (1981) original conceptualizations of how the left and right hemispheres differed in terms of their neuropsychological functions. Denckla (1991) elaborates on this stating "in fact, the frequent association of an attentional/executive functional component and a visuoperceptual/simultaneous information processing component has made the term 'right hemisphere LD' seem more appealing in terms of the parsimony afforded by an anatomical expression that captures the affiliation of its behavioral manifestations" (p. 718), although she also cautioned that her conclusion may have been a bit premature.

Moving on from the right hemisphere model, Rourke (1995) postulated that it is more likely that deficits in subcortical white matter are responsible for the symptoms seen in NVLD. Rourke and colleagues (Rourke, 1995; Rourke, Ahmad, Collins, Hayman-Abello, & Warriner, 2002) have written about the neuropsychological symptoms that develop from damage to or a disturbance in white matter, as opposed to gray matter. Hale and Fiorello (2004) describe and have a useful metaphor for the differences between the two. "Recall the central nervous system is primarily composed of gray matter (the nerve cells) and white matter (mylenated axons that speed transformation of information). We like to think of the gray matter as the houses and neighborhoods, and the white matter pathways as the streets and highways" (p. 45). The white matter then is the means by which information is generally transmitted within and between the two hemispheres. It is commonly believed that these white matter disruptions can be from a myriad of different causes but ultimately all create somewhat consistent sets of difficulties. To borrow Rourke et al.'s own words (2002):

> The syndrome of NLD [which here is referred to as NVLD] is characterized by significant primary deficits in some dimensions of tactile perception, visual perception, complex psychomotor skills, and in dealing with novel circumstances. These primary deficits lead to secondary deficits in tactile and visual attention and to significant limitations in exploratory

> behavior. In turn there are tertiary deficits in tactile and visual memory and in concept-formation, problem-solving, and hypothesis-testing skills. Finally, these deficits lead to significant difficulties in the content (meaning) and function (pragmatics) dimensions of language. (pp. 310–311)

This approach to understanding how these disorders manifest has often been referred to as a *cascade* (Schultz, Romanski, & Tsatsanis, 2000) or *downstream* (Fine & Semrud-Clikeman, in press) effect whereby all the deficits that develop, including some neuropsychological, executive function, academic, linguistic, and social difficulties, are the *result* of the initial or *core* difficulties of tactile perception, visual perception, and complex psychomotor skills, and in dealing with novel circumstances. However, here as well, findings can be somewhat inconsistent. For instance, in Wilkinson and Semrud-Clikeman's (2008) study of motor speed in children and adolescents with nonverbal learning disabilities, they found no evidence of tactile perceptual difficulties. As of yet we do not have enough consistent empirical support to either endorse or refute the remainder of this theory, but more data is accruing. In addition, we have yet to find research which might determine the genetic contribution to the more idiopathic form of NVLD and no theory has been proven. It is clear, however, that NVLD *can* result from medical conditions that seem to cause more damage to right than left hemisphere regions. The Australian Government's Website dedicated to nonverbal learning disorders (http://www.nld-line.com/childdrema2.htm) lists the following disorders that result in NVLD-like symptoms:

- *Hydrocephalus*—where increased fluid pressure inside the brain may damage white matter more than gray.
- *Turners syndrome*—a genetic problem in girls with only one X chromosome instead of two. This can alter brain development, leading to an NVLD pattern of problems.
- *Fragile X syndrome*—another genetic disorder of the X chromosome, usually manifests in males. It can alter brain development, leading to different patterns of developmental problems including NVLD.
- *Tumors*, *calcification*, *cysts*, and *brain injury*—any process that selectively damages the right side of the brain can lead to the clinical picture of NVLD. Rare cases have been described where damage was on the left side in fetal development. Somehow, the left-brain functions were taken over by the right side, enabling children to develop language skills, and normal right-side functions were impaired.
- *Multiple sclerosis, and other disorders of white matter*—though very rare in childhood, these disorders cause many neurological problems.
- *Agenesis of the corpus callosum*—where the major communication fibers between the left and right side of the brain fail to develop correctly.
- *Congenital hypothyroidism*—occurs when the fetus is deprived of normal amounts of thyroid hormone during the pregnancy.
- *Fetal alcohol syndrome*—is caused by alcohol damage to the developing fetus.

- *Treatment for leukemia and brain tumors*—the radiation used to treat leukemia and tumors in the brain can damage white matter (Teeter & Semrud-Clikeman, 1997).
- *Others*—including velocardiofacial syndrome, Williams syndrome, de Lange syndrome, and Sotos syndrome.

Despite this list, we do not find medical causes in most of the children with NVLD. For this reason we will next present NVLD primarily as a developmental disorder.

NVLD: A Developmental Orientation

In this section we offer a look at how a child with NVLD can manifest at different developmental stages. We briefly address signs of NVLD in early (preschool) development, early schooling, later elementary and middle school, and high school. It is important to note that the presenting symptoms change across development and are often difficult to identify.

Early Developmental Signs of NVLD

Piaget (Inhelder & Piaget, 1964) refers to the first stage of development as the sensorimotor stage, whereby much of learning is about the child's interactions with his/her environment and on a sensory level. However, the usual amount of or exposure to sensorimotor learning is less for an NVLD child. As Rourke (1995) notes, in describing NVLD children, "these children remain essentially sedentary, exploring the world not through vision or locomotion, but rather through receiving verbal answers to questions posed about the immediate environment" (p. 8). The disparity between precocious language development, especially vocabulary, and the delays in motor development in the child are most notable in the early years.

Anecdotal reports from parents of children with NVLD often state that their child would sit and point at an object, saying what they wanted rather than crawling towards it. In anticipation of normal exploration, one parent spoke of how she *baby-proofed* her house to protect her child, yet her child never crawled to or tried to open anything. Many of these children do not use typical toddler toys or enjoy coloring or drawing. They are usually disinterested in or unable to put puzzles together (Johnson, 1987). Parents are often confused when their extremely verbal child is not developing consistently across developmental lines. They may create unwarranted and inaccurate expectations, based upon inappropriate assumptions about their child's superior language development. Problems for the child can become exacerbated when poor motor and spatial development can disappoint and confound the parents. Early sensorimotor exploration is important in the child's development, since learning depends upon the interaction of the child with the environment

(Piaget, 1972). The brain develops secondary to its interactions with the environment, developing neural networks that then create neural efficiency. Although NVLD children are interacting with their environment, it is often more verbal and observational and less motoric and spatial, which alters development of the neural networking. As the old saying goes, *neurons that fire together wire together*. It is likely that less interaction and practice exploring the environment with the body may lead to less efficiency in motor skills compared to children with many more hours of practice. In turn, as they grow older, children with less confidence in their motor skills may be less inclined to engage in activities demanding it, further reducing their skill growth and development.

Early Schooling

Kindergarten teachers may notice problems in fine motor skills that have not been noted earlier in a child with NVLD. The child may struggle more than his peers with items such as scissors, crayons, or pencils. As demands for writing and drawing increase, the teacher may notice immaturity in children with NVLD compared to typically developing peers.

The teacher may turn to an occupational therapist (OT) for consultation and guidance. After observing the child, the OT might provide an evaluation or offer treatment. Sensory integration therapy (Ayres, 1994) might be offered to treat what the OT views as a sensory integration disorder, although this is still considered a somewhat controversial intervention (see Chap. 3). If the child's issues are in the mild to moderate range, this may be all that is offered.

Sometimes children with NVLD may be referred for help with non-phonological reading difficulties (Pennington, 1991), but intervention may be a premature. Rourke (1995) notes that these difficulties may well be developmental for children with NVLD and most children with NVLD develop basic reading skills without intervention. However, Griffin and Gresham (2002) theorize that these reading problems are often associated with difficulties in visual processing problems, like tracking. Tracking refers to the ability of the child to stay on the correct line of reading or math without veering off course creating confusion and extra time for the student to reorient oneself. They further theorize that these problems are due to visual–spatial processing difficulties and claim that NVLD children frequently require tracking training with as many as thirty percent needing to be retrained in order to read fluently. He suggests performing a thorough optometric examination that includes an assessment of visual tracking.

Often children with NVLD develop early math difficulties, although some use their verbal memory strengths to help them compensate through third grade, and occasionally beyond. If not earlier, during this period concerns begin to develop about social perception and pragmatic language development. Further, boys and girls with NVLD can present with clinical signs of anxiety, depression, attention problems, obsessional preoccupations, and self-esteem problems (Palombo &

Berenberg, 1999). It remains unclear whether children with NVLD experience difficulties with peers because of processing issues, for example: difficulty processing facial expressions and social signals, executive function difficulties, novel problem solving, or due to another yet unknown reason. They might even result from reduced interaction with peers due to their sensorimotor issues (Hale & Fiorello, 2004). Clearly further research is required to evaluate these hypotheses.

With difficulties in the social area, especially with pragmatic language problems, the next professional to become involved is most often a speech and language therapist. During earlier stages these children might have been seen for articulation issues connected with poor oro-motor functions, while in early elementary school they are more likely seen for pragmatic language difficulties in social discourse. Children with NVLD often do not use appropriate vocal intonations. They might speak in a flat monotone or with a singsong voice. It can be difficult to read their mood from their facial expressions and they may seem wooden and constricted (Palombo & Berenberg, 1999). In speech and language nomenclature these issues are often called *semantic–pragmatic* disorders (Volden, 2004). It is believed to bode well for youngsters if these issues are identified early and intervention begins before the child falls behind allowing secondary features, especially anxiety, to develop (Palombo & Berenberg, 1999).

Even though children with these processing difficulties may struggle and become frustrated by math and written expression, they tend not to be referred to special educators because they perform *well enough*. Their superior verbal skills often cause educators and parents to assume that their difficulties arise from insufficient effort, or difficulty paying attention. Rourke (1995) wrote that young children with these symptoms are often misdiagnosed with ADHD. Unfortunately such misdiagnoses can lead to a host of self-esteem problems and psychological issues, particularly when appropriate interventions are withheld.

Later Elementary and Middle School Signs

As academic subjects become more abstract, and more independent work is expected, children with NVLD often begin to experience greater difficulties. Executive function problems increase. At the same time more demands are placed on social skills creating significant additional stress and frustration that can elevate anxiety which also makes academic progress difficult.

At this point academically oriented professionals often become involved in the lives of children with NVLD. Teachers become alarmed and mention their concerns at parent conferences. Parents ask for help for their children, and public or private school wheels are set in motion. Student Study Team (SST) meetings are called or Individualized Educational Plans (IEP) are developed, the latter based upon psychoeducational evaluations in order to develop appropriate interventions (Hale & Fiorello, 2004; Telzrow & Bonar, 2002).

Providing the best assistance for the student can become problematic because so much depends upon who gets involved and what they already know. The child's parents also need to educate themselves to become more knowledgeable as they will become increasingly involved in their child's treatment team. Helpful books for parents include Sue Thompson's *The Source for Nonverbal Learning Disorders* (1997); Pamela Tanguay's *Nonverbal Learning Disorders at Home* (2001) or *Nonverbal Learning Disorders at School* (2002); Kathy Allen's *Star Shaped Pegs, Square Holes: Nonverbal Learning Disorders and the Growing Up Years* (1998); and Rondalyn Whitney's *The Nonverbal Learning Disorder Guide for Teachers, Parents, Employers, and Therapists* (2000). The SST or IEP teams could advise them to join the Nonverbal Learning Disorders Association (www.nlda.org) or to become familiar with websites such as Judy Lewis's www.nldline.com, Pam Tanguay's www.NLDontheweb.org, or the Charles Schwab Web site, www.schwablearning.org. More information related to working with the families will be provided in a later chapter.

High School Signs

If the child with NVLD has managed to navigate the comprehensive middle school environment, the high school experience becomes the next challenge. During high school, social skills can become a source of even greater concern, as social stresses, such as the demands of dating, are increased. Advanced math and sciences will also be more challenging. Increased demands on executive functioning, as in written expression and advanced reading skills, can present major challenges.

Research is mixed regarding whether students with NVLD are more at risk for psychiatric disorders, like depression, with some finding increased levels of depression (Brumbach, 1985; Fletcher, 1985; Rourke, Young, & Leenaars, 1986) and others not finding that children with NVLD are at increased risk for psychiatric disorders (Forrest, 2004; Mokros, Poznanski, & Merrick, 1989). It is possible that these contradictory findings are due to the significant differences in age groups, race, and income among the different studies or differing definitions for diagnosis given the wide range of diagnostic criteria used in research on NVLD.

However, with interventions, accommodations, and modifications students with NVLD are often able to tap into their skill sets and experience success as emphasized by Brooks (1991) and his concept of *islands of competence*. By this he is referring to the fact that students with learning disabilities have relative strengths and weaknesses and it is at least equally important that the student's strengths get recognized and enhanced as it is to remediate any relative weaknesses or deficits. Skill sets might include acquisition of a second language, drama, certain aspects of the arts, language arts, and some of the language-based sciences.

Generally the support team continues to be involved in the student's program if not via the Individual Educational Plan (IEP) process then sometimes utilizing the Section 504 laws. Transition planning becomes essential and decisions about further education need to be made. In our experience, students who have not become too de-motivated, depressed, or demoralized can move on to successful adulthood if they, with the help of their parents and coaches, choose wisely with special regard for their strengths. Students with NVLD often interact better with adults than with their peers. Personal accounts written by people with NVLD suggest that adulthood may bring more successful interactions and relationships. Debbie Green, for example, in *Growing Up with NLD* (1999) writes of her joys as a teacher. Laurie E. Reed talks of her career as an occupational therapist in *Unaware*: *Living with Non-Verbal Learning Disabilities* (2001). These authors emphasize that early accurate diagnosis and appropriate intervention is crucial to the well-being of the person with NVLD. To add in that process we next suggest broadening our understanding of NVLD to consider it a neurobiologically based learning disorder and by looking at it through the clinical lens of multiple subtypes.

NVLD Subtypes

Historically, Rourke (1985, 1991) and others (Drummond, Ahmad, & Rourke, 2005; Harnadek & Rourke, 1994; Johnson & Myklebust, 1967; Pennington, 1991) spent a significant amount of time clarifying the differences between what are often referred to as verbal or phonologically based learning disorders and nonverbal learning disorders. More recently, some theorists are suggesting that, as with many developmental disorders, NVLD should be considered as a disorder with different subtypes (Davis & Broitman, 2007; Grodzinsky, 2003; Mamen, 2006; Palombo, 2006). This notion fits with our clinical experience. This section reviews the most recent developments in the understanding of NVLD as a disorder with multiple subtypes or components.

Researchers such as Semrud-Clikeman (2001) and others (Forrest, 2004, Myklebust, 1975) continue to view NVLD somewhat differently than Rourke. Without citing specific numbers Semrud-Clikeman suggests that only some of the strengths and weaknesses proposed by Rourke need to be present for a child to be diagnosed with NVLD. More recently, a study by Wilkenson and Semrud-Clikeman (2008) found no differences between children with NVLD and those without NVLD on measures of sensory and tactile measures. Further, Semrud-Clikeman and her group are finding that other measures such as social perception (Fine, Semrud-Clikeman, Reynolds, & Smith, unpublished manuscript), cognitive flexibility, and fluid reasoning can also contribute to a differential diagnosis (Semrud-Clikeman & Glass, 2008). Thus, it appears that all symptoms listed by earlier studies do not carry the same weight for a diagnosis of

NVLD. This supports our view that various permutations with these symptoms may result in different behavioral manifestation of the disorder, or subtypes, and that the diagnostic criteria are still evolving. Further study is needed to better understand whether these possible subtypes are phenotypically distinct or whether there is overlap among them.

Grodzinsky (2003; Grodzinsky, Forbes, & Bernstein, 2010), Mamen (2002), and Palombo (2006) suggest that there are specific clinical symptoms or subtypes of NVLD that are important to understand in order to diagnose and treat the child or adult appropriately. An example of a similar situation can be found with the current definition of ADHD, which has evolved to include the inattentive, hyperactive/impulsive, and combined types. For a more detailed description of their perspectives we refer the reader to *Nonverbal Learning Disabilities in Children: Bridging the Gap Between Science and Practice* (Davis & Broitman, 2011). Rourke (2006), however, disagrees, suggesting that what are being referred to as subtypes are really just different symptom clusters within in unitary disorder (Rourke, http://www.NLD-BPROURKE.CA). Or in other words, these subtypes are really just variations in the expression of NVLD. As we have no available data documenting that visual–spatial issues alone are responsible for these differences, multiple lines of development, along the lines proposed by Howard Gardner (1999), could prove to be another valuable model from which to conceptualize the various manifestations of NVLD. We therefore suggest that it is important to expose school and other clinical personnel who are diagnosing, treating, and educating children with NVLD to viable alternatives of ways of understanding NVLD. We believe this would help ensure that the NVLD student is getting appropriate interventions for success in school and in life.

Our Subtype Model

From our review of the existing models and the current available empirical evidence base, along with our clinical experience, we believe that a four-subtype model has the most clinical relevance. We also believe that NVLD can best be viewed as a *spectrum* disorder. Children can have mild versions of some problems, for example, present without a specific functional impairment. Our observations suggest that the lack of functional impairment is mediated by overall intellectual potential, level of discrepancies between verbal and nonverbal measures, and parenting/intervention strategies which have enhanced coping mechanisms. It is our contention that all children who present with NVLD have visual–spatial and executive function difficulties relative to their non-impacted peers. Therefore we consider these deficits to be the primary components of NVLD, constituting our first and core subtype. In Table 2.2 we list most of the available research which contributed to our viewing

Table 2.2 Researchers supporting visuospatial reasoning difficulties

- Cornoldi, Dalla-Vecchia, and Tressoldi (1995)
- Cornoldi, Rigoni, Tressoldi, and Vio (1999)
- Cornoldi, Marconato, and Molin (2003)
- Denckla (1991)
- Forrest (2004, 2007)
- Grodzinsky et al. (2010)
- Hain (2008)
- Mammarella, Lucangeli, and Cornoldi (2010)
- Semrud-Clikeman, Fine, and Bledsoe (2008a)
- Semrud-Clikeman, Walkowiak, Wilkinson, and Christopher (2010)

visuospatial functioning as central to this disorder. Cornoldi, Venneri, Marconato, Molin, and Montinari (2003) have gone so far as to suggest that nonverbal learning disorders be replaced by visuospatial learning disability (VSLD), with which we would also be comfortable. In Table 2.3 we list most of the available research which contributed to our viewing executive functioning as a core aspect of this disorder. Aspects of organization, attention, and working memory are the most supported of the executive functions in the current research.

Children in this subtype may also have mild social and academic deficits which do not necessarily rise to the level of a significant discrepancy or a functional impairment needed for eligibility or diagnostic purposes.

Our second subtype includes children with visual–spatial and executive function difficulties that significantly impact their social functioning. These children need formal evaluations and treatment programs, e.g., pragmatic language therapy and social skills training, and would be likely to meet some form of eligibility or diagnostic criteria (Table 2.4).

The third subtype is characterized by children with significant visual–spatial and executive function difficulties which are functionally impacting their academic work and again are likely to meet some formal eligibility or diagnostic criteria and would be in need of academic supports and interventions. These academic problems are most likely to be math related but can also be in areas like advanced reading comprehension, written expression (especially expository), geography, and math-related sciences (Table 2.5).

The fourth and final subtype is characterized by children with visual–spatial, executive function, social difficulties, and academic deficits, wherein all areas are functionally impaired. We do not believe that these are the only possible subtypes of NVLD but we do feel that all are justified at this state of our knowledge base, and ongoing research should pursue other possible models (Fig. 2.1).

Table 2.3 Researchers supporting executive functioning

- Cornoldi et al. (1999)
- Cornoldi et al. (2003)
- Denckla (1991)
- Fine, Semrud-Clikeman, Butcher, and Walkowiak (2008)
- Fine et al. (unpublished Manuscript)
- Hain (2008)
- Mammarella et al. (2006)
- Mammarella, Lucangeli, and Cornoldi (2010)
- Semrud-Clikeman, Walkowiak, Wilkinson, and Minne (2010)

Table 2.4 Researchers supporting social difficulties

- Bloom and Heath (2010)
- Fine, Semrud-Clikeman, Butcher, and Walkowiak (2008)
- Fine et al. (unpublished Manuscript)
- Palombo (2006)
- Petti, Voelker, Shore, and Hayman-Abello (2002)
- Schafer and Semrud-Clikeman (2008)
- Semrud-Clikeman and Glass (2008)

Table 2.5 Researchers supporting academic functioning difficulties

• De Smedt et al. (2007)	• Math
• Forrest (2004)	• Written math
• Humphries, Cardy, Worling, and Peets (2004)	• Narrative comprehension
• Mammarella, Lucangeli, and Cornoldi (2010)	• Math
• Mammarella et al. (2010)	• Math
• Rourke and Tsatsanis (1996)	• Reading comprehension
• Worling, Humphries, and Tannock (1999)	• Reading comprehension

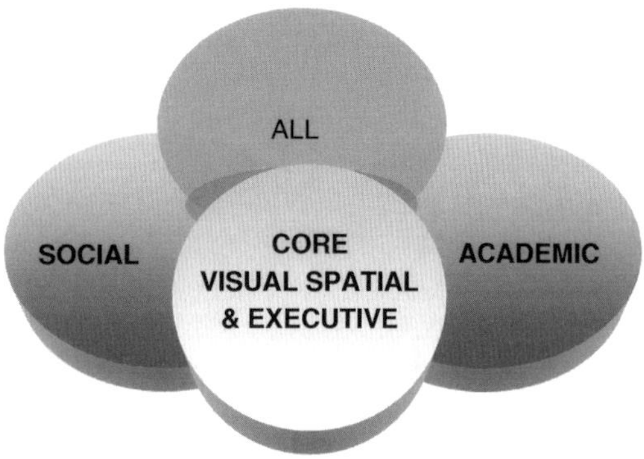

Fig. 2.1 Davis-Broitman model of NVLD

Conclusion

In this chapter we have offered an overview of the history of the development and understanding of nonverbal learning disorders. The most commonly used definition has been reviewed and we have considered how the child with NVLD might appear at different developmental stages. We have offered several ways to understand the varied roads to acquiring NVLD. Clinical observation suggests that at this time most NVLD children present without a clear cause (idiopathic). Hopefully future studies will offer more definitive answers to these important questions. The most important concept we would like for the reader to take from this chapter is that nonverbal learning disorders are complex and not necessarily as *specific* as the term specific learning disability might suggest. In our view, any assessment or remedial plan for a child with NVLD has to account for all potential symptom areas identified. However, we also believe that as more data accumulates a multidimensional model may at some time seem a more appropriate metaphor for NVLD than a subtyping model. Therefore, the SST or IEP teams for children with suspected NVLD should consist of a school psychologist, or his or her private practice alternative like an educational psychologist or neuropsychologist to look at the intellectual, neuropsychological/information processing, and executive function; a special education teacher for the academic concerns; a speech and language pathologist for the semantic–pragmatic difficulties; and an occupational therapist for possible fine/gross motor difficulties. Other professionals might include a school counselor for social skills interventions and/or a referral to a child psychiatrist or developmental pediatrician for possible medication if needed. In the chapters that follow you will hear from each of these professionals. They will describe how they diagnose and work with children and adults with NVLD.

References

Allen, K. (1998). *Star shaped pegs, square holes: Nonverbal learning disorders and the growing up years*. Livermore, CA: Good Enough Books.

American Psychiatric Association. (2000). *Diagnostic and statistical manual of mental disorders—text revision* (4th ed.). Washington, DC: American Psychiatric Association.

Ayres, J. (1994). *Sensory integration and learning disorders*. Los Angeles, CA: Western Psychological Services.

Bloom, E., & Heath, N. (2010). Recognition, expression, and understanding facial expressions of emotion in adolescents with nonverbal and general learning disabilities. *Journal of Learning Disabilities, 43*(2), 180–192. doi:10.

Brooks, R. (1991). *The self-esteem teacher*. Loveland, OH: Treehaus Communications.

Brumbach, R. A. (1985). Wechsler performance IQ deficit in depression in children. *Perceptual and Motor Skills, 61*, 331–335. 1992-72720-001.

Cornoldi, C., Rigoni, F., Tressoldi, P. E., & Vio, C. (1999). Imagery deficits in nonverbal learning disabilities. *Journal of Learning Disabilities, 32*(1), 48–57.

Cornoldi, C., Vecchia, R. D., & Tressoldi, P. E. (1995). Visuo-spatial working memory limitations in low visuo-spatial high verbal intelligence children. *Journal of Child Psychology and Psychiatry, 36*(6), 1053–1064.

Cornoldi, C., Venneri, A., Marconato, F., Molin, A., & Montinari, C. (2003). A rapid screening measure for the identification of visuospatial learning disability in schools. *Journal of Learning Disabilities, 36*(4), 299–306.

Davis, J., & Broitman, J. (2007). Nonverbal learning disabilities: Models of proposed subtypes, part II. *The Educational Therapist, 27*(4), 5–10.

Davis, J., & Broitman, J. (2011). *NVLD in children: Bridging the gap between science and practice*. New York: Springer.

De Smedt, B., Swillen, A., Devriendt, K., Fryns, J. P., Verschaffel, L., & Ghesquière, P. (2007). Mathematical disabilities in children with velo-cardio-facial syndrome. *Neuropsychologia, 45*(5), 885–895. doi:1177/0022219409345014.

Denckla, M. B. (1991). Academic and extracurricular aspects of nonverbal learning disabilities. *Psychiatric Annals, 21*, 717–724.

Duane, D. D. (1991). Neurobiological issues in dyslexia. In M. Snowling & M. Thomson (Eds.), Dyslexia: Integrating theory and practice (pp. 21– 30). London: Whurr.

Drummond, C. R., Ahmad, S. A., & Rourke, B. P. (2005). Rules for the classification of younger children with nonverbal learning disabilities and basic phonological processing disabilities. *Archives of Clinical Neuropsychology, 20*, 171–182.

Fine, J. G., Semrud-Clikeman, M., Butcher, B., Walkowiak, J. (2008). Brief report: Attention effect on a measure of social perception. *Journal of Autism and Developmental Disorders, 38*, 1797–1802.

Forrest, B. (2004). The utility of math difficulties, internalized psychopathology, and visual-spatial deficits to identify children with the nonverbal learning disability syndrome: Evidence for a visual-spatial disability. *Child Neuropsychology, 10*(2), 129–146.

Forrest, B. J. (2004). The utility of math difficulties, internalized psychopathology, and visual-spatial deficits to identify children with nonverbal learning disability syndrome: Evidence for a visual spatial disability. *Child Neuropsychology, 10*(2), 129–146.

Forrest, B. (2007). Diagnosing and treating right hemisphere disorders. In S. J. Hunter & J. Donders (Eds.), Pediatric neuropsychological intervention (pp. 175–192). UK: Cambridge University Press.

Fletcher, J. M. (1985). External validation of learning disability typologies. In B. P. Rourke (Ed.), Neuropsychology of learning disabilities: Essentials of subtype analysis (pp. 187–211). New York: Guilford Press.

Gardner, H. (1999). *Intelligence reframed: Multiple intelligences for the 21st century*. New York: Basic Books.

Gerstmann, J. (1940). Syndrome of finger agnosia, disorientation for right and left, agraphia and acalculia. *Archives of Neurology and Psychiatry, 44*, 389.

Goldberg, E., & Costa, L. D. (1981). Hemisphere differences in the acquisition and use of descriptive systems. *Brain and Language, 14*, 144–173.

Green, D. (1999). *Growing up with NLD*. Albuquerque, NM: Silicon Heights.

Griffin, J., & Gresham, D. (2002). *Binocular anomalies: Diagnosis and vision therapy* (4th ed.). London: Butterworth-Heinemann.

Grodzinsky, G. M. (2003). *Subtypes of nonverbal learning disability: A neuropsychological analysis*. Presented at the 13th Annual Nelson Butters' West Coast Neuropsychology Conference, March 20–23, San Diego, CA.

Grodzinsky, G. M., Forbes, P. W., & Bernstein, J. H. (2010). A practice-based approach to group identification in nonverbal learning disabilities. *Child Neuropsychology, 16*, 433–460.

Hain, L. A. (2008). Exploration of specific learning disability subtypes differentiated across cognitive, achievement, and emotional/behavioral variables. Unpublished doctoral dissertation, Philadelphia College of Osteopathic Medicine, Philadelphia.

Hale, J. B., & Fiorello, C. A. (2004). *School neuropsychology: A practitioner's handbook*. New York: Guilford Press.

Harnadek, M., & Rourke, B. P. (1994). Principal identifying features of the syndrome of nonverbal learning disabilities in children. *Journal of Learning Disabilities, 27*, 144–154.

Humphries, T., Cardy, J. O., Worling, D. E., & Peets, K. (2004). Narrative comprehension and retelling abilities of children with nonverbal learning disabilities. *Brain and Cognition, 56*, 77–88.

Inhelder, B., & Piaget, J. (1964). *The early growth of logic in the child*. New York: W. W. Norton & Company.

Johnson, D. J. (1987). Nonverbal learning disabilities. *Pediatric Annals, 16*, 133–141.

Johnson, D. J., & Myklebust, H. R. (1967). *Learning disabilities: Educational principles and practices*. New York: Grune & Stratton.

Landau, Y., Gross-Tsur, V., Auerbach, J., Van deer Meere, J., & Shalev, R. (1999). Attention-deficit hyperactivity disorder and development right-hemisphere syndrome: congruence and incongruence of cognitive and behavioral aspects of attention. *Journal of Child Neurology, 14*, 209–303.

Mamen, M. (2002). *Nonverbal learning disabilities and their clinical subtypes: Assessment, diagnosis and management*. Ottawa, ON: Centrepointe Professional Services.

Mamen, M. (2006). *Nonverbal learning disabilities and their clinical subtypes: A handbook for parents and professionals—new edition*. Ottawa, ON: Centrepointe Professional Services.

Mammarella, I. C., Cornoldi, C., Pazzaglia, F., Toso, C., Grimoldi, M., & Vio, C. (2006). Evidence for a double dissociation between spatial-simultaneous and spatial-sequential working memory in visuospatial (nonverbal) learning disabled children. *Brain and Cognition, 62*(1), 58–67.

Mammarella, I. C., Lucangeli, D., & Cornoldi, C. (2010). Spatial working memory and arithmetic deficits in childrne with nonverbal learning difficulties. *Journal of Learning Disorders, 43*(5), 455–468.

Mokros, H. B., Poznanski, E. O., & Merrick, W. A. (1989). Depression and learning disabilities in children: A test of an hypothesis. *Journal of Learning Disabilities, 22*, 230–244.

Myklebust, H. R. (1975). Nonverbal learning disabilities: Assessment and intervention. In H. R. Myklebust (Ed.), *Progress in learning disabilities* (Vol. III, pp. 85–121). New York: Grune & Stratton.

Ozols, E. J., & Rourke, B. P. (1988). Characteristics of young learning-disabled children classified according to patterns of academic achievement: Auditory-perceptual and visual-perceptual abilities. *Journal of Clinical Child Psychology, 17*, 44–52.

Ozonoff, S., & Rogers, S. J. (2003). From Kanner to the millennium: Scientific advances that have shaped clinical practice. In S. Ozonoff, S. J. Rogers, & R. L. Hendren (Eds.), Autism spectrum disorders: A research review for practitioners (pp. 3–33). New York: American Psychiatric Publishing Inc.

Palombo, J. (2006). *Nonverbal learning disabilities: A clinical perspective*. New York: WW Norton.

Palombo, J., & Berenberg, A. H. (1999). Working with parents of children with nonverbal learning disabilities: A conceptual and intervention model. In J. A. Incorvaia, B. S. Mark-Goldstein, & D. Tessmer (Eds.), *Understanding, diagnosing, and treating AD/HD in children and adolescents: An integrated approach* (pp. 389–441). Northvale, NJ: Aronson.

Pelletier, P. M., Ahmad, S. A., & Rourke, B. P. (2001). Classification rules for basic phonological processing disabilities and nonverbal learning disorders. *Child Neuropsychology, 7*, 84–98.

Pennington, B. F. (1991). *Diagnosing learning disorders: A neuropsychological framework*. New York, NY: Guilford Press.

Pennington, B. F. (2009). *Diagnosing learning disorders* (2nd ed.). New York: Guilford Press.

Petti, V. L., Voelker, S. L., Shore, D. L., & Hayman-Abello, S. E. (2002). Perception of nonverbal emotional cues by children with nonverbal learning disabilities. *Journal of Developmental and Physical Disabilities, 15*(1), 23–36.

Piaget, J. (1972). *The psychology of intelligence*. Totowa, NJ: Littlefield Adams.
Reed, L. E. (2001). Unaware: Living with non-verbal learning disabilities. Self published.
Rourke, B. P. (Ed.). (1985). *Neuropsychology of learning disabilities: Essentials of subtype analysis*. New York: Guilford Publications.
Rourke, B. P. (1988). The syndrome of nonverbal learning disabilities: Developmental manifestations in neurological disease and dysfunction. *The Clinical Neuropsychologist, 4*, 293–330.
Rourke, B. P. (1995). The NLD syndrome and the white matter model. In B. P. Rourke (Ed.), *Syndrome of nonverbal learning disabilities: Neurodevelopmental manifestations*. New York: Guilford Press.
Rourke, 2006. http://www.NLD-BPROURKE.CA
Rourke, B. P., Ahmad, S. A., Collins, D. W., Hayman-Abello, S. E., & Warriner, E. M. (2002). Child clinical/pediatric neuropsychology: Some recent advances. *Annual Review of Psychology, 53*, 309–339.
Rourke, B. P., & Tsatsanis, K. D. (1996). Syndrome of nonverbal learning disabilities: Psycholinguistic assets and deficits. *Topics in Language Disorders, 16*(2), 30–44.
Rourke, B. P., Young, G. C., & Leenaars, A. A. (1986). A childhood learning disability that predisposes those afflicted to adolescent and adult depression and suicide risk. *Journal of Learning Disabilities, 22*(3), 169–175.
Schafer, V., & Semrud-Clikeman, M. (2008). Neuropsychological functioning in subgroups of children with and without social perception deficits and/or hyperactivity-impulsivity. *Journal of Attention Disorders, 12*(2), 177–190.
Schultz, R. T., Romanski, L. M., & Tsatsanis, K. D. (2000). Neurofunctional models of autistic disorder and Asperger syndrome: Clues from neuroimaging. In A. Klin, F. R. Volkmar, & S. Sparrow (Eds.), *Asperger syndrome*. New York: Guilford Press.
Semrud-Clikeman, M. (2001). *Traumatic brain injury in children and adolescents*. New York: Guilford Press.
Semrud-Clikeman, M., & Hynd, G. W. (1990). Right hemispheric dysfunction in nonverbal learning disabilities: Social, academic, and adaptive functioning in adults and children. *Psychological Bulletin, 197*, 196–209.
Semrud-Clikeman, M., Fine, J. G., & Bledsoe, J. (2008a). Meta-analysis of empirical literature on NVLD. Paper presented at the International Neuropsychological Hawaii, August 2008.
Semrud-Clikeman, M., Fine, J. G., & Bledsoe, J. (2008b). Meta-analysis of empirical research in assessment and diagnosis in NVLD. Paper presented at the International Neuropsychological Hawaii, August 2008.
Semrud-Clikeman, M., & Glass, K. L. (2008). Comprehension of humor in children with nonverbal learning disabilities, verbal learning disabilities and without learning disabilities. *Annals of Dyslexia, 58*, 163–180.
Semrud-Clikeman, M., Walkowiak, J., Wilkinson, A., & Christopher, G. (2010). Neuropsychological differences among children with Asperger syndrome, nonverbal learning disabilities, attention deficit disorder, and controls. *Developmental Neuropsychology, 35*(5), 582–600.
Semrud-Clikeman, M., Walkowiak, J., Wilkinson, A., & Minne, E. P. (2010). Direct and indirect measures of social perception, behavior, and emotional functioning in children with Asperger's disorder, nonverbal learning disability, or ADHD. *Journal of Abnormal Child Psychology, 38*, 509–519.
Tanguay, P. B. (2001). *Nonverbal learning disabilities at home*. London: Jessica Kingsley.
Tanguay, P. B. (2002). *Nonverbal learning disabilities at school*. London: Jessica Kingsley.
Teeter, A. T., & Semrud-Clikeman, M. (1997). *Child neuropsychology: Assessment and interventions for Neurodevelopmental disorders*. Needham Heights, MA: Allyn & Bacon.
Telzrow, C. F., & Bonar, A. M. (2002). Responding to students with nonverbal learning disabilities. *Teaching Exceptional Children, 34*, 8–13.
Thompson, S. (1997). *The source for nonverbal learning disorders*. East Moline, IL: Linguisystems.

Voeller, K. K. S. (1986). Right-hemisphere deficit in children. *The American Journal of Psychiatry, 143*, 1004–1009.

Volden, J. (2004). Nonverbal learning disability: A tutorial for speech-language pathologists. *American Journal of Speech-Language Pathology, 13*, 128–141.

Weintraub, S., & Mesulam, M. M. (1983). Developmental learning disabilities of the right hemisphere. *Archives of Neurology, 40*, 463–468.

Whitney, R. V. (2000). *The nonverbal learning disorder guide for teachers, parents, employers, and therapists*. Campbell, CA: Lighthouse Project.

Wilkinson, A., & Semrud-Clikeman, M. (2008). Motor speed in children and adolescents with nonverbal learning disabilities. Paper presented at the International Neuropsychological Society.

Worling, D. E., Humphries, T., & Tannock, R. (1999). Spatial and emotional aspects of language inferencing in nonverbal learning disabilities. *Brain and Language, 70*(2), 220–239.

Chapter 3
The Role of the Occupational Therapist

Rebecca Schatz

Background

While there is very little research to date in the occupational therapy field on nonverbal learning disorders (NVLD), many children with similar motor and sensory profiles may be diagnosed with other learning disabilities, developmental coordination disorder (DCD), and/or sensory processing disorder (SPD). These children, due to their identified challenges in the areas of fine motor and gross motor coordination, sensory processing, and writing, may be referred to an occupational therapist (OT) both in schools and outpatient facilities.

It should be noted that these children are identified for occupational therapy due to their motor or sensory issues not because it has been recognized that they have NVLD specifically. The challenge today is to accurately identify children with NVLD apart from children who fit the profile but do not have NVLD.

This chapter highlights the intervention areas that are relevant for a child with NVLD (whether or not they have received an official diagnosis) so they will receive the full complement of appropriate treatment that they require to function successfully in the school, home, and social environments. The intervention therapies, strategies, and suggestions outlined in this chapter are drawn from my own experiences as well as those of other colleagues, working as a pediatric OT for the last 17 years.

R. Schatz, M.S., OTR/L (✉)
Rebecca Schatz & Associates, Inc., 2000 N. Racine #3600,
Chicago, IL 60614, USA
e-mail: rebecca.schatz@comcast.net

J. Broitman and J.M. Davis (eds.), *Treating NVLD in Children: Professional Collaborations for Positive Outcomes*, DOI 10.1007/978-1-4614-6179-1_3,

Introduction

Children with NVLD present with various challenges including those associated with motor, visual–spatial organization, social skills, and academic skills. Children with NVLD may appear awkward or clumsy in their motor coordination in tasks such as ball throwing and catching, riding a bike, tying shoes, cutting, and writing (Stewart, 2007). Atypical sensory processing, including high or low sensory thresholds, is commonly seen (Whitney, 2008). In addition, NVLD children are often challenged in perceiving and interpreting social situations accurately (see Chap. 10 for more information). The occupational therapist plays a key role in working with these children on their gross and fine motor, sensory, written expression skills, organization, and social processing.

The occupational therapist completes a thorough evaluation to assess current levels of functioning in a wide range of motor and sensory areas and then determines whether occupational therapy is warranted for the child.

The Assessment Process

When assessing children with NVLD, there are a number of different areas that require evaluation before an appropriate treatment plan can be determined. As part of the assessment process, an occupational therapist utilizes motor skills assessments, handwriting and visual–motor evaluations, sensory processing, visual processing, and clinical observations (Bowyer & Cahill, 2009). The following assessment tools may be included in the evaluation process.

Motor Assessments

1. Bruininks-Oseretsky Test of Motor Proficiency, second edition (BOT-2: Bruininks & Bruininks, 2005), is an assessment tool that is administered individually to children ranging in age from four and a half to twenty-one years. There are eight subtests including fine motor precision, manual dexterity, bilateral coordination, balance, running speed and agility, upper-limb coordination, and strength. There are five composite scores which include fine motor control, manual coordination, body coordination, strength, and agility. This test battery has high reliability and concurrent validity.
2. Miller Function and Participation Scales (Miller, 2006) is a standardized assessment scale that examines children's (2 years and 6 months to 7 years and 11 months) fine, gross, and visual–motor skills using hands-on functional activities.
3. School Function Assessment (SFA: Coster, Deeney, Haltiwanger, & Haley, 1998) is an assessment tool that evaluates a child's performance (kindergarten through sixth grade) on functional tasks and activities. The three scales—Participation, Task Supports, and Activity Performance—provide criterion cutoff scores that are helpful in determining eligibility for services.

4. Peabody Developmental Motor Scales, second edition (PDMS-2: Folio & Fewell, 2000), is a norm-referenced tool to assess motor skills for younger children (birth to 6 years). Motor skills assessed include reflexes, stationary postures, object manipulation, grasping, and visual–motor integration. Fine motor, gross motor, and total motor quotients are completed. This tool has high reliability and adequate concurrent validity.

Visual–Motor Integration (VMI)

1. Beery-Buktenica Developmental Test of Visual–Motor Integration—sixth edition (Beery, Buktenica, & Beery, 2010). The VMI is a standardized tool that evaluates visual–motor integration, visual perception, and motor coordination abilities in children from 2 to 18 years. The short and full format tests have proven to have high reliability and validity. Norms are provided as young as 2 years of age.
2. Test of Visual–Motor Skills (TVMS-3: Martin, 2006a). This standardized test assesses visual–motor integration skills in children from 3 years to 13 years and 11 months with norms.
3. Evaluation Tool of Children's Handwriting (ETCH: Amundson, 1995). This criterion-referenced tool is used to evaluate both manuscript and cursive handwriting in children from first through sixth grade. Results from this test are helpful in designing treatment goals related to handwriting.

Visual Processing

1. Developmental Test of Visual Perception-2 (DTVP-2: Hammill, Pearson, & Voress, 1993). This assessment tool is for children 4–9 years of age. Areas assessed include eye-hand coordination, spatial relations, figure ground, visual–motor speed, copying, position in space, visual closure, and form constancy.
2. Motor-Free Visual Perception Test, third edition (MVPT-3: Colarusso & Hammill, 2003). This tool assesses a child's visual perceptual ability with no motor involvement. It includes spatial relationships, visual closure, visual discrimination, visual memory, and figure ground.
3. Test of Visual Perception (non-motor), third edition (TVPS-3: Martin, 2006b). This assessment tool evaluates visual processing with no motor components. It includes visual discrimination, visual memory, visual–spatial relationships, form constancy, visual sequential memory, visual figure ground, and visual closure.

Sensory Processing

Since children with NVLD present with various sensory processing challenges it is important to determine the sensory systems involved in order to plan treatment goals for occupational therapy services as well as parent and teacher consultations.

Accommodations given to a child's teachers may have numerous sensory-related activities that will be helpful during the school day.

An OT investigates numerous sensory systems including tactile, proprioceptive, vestibular, auditory, and visual:

- Tactile: This system gives information important for many everyday skills such as tactile perception, motor planning, and academic learning (Kranowitz, 2005).
- Proprioceptive: This system provides unconscious information from muscles and joints regarding movement and position. The proprioceptive system works closely with the tactile and vestibular systems; therefore many of the functions are similar including body awareness and grading of movement (Kranowitz, 2005).
- Vestibular: This system provides information from the inner ear regarding movement and position in space. The vestibular sense gives us information that is critical for many everyday skills such as gravitational security, muscle tone, and bilateral coordination (Kranowitz, 2005).
- Auditory: This system provides stimulation to auditory receptors in the inner ear from sound waves (Ayres & Robbins, 2005).
- Visual: This system provides stimulation to the retina from light. It sends input to the visual processing centers in the brain (Ayres & Robbins, 2005).

Keeping these sensory systems in mind, an OT will utilize various sensory assessments (some of which rely on parent and teacher observations and reports) to determine whether the child is experiencing sensory processing challenges that are affecting them in their school and home environments:

1. Sensory Profile (Caregiver Questionnaire) is a standardized assessment tool that evaluates children's (3–10 years) sensory processing in everyday situations. Results from this assessment provide helpful information for diagnosis and intervention planning. The Sensory Profile Supplement provides up-to-date research regarding sensory processing with expanded cut scores and quadrant cut scores (Dunn, 2006b).
2. Sensory Profile School Companion is a standardized assessment tool that provides information regarding a child's level of responsiveness to stimulation in the classroom environment, a factor affecting behavior and performance. The profile is organized into different sensory sections. It takes approximately 15 min to complete and helps the occupational therapist and teacher plan effective strategies for the student within the classroom (Dunn, 2006a).
3. Sensory Processing Measure (SPM) developed by Parham, Ecker, Kuhaneck, Henry, and Glennon (2007) assesses sensory processing in children from kindergarten through sixth grade. Test items relate to sensory processing, social participation, and motor performance (balance and motion, planning and ideas) and yield norm-referenced standard scores. In addition, the school environment forms assess a child's sensory processing in art class, music, P.E., cafeteria, at recess/playground, and on the school bus.

These sensory profiles (Sensory Profile Caregiver Questionnaire (Dunn, 1999), Sensory Profile Supplement (Dunn, 2006b), and Sensory Profile School Companion

(Dunn, 2006a)) characterize children's behaviors and performance in relation to their sensory processing. The profiles that are developed from these questionnaires are purported to expand information regarding the interaction of neurological thresholds and behavioral responses. Neurological thresholds are the amount of stimuli required for a neuron system to respond. Low-registration children have high thresholds and are passive self-regulators. It takes a great deal of sensory information within their environments to garner a response; that is, these children let things happen and then respond.

Sensation-seeking children also require a significant amount of sensory input to respond, but at the same time these children are actively trying to control their environments.

Sensory-sensitive children need very little sensory inputs to respond and are passive self-regulators; that is, they allow things to happen and then respond.

Finally, sensation-avoiding children need very little sensory inputs in their environments to respond and actively try to control their situation (Dunn, 1999).

OT Report and Recommendations

Following the evaluation process outlined, a complete report is written including test results, interpretation, intervention plan consisting of goals for home and school, classroom accommodations, and reevaluation. Important areas to include in the report:

Background Information

This includes any birth-related information, family history, previous therapies, or interventions.

Developmental Milestones

This section covers motor skill acquisition such as rolling, sitting, crawling, standing and walking, tricycle/bike riding, and handedness. Other areas to incorporate in the report include language acquisition, following directions, play skills, dressing, eating, toileting, and peer interactions.

Initial Observations

This section covers observations made during the evaluation such as behavior, attention, regulation, and following directions.

Example of OT's report of initial observations:

"Jack, a 7 year old boy, entered the therapy room excited and quickly established good rapport with this examiner. Some difficulties were seen with attention and distractibility. Jack was seen to move around and fidget in his chair frequently by the table. It was difficult for him to complete tasks sitting in his chair and he was seen to stand during many table tasks he engaged in. Eye contact was inconsistent. Jack demonstrated auditory sensitivities by frequently stopping the activity he was engaged in each time he heard a noise from outside or inside the room."

Gross Motor Skills of Child

This section covers strength, muscle tone, bilateral coordination, balance, and multistep motor sequencing. In addition to including a table with all raw and converted scores, a summary of observed motor skills coordination is helpful for both parents and teachers.

Example of OT's report of gross motor skills:

"Nathan, an 8 year old child, completed various motor coordination activities using both standardized and non-standardized assessment tools. While many of the motor tasks presented were challenging for Nathan, he did try his best. Nathan experienced challenges with coordinating left and right sides of his body together with both his upper and lower extremities. Balance activities were equally as challenging on both right and left sides especially with vision occluded. Nathan was unable to complete the motor sequencing patterns on his first try (e.g. hopping patterns). Nathan attempted to complete the eye-hand coordination activities with little success. Strength and agility were all within normal limits.

Nathan also completed various motor coordination activities using suspended equipment in the clinic. When given some verbal and visual prompting and breaking down the task, Nathan experienced greater success. Step by step instructions were needed in order to successfully complete the motor activity. This is very important to keep in mind for Nathan's participation in physical education classes at school. He will benefit from all motor tasks being broken down into simple, concrete steps to help further his motor planning. Nathan was tentative for many of the motor activities presented and this may be stemming from the challenges he experiences in motor planning out the necessary steps."

Fine Motor/Visual–Motor Skills of Child

This section covers strength and manual dexterity with both dominant and non-dominant hands, motor speed, fine motor control, and visual–motor integration. Summary of observations and scores should be provided in this section.

Example of OT's report of fine motor/visual skills:

"Andrew demonstrated strengths and weaknesses with his fine and visual motor abilities. Andrew was able to construct sophisticated lego designs and could duplicate block and puzzle patterns given to him. While stick designs appeared easy to complete, the fine motor manipulation of these sticks impacted overall success with this task. Copying figures and drawing from memory all scored below age expectations. It appears that Andrew needs to learn strategies of where to start and what the steps are to complete these types of activities. Forms that involve midline crossing were also challenging at this time for Andrew. Tongue protrusion (an overflow movement seen when a motor task is difficult) was observed during many of the visual motor tasks.

It appears that Andrew may become overwhelmed when too much visual information is presented to him. Within the school setting, worksheets with lots of visual information may be challenging for Andrew at this time. It is recommended that Andrew be given worksheets that have some parts covered up and/or the amount of visual information reduced. Again, Andrew needs visual motor tasks broken down into simple concrete steps so that he can successfully complete them."

Visual Processing

This section includes reporting on the child's visual perceptual abilities, visual problem solving, copying, spatial relations, visual closure, visual–motor speed, and eye-hand coordination skills.

Example of OT's report of visual processing:

"Strengths and weaknesses in the visual processing area may correlate with performance in writing and spelling. Jonathan was able to discriminate left and right on himself however when he needed to complete this task pointing (to left or right) on this examiner, he was unable to do so. While copying a form given to him on graph paper, Jonathan was able to complete all details and size of the form but was challenged with placing it in the correct place on the paper. In addition, his decreased fine motor control hindered his performance on this task. While Jonathan demonstrated strengths with visual pattern recognition, figure-ground and spatial relations, he worked at these tasks randomly, without using an organized approach. This lengthened the time needed to complete them. Visual tasks involving a motor component were completed with difficulty."

Written Expression of Child

This section includes reporting on pencil grip, writing posture, letter, and sentence formation.

Example of OT's report of written expression:

"Sara utilized an appropriate right handed tripod pencil grasp with left hand stabilization. Letter formation was slow and laborious for Sara. Sentence copying scored well below age expectations. When writing a story, Sara experienced challenges in organizing her thoughts (forming a logical sequence of events), figuring out how to start, and physically putting words and sentences down on paper."

"While completing writing activities, Sara would benefit from using a slant board to provide a better sitting posture for her. In addition, Sara may benefit from sitting on a ball chair to complete writing activities. This will provide her with both gentle sensory motor inputs and assist with posture during table tasks. Sara needs reminders to space her words when writing sentences (at times she will use a space stick). While Sara utilizes an appropriate grip pattern, she may benefit from using thick triangular pencils or mechanical pencils when writing to decrease overall fatigue. Sara also benefits from planning and organizing her thoughts using visual planners and visual maps before writing paragraphs or stories. Organizing ideas is critical before beginning any written expression task. Sara will benefit from a handwriting program that provides visual and verbal cueing in letter formation so she can learn correct direction and orientation when forming letters. Writing paper should be carefully selected (some examples include handwriting without tears, highlighted lined paper, and raised line paper)."

Sensory Processing Abilities of the Child

While there are many examples outlined in the Intervention section, included here is a brief summary that can be incorporated in the occupational therapy report.

Example of OT's report of sensory processing:

"According to the sensory profile filled out by Sheri's parents and by examiner observation, Sheri exhibits many behaviors seen in Sensory Processing Disorder. Sensory processing disorder occurs when the nervous system is not able to process and modulate the sensations in the environment in a calm, organized, and meaningful way. The nervous system may be taking in too much or too little sensory information. The child who is not getting enough sensory information/input may need more stimulation to be alert and aroused. Behaviors commonly observed are a great deal of touching, feeling, bumping, and crashing.

Sheri's nervous system at times is unable to regulate itself properly because it has become overwhelmed with the sensory input in the environment. Other times, her nervous system needs more input and Sheri can be observed seeking out more input in different ways. It is important to observe closely how Sheri's nervous system is responding, whether she is over stimulated and challenged with her regulation or whether the amount of sensory input is just right. In addition, it is important to pay close attention to the occasions when Sheri seeks out more input in her environment and see what kinds of sensory experiences might be helpful for her at that moment in order to stay regulated and focused."

Summary of Findings

This section of the OT report covers both strengths and weaknesses of the child, assessments results, discussion, and goals.

Occupational Therapy Goals

Occupational therapists work with children and youth at different stages in development. It is important for the OT to determine how best to further a child's development given the challenges presented and enhance their activity performance and their overall participation in daily life. As an OT evaluates and begins to determine appropriate goals for the student, successful occupational performance remains the forefront of occupational therapy practice (Bendixen & Kreider, 2011).

The OT report and recommendations should address the various areas discussed including fine motor, gross motor, writing, keyboarding, and sensory processing goals.

Intervention

Once the report has been completed, the occupational therapist writes up specific goals for the intervention program. Typically, children with NVLD require treatment for the following areas: gross motor skills development, fine motor skills development, handwriting, sensory processing, and social skills development.

Motor Development Interventions

Students with NVLD typically present with motor challenges in the areas of bilateral coordination (i.e., using both sides of the body in a coordinated manner), balance, motor sequencing, body awareness, postural control, and fine motor.

Activities such as bike riding, scootering, swimming, ball throwing, and catching may present challenges and are often avoided by children with NVLD. These children benefit from working on these motor coordination activities while having each step of the activity broken down and verbalized to them. If the child repeats back directions before executing the necessary actions, it reinforces the motor sequence. Therapeutic interventions such as Brain Gym® (Dennison & Dennison, 1994) teach children to "learn through movement" by coordinating eyes, ears, hands, and entire body. Changes that have been documented with Brain Gym include improvements in attention, focus, memory, physical coordination, organizational skills, and academic skills (www.braingym.org/studies). Sensory motor activities (work on suspended equipment) benefit the child with both sensory and motor challenges. The Integrated Listening Systems (iLs: Minson, 2007) is a multisensory program that effectively combines auditory stimulation with balance, movement, and visual–motor tasks. The iLs program utilizes many of the principles of Dr. Tomatis' method which identified relationships between sound frequencies and the effect on mind and body. "The Tomatis Effect" identified three frequency zones. Zone 1, lower frequency sounds, is at the level of sensory integration which includes such skills as rhythm, coordination, balance, sense of direction, laterality, body awareness, and right/left discrimination (Gerritsen, 2009). Many of the music selections in the iLs program target this auditory integration zone.

Handwriting Development Interventions

Children need successful development of fine motor control, motor planning, concepts of directionality, visual memory, and visual perceptual skills in order to write effectively. Case-Smith (2002) conducted a study to determine the effectiveness of school-based OT services on students' handwriting. Students that received OT services that focused on visual–motor skills and handwriting practice demonstrated improved letter legibility; however speed and numeral legibility did not demonstrate improved effects.

There are many handwriting programs used by OTs including Olsen's Handwriting Without Tears® (2012), Benbow's Kinesthetic Writing System (1999), and Write-On Handwriting LLC (Ford, 2003). Many components are addressed within OT therapy sessions to improve handwriting abilities:

- Visual memory for letter formation
- Orientation, direction, sequence, and starting point of letters
- Placement of letters on paper
- Size of letters
- Fine motor control-strengthening activities, individual finger movements, pressure and grading of movements
- Spacing of letters

The older child with NVLD may require additional accommodations within the classroom to assist with handwriting and written expression activities. Letter strips that are placed either on the student's desk or close by allow for quicker visual recognition of letters. Creating visual boundaries for the student promotes greater success when navigating math work or other handwriting activities. The older student who writes more sophisticated and lengthy stories might try more detailed graphic organizers/story maps to outline ideas before writing. The occupational therapist, however, may have to customize a visual organizer for the student depending on individual needs. Children with NVLD present with organizational challenges and therefore tools that the occupational therapist provides the student will promote greater success in written expression.

Keyboarding Development Interventions

Initially, an early focus should be given on handwriting (print and cursive) for children in kindergarten through third grade. Cursive writing is often a frustrating and challenging experience and therefore it is important to begin to evaluate other modes of written communication. Children should be introduced to keyboarding when the act of writing becomes too cumbersome and laborious (Stewart, 2007). There are many keyboarding programs students can use including Type to Learn® 4 (Sunburst Digital, 2010), UltraKey® 5 (Bytes of Learning Inc., 2006), Typing Instructor for Kids (2009), and Typing Quick & Easy 17 (Individual Software Inc., 2007). Once a student is proficient in keyboarding, many online organizational tools can be introduced for written expression assignments such as Inspiration® 9 (Inspiration Software Inc., 2011) or Kidspiration® 3 (Inspiration Software Inc., 2008). Kidspiration software program is intended for kindergarten through fifth grade. These programs can be modified and individually created to meet the demands of different learning styles and abilities.

Sensory Processing Intervention

Sensory integration (SI) organizes information received from a child's senses including taste (gustatory sense), sight (visual sense), hearing (auditory sense), smell (olfactory sense), touch (tactile sense), movement and position (proprioceptive sense), head movement, balance, and gravity (vestibular sense). SI intervention focuses on assisting the child to become an active participant, which leads to an adaptive response. SI theory asserts that an adaptive response (a purposeful and goal-directed response) leads to increased sensory integration, which in turn results in the brain achieving a more organized state (Ayres & Robbins, 2005).

The Alert Program® (Williams & Shellenberger, 1996) helps children become more aware of their internal arousal states and organization. Their program "How Does Your Engine Run?"® teaches strategies children can use in moments of sensory regulation challenges at home, at school, and in other environments.

A number of studies and case studies have been conducted determining the efficacy of SI therapy. However, SI treatment remains controversial. Empirical studies have determined varying results in part due to a lack of consistency in principles of SI theory and treatment, heterogeneity of populations studied, and varying outcome measures (Schaaf & Nightlinger, 2007).

Sensory processing challenges can be differentiated into four quadrants—poor registration, sensitivity to stimuli, sensation seeking, and sensation avoiding (Dunn, 1999). It is important to understand a child's sensory profile so that appropriate environmental modifications can be made (Whitney, 2008). Koenig and Rudney (2010) completed a systematic review of the challenges experienced by children and adolescents with sensory processing challenges.

Sensory Processing Challenges

1. Poor registration characteristics are seen in children who miss or notice fewer sensory cues that occur. They may not respond to their teacher calling to them,

or may not notice if their clothes are twisted or not positioned on their body correctly. In addition, difficulties in noticing cues result in attention drifting during activities and/or experiencing a more difficult time completing tasks in a timely manner. It is important that all experiences are more concentrated with sensory information so children will be able to notice and respond to cues within their environment. Activities that give strong feedback, such as deep touch instead of light touch, help children respond more appropriately (Dunn, 1999).

(a) Home suggestions to improve poor registration:
In the home, parents can provide increased sensory inputs for their child by providing greater opportunities to move about during bath time, mealtime, or playtime.

Playing with textured materials (e.g., rough sponges, washcloths, rough handmade soaps, sprayers, squishy or bumpy balls) gives added tactile input to the child. Playing catch or bowling with weighted balls provides greater proprioceptive inputs (i.e., greater awareness into the child's muscles and joints promoting a response).

During mealtime, the child may benefit from standing up to eat, actively participating in setting the table (heavier plates and bowls again provide increased inputs), and dishing out the food (i.e., using tongs or spatulas).

Building forts during playtime that allow for climbing and crawling provide greater inputs. Heavy pillows, blankets, or old mattresses can be easily used within this type of play. When playing outdoors, sensory motor activities that the low registration child may benefit from include climbing structures, crawling through narrow spaces, swinging, riding bicycles, or scootering.

(b) School suggestions to improve poor registration:
During the school day, the child may benefit from movement breaks after a table task, before sitting down for rug/learning times, or before transitioning to another class. These children need paper and materials highlighted or bolded. For example, writing paper lines can be highlighted at the top and bottom to allow for greater visual focus.

It is important for the teacher to frequently check in with the child to make sure they understand and process directions accurately. Written and pictorial schedules posted in close proximity to the child help the child to stay on task. Teachers may initially need to cue the child on when to check in or look at their schedule, until it becomes an automatic response. A teacher may tap a child on his/her shoulder when noticing that their attention is drifting. Lastly, a child may benefit from a change in their seat location.

2. Sensitivity to stimuli behavioral indicators may include distractibility and hyperactivity. Children may show sensitivities to sensory input such as exhibiting strong reactions to loud noises or eating very selectively. Children who are sensitive tend to notice more things than children who are not. Because of this characteristic these children become more easily distracted than other children and

notice changes in their environment very quickly. As a result, they may be frequently interrupted from completing tasks in a timely manner. Again, it is important to monitor the sensory experiences that support the child's ongoing performance and continuation of a task. It is important to determine elements within the environment that may impede participation. Sensitivities to touch input and sensitivities to sounds must all be taken into consideration within the environment (Dunn, 1999).

Children with sensory modulation disorders (SMD) frequently exhibit similar characteristics to children diagnosed with attention deficit hyperactivity disorder (ADHD), which can complicate assessments and intervention. A recent study by Miller, Nielsen, and Schoen (2012) found that these children (those with ADHD and SMD) are more distinct than previously thought and differed in measures of emotion-, attention-, and sensory-related behaviors. This is important to keep in mind when determining intervention plans for children that may exhibit both sensory and attention challenges.

(a) Home strategies to improve sensitivity to stimuli:
Children who present with sensitivities to stimuli typically need greater predictability within their daily routines. Sensitivity to clothing may be addressed by having the child wear well-fitted clothing or removing tags. Typically, these children prefer to wear the same clothes each day. Slowly introducing new textures of clothing (when these sensory sensitivities begin to show improvements) is received with greater comfort.

These children may require a consistent spot to sit and eat meals (a place with fewer distractions/things going on). Play that incorporates heavy movement activities (weighted materials, crawling through tight spaces, pushing and pulling) provides an appropriate amount of input. Bedtime routines that are comfortable for the sensitive child may include gentle movement in a rocking chair and using weighted blankets or lap weights while sleeping.

(b) School strategies to improve sensitivity to stimuli: Strategies include limiting the number of steps involved when teaching the child a new movement activity, during classes such as physical education. Having a teacher physically move through each step slowly with child may also be helpful.

Choosing a desk or work area with minimal visual distractions (i.e., front of the class or in a corner spot) and providing written instructions or pictures to supplement verbal information are useful. This child may benefit from working at a back table where no other students are present or an area that has little visual and auditory stimulation. The child may also benefit from wearing a weighted vest or using small lap weights during seated work time.

3. Sensation-seeking behavioral indicators include active, continuously engaging, fidgety, and an excitable demeanor. Children are continuously working to obtain more sensory input such as touching things, tapping their pencils, or chewing on things during class (Dunn, 1999).

(a) Home suggestions to improve sensation seeking: Beneficial playtime sensory activities include engaging in "roughhouse" play with weighted materials, pillows and/or blankets, wheelbarrow, or animal walks; carrying heavy objects in the house (boxes, grocery bags, laundry basket); jumping on a mini-trampoline (it is important to pay careful attention that the movement is not too much for the child's nervous system to handle); movement activities on therapy balls; swinging; biking; and running outdoors.

(b) School suggestions to improve sensation seeking: Effective strategies include incorporating movement in activities, allowing the child to step out of the class to get a drink of water, climbing stairs outside of the classroom, selecting the child to pass out materials, putting away chairs or tables, selecting the child to clean tables or boards, providing bumpy or raised cushions to sit on during seated work, offering drinks from water bottles with thick straws, and offering gum or dried fruit snacks to chew on.

4. Sensation-avoiding behavioral indicators include resistance to change and reliance on rigid rituals. These children are frequently bothered by sensory input so they will move away from activities or choose to work alone. It is important to honor a child's need to limit unfamiliar input while at the same time broadening his/her sensory processing range (Dunn, 1999). Schedules are critical for these children so that they are able to predict with assurance what is coming next. Once children are comfortable with their written or visual schedule, it would be beneficial to slowly change one thing at a time in the schedule. This needs to be done slowly and comfortably for the child.

(a) Home strategies to improve sensation avoiding:
At home, it is important to provide the child with consistent and comfortable routines in bathing, dressing, and mealtime. This child does best when their morning and evening routines remain the same. While they benefit from this predictability, it is important to slowly change the routine at a pace that is comfortable for the child (e.g., making one small change in the schedule once a week). This child may benefit from a consistent spot to eat. They may struggle when new textures of food are introduced so it is important to introduce these foods slowly and comfortably for the child.

(b) School suggestions to improve sensation avoiding: Strategies include limiting the amount of information or steps provided to the child at one time (e.g., giving one direction at a time when completing a new activity), having the child sit at a desk that has minimal visual and auditory distractions (perhaps at the back of the classroom), and establishing a routine that feels comfortable and supportive for the child.

It is important for the teacher to process with the child when changes in the schedule will be happening. Working on concrete strategies to use in these moments of change in the school day will be helpful. These strategies may include deep breathing or counting.

This child may struggle with large group work and may therefore benefit from beginning in a smaller, more manageable size group. Lastly, it is important for both teacher and therapist to work on the language a child can use such as "I am not feeling comfortable working here. Can I work in a different place?" or "Can you please help me, I am not sure what to do in this situation." Role-playing with the child can help when sensations or experiences within their environment feel uncomfortable.

Therapeutic Listening Programs

Children with NVLD often benefit from a therapeutic listening program to address auditory sensitivities, visual–motor abilities, and balance. Various listening programs are available for occupational therapists who complete training and certification. Programs include Therapeutic Listening® (Frick & Young, 2009) and Integrated Listening Systems (iLs: Minson, 2007). Typically these auditory programs involve equipment such as headphones, tune belts, CDs, and manuals and therefore must be carefully considered in an appropriate home or school treatment program. A 2007 study evaluated the effectiveness of therapeutic listening on children with sensory processing disorders and visual–motor delays. Results from this study found positive changes when children were given a combination of specific sensory experiences throughout their day while following the protocol of the therapeutic listening program. The children's behavior with regard to their sensory processing changed along with improvements in visual perception and handwriting (Hall & Case-Smith, 2007).

Visual–Spatial

Children with NVLD often present with visual–spatial challenges including right/left discrimination, directionality, and organization. The OT can provide a number of playful gross motor activities (e.g., obstacle courses, hopscotch, Twister®, ball activities) that target these areas. Board games that focus on visual problem solving and organizational skills include Mighty Mind (MightyMind), Rush Hour Traffic games (Think Fun), Labyrinth and Labyrinth Jr. (Ravensburger), Qwirkle (Mindware), Blokus (Mattel), and Rumis (Educational Insights). Additionally, the OT can provide support to the classroom teacher on how to modify worksheets and other materials (e.g., graph paper, highlighted paper).

Social Processing

An OT treatment program for a student with NVLD should take social processing into consideration. While this area will most likely be addressed by other members of the team, occupational therapists should be acutely aware of activities or strategies to assist in this area. While working on motor and sensory activities, the child with NVLD can also work on identifying nonverbal cueing (from both the therapist and other children who may be present within the therapeutic environment).

Within the clinic setting, opportunities to problem solve social situations are easily integrated and woven into a therapy session. Sensory motor activities assist the NVLD child to gain greater awareness into their own nonverbal cueing and body in space when they are on their own or with others with whom they come into contact. During this time, it is ideal to integrate discussions surrounding playground and other school environments into the therapy since the child's nervous system is well regulated and organized. Oftentimes, these moments of sensory regulation bring a greater openness and sharing into those situations or environments that can be challenging for the child with NVLD.

Lastly, if the child with NVLD is participating in a sensory motor occupational therapy group, multiple social problem-solving opportunities are created. Processing these situations "in the moment" helps the child with NVLD to gain greater awareness of nonverbal cues, social communication, and negotiation.

There are many social skills programs designed for children with NVLD (and other social communication disorders) including Michelle Garcia Winner's Social Thinking® (2005), Jed Baker's Social Skills Training (2003), and Carol Gray's Social Stories (2010). Some of the numerous board games that occupational therapists find effective when working with NVLD students include "What Do you Say … What do you do?® … at school?", which challenges students with questions to answer or situations to problem solve in various places in school including home room, library, playground, and lunchroom. "My School Day" (Social Skill Builder, 2000) is a computer software program for children (6–12 years) that teaches appropriate interactions and classroom social skills. Areas covered include responding to teasing, compromising, resolving conflicts, and following rules. Important areas to address in therapy include working on nonverbal cueing, increasing awareness in social situations, social negotiations, and developing skills in perceiving and interpreting social situations.

Individualized Education Plan Process

A student in the public school system is eligible for testing and evaluation by an occupational therapist. Many school districts are utilizing a newer model of intervention, response to intervention (RTI) (Bradley et al., 2011). A teacher will initially fill out a referral stating their concerns with the student's ability to learn. The teacher and RTI team will develop a new plan of how to address the student's needs through evidence-based interventions for 6 weeks and then retest to see if the issue has been resolved.

After a lengthy RTI process, and proof that the student's issues were NOT due to the methods of teaching, the student is then referred to the special education process.

A domain meeting is then held. The entire team (psychologist, speech language pathologist, occupational therapist, physical therapist, social worker, teacher, case manager, parent) meets with the teacher to discuss the student's issues. If it appears that there is a problem with the student's learning related to OT concerns, the OT will complete an evaluation.

The final step in the process is an eligibility meeting where all team members discuss results. If the student qualifies for special education, he/she will receive an individualized education plan (IEP). If the student qualifies for OT as a related service (related to access to curriculum), this will go on the IEP as well. If a student does not qualify for special education services, but does qualify for OT, a 504 plan may be written. Challenges are experienced when a student does not receive an NVLD diagnosis and therefore is ineligible for OT services or is placed under a different label that may make it harder to receive support services. An OT will use specific "OT Guidelines" outlined by the school district that direct observations and assessments to determine what the student can or cannot do in their specific environment.

Occupational Therapist Assessment

An OT will typically assess the following areas through a teacher interview, student interview, and student observation—all of his/her routines, standardized testing, and review of current academics:

- Behavioral organization: assessment of attention and arousal levels of the student. How does the student respond to visual and auditory stimulation in the classroom? Is the student able to listen to and follow directions given by the classroom teacher?
- Task organization: assessment of some executive functioning areas including organization of materials for tasks given and organization for completing them. It is especially important to carefully evaluate both the initiation and completion of work-related tasks. How does the student follow classroom schedules and transitions?
- Sensory integration: assessment/evaluation of all sensory systems including vestibular, proprioceptive, tactile, auditory, and visual systems. Within the sensory evaluation, attention is given to how a student registers, processes, and modulates these incoming sensory inputs within the school setting and the resulting output in motor, visual, and social areas. Careful attention should be given to body awareness in classroom and motor coordination including balance, eye-hand and postural control, task and work completion, visual processing, and social negotiations.
- Fine motor control/written expression: assessment/evaluation of a student's grasp pattern, manipulation and use of writing tools, and written expression abilities (e.g., note taking, creative story writing).

1. Summary of questions to consider for the younger student with NVLD:
   - Does the student avoid manipulation of tools such as crayons, markers, or scissors?
   - Does the student have difficulty with cutting, coloring, drawing, or painting?
   - Does the student have poor posture or slump by the table when sitting?
   - Does the student have a poor pencil grasp or drop their pencil frequently?
   - Does the student write really faintly or very darkly on the paper?
   - Does the student hold their pencil tightly or fatigue quickly?
   - Was the student slow to show a clear and consistent hand preference?
   - Does the student exhibit other motor difficulties such as dressing, undressing, negotiating zippers, or putting on shoes?
2. Summary of questions to consider for the older student with NVLD:
   - Does the student frequently try to avoid writing activities?
   - Does the student have difficulties knowing where to start their sentence?
   - Does the student have difficulties spacing words within their sentence?
   - Does the student experience difficulties remembering how to form individual letters within words?
   - Does the student have difficulties writing their words or sentences within the spaces provided on the paper?
   - Does the student have difficulties coming up with ideas for their stories?
   - Is the student able to organize their ideas before writing their stories? Do they use a story map/visual organizer?
   - Does the student fatigue quickly when writing a story?
   - Does the student stop frequently when writing a story so that it appears to take an exceptionally long time to complete the written activity?

Services

Results of these assessments will determine eligibility for *direct* or *consult OT services*.

1. Direct OT services
   An OT will typically provide direct service minutes if a strong visual–motor component is affecting and inhibiting the writing process for a student. For the younger student, initiation of a fine motor/handwriting program will begin. For the older student who demonstrates poor handwriting abilities, an OT may move directly to keyboarding and assistive technology since it may be difficult to change a student's motor memory for handwriting.
2. Consult OT services
   If a student is experiencing challenges with completing work assignments and their handwriting is legible, consult services may be recommended. The OT will provide both teachers and students with information on executive functioning

areas and organizational strategies including timers, visual aids on desks for reminders, peer mentoring/modeling, copying task strategies, and accommodations for departure routines (e.g., having assignments already written down for the student, making any necessary changes to homework planners).

Various accommodations can be written into the IEP even if a student has not received an official NVLD diagnosis. These students may have received a different diagnosis but fit the NVLD profile.

Sample IEP Goals

Annual goals with individual benchmarks are written for the student. These benchmarks are evaluated quarterly in order that goals may be added, updated, or continued depending on a student's success in completing them.

1. Handwriting:
   "Student will be able to initiate and complete an in-class writing assignment, using available technology, within 30 min, provided with minimal verbal/visual cues from an adult, 3/5 days per week."
   "Student will be able to complete an in-class writing assignment when provided a graphic organizer and moderate cues from an adult, 2/5 days per week."
   "Student will be able to complete an in-class writing assignment that is legible to teacher and a peer using minimal verbal/visual cueing."

   These goals may be adjusted by an OT: for example, number of therapy days per week, how many classroom assignments are needed to meet the goal, and how much support or cueing is needed. It may be important for the OT to slowly decrease the amount of support required (i.e., verbal and visual cueing) to complete the task.
2. Motor goals:
   "Student will be able to complete an adult-directed table top fine motor activity with maximum verbal and visual cueing, 3/5 days per week."
   "Student will be able to independently complete an adult-directed table top fine motor activity for 15 min, 4/5 days per week."

   Within these motor goals, benchmarks may include a cutting goal, a stringing goal, and/or a grasping objects goal. An OT may also modify goals to include attention to task (with or without cueing).
3. Organization goals:
   "Using organizational systems/strategies, Student will turn in 80 % of homework assignments throughout the quarter, provided only visual cues and reminders."
   This goal can be adjusted by modifying the cueing provided to the student to minimal verbal reminders from an adult.
4. Sensory organization goals:
   "Student will utilize sensory strategies for self-calming in classroom setting, provided with only visual cues and reminders."
   "Student will utilize sensory strategies for calming when participating in music class."

"Student will utilize sensory strategies for calming when participating with a variety of classroom textures and materials."
"Student will attend to class task and complete task with verbal and visual cueing provided."
"Student will maintain appropriate regulation when walking through hallways between classes with minimal verbal prompting."

Sample Accommodations

Sample accommodations that may be included in an IEP:

- Provide preferential seating.
- Allow additional minutes for departure and/or arrival routines.
- Allow for the use of adaptive seating (e.g., air cushions, T-stools, and therapy ball chairs).
- Provide the use of a portable word processor and/or laptop in school computer lab for written assignments.
- Repeat directions or provide physical prompts as necessary in order to secure student's attention.
- Provide externally imposed structure and frequent reminders to sustain attention to task and reduce distractibility.
- Provide sensory motor breaks as needed (refer to list).

Classroom Strategies

Classroom strategies teachers can implement for children with NVLD who demonstrate sensory processing challenges include:

- Incorporate movement in activities: allow student to move about before classroom meeting time or before any table work.
- Select student to pass out materials in the classroom.
- Send student on errands throughout the day.
- Encourage student to move or put chairs away.
- Select student to help in rearranging desks in the classroom.
- Choose student to carry heavy books or boxes.
- Ask student to staple paper onto bulletin boards.
- Choose student to help gym teacher move mats or hand them out.
- Engage student in physical activity before a challenging work task.
- Ask student to stack chairs.
- Vary where student sits in the classroom.
- Play background music when student is completing table work.
- Ask student to sharpen pencils with a manual sharpener.
- Choose student to help to clean desks and tables.

- Encourage student to look frequently at the written schedule for the day in order to reinforce the sequence of activities for the day.
- Designate areas within the classroom for frequently occurring information.
- Provide a quiet corner in the classroom.
- Permit student to chew gum when required.
- Permit student to step out of the classroom to get a drink of water.
- Encourage students to climb up the stairs.
- Encourage students to do chair push-ups.

Reevaluation

Reevaluations by a school OT are typically completed at different points within the school year. Benchmarks are evaluated quarterly while main goals are determined annually. In a private or outpatient setting, goals can be continuously updated as therapy progresses.

Formal reevaluations depend on goals outlined for the child and expected completion of them. There are some formal assessments that do require a certain length of time to lapse before they can be repeated (e.g., 6 months). It is important for occupational therapists to keep ongoing communication with both teacher and parent as the therapy progresses in order to determine ideal times to reevaluate and update goals and expectations.

Conclusion

Since there is no typical picture of a child with nonverbal learning disorder, a scrupulous assessment process is an essential first step in accurately diagnosing the child suspected to have NVLD and to providing effective intervention.

Utilizing the assessment process outlined in this chapter assists the occupational therapist to successfully identify the NVLD child.

Once identified, the recommendations discussed in this chapter focus specifically on the skills in need of improvement and the environment which is optimal for this improvement to take place.

The lengthy list of interventions included open for the therapist a wide variety of treatment options.

While the occupational therapist plays a significant role in assisting NVLD children, they do so in tandem with other professionals (whose roles are outlined in other chapters). Together these professionals provide the interventions best suited for each individual child.

With such a large and detailed battery of assessment tools and therapeutic interventions available today, no child needs to be left without the assistance they deserve to enable them to function productively in the classroom environment as well as in their social environment.

References

Amundson, S. (1995). *Evaluation tool of children's handwriting*. Homer, AL: OT KIDS.

Ayres, A. J., & Robbins, J. (2005). *Sensory integration and the child: Understanding hidden sensory challenges*. Los Angeles, CA: Western Psychological Services.

Baker, J. (2003). *Social skills training for children & adolescents with Asperger syndrome and social-communications problems*. Overland Park, KS: Autism Asperger.

Beery, K. E., Buktenica, N. A., & Beery, N. A. (2010). *Beery-Buktenica developmental test of visual-motor integration* (6th ed.). Bloomington, MN: Pearson.

Benbow, M. D. (1999). *Benbow's kinesthetic writing system*. San Antonio, TX: Pearson.

Bendixen, R. M., & Kreider, C. M. (2011). Centennial vision-review of occupational therapy in the practice area of children and youth. *The American Journal of Occupational Therapy, 65*, 351–359.

Bowyer, P., & Cahill, S. M. (2009). *Pediatric occupational therapy handbook*. St. Louis, MO: Mosby.

Bradley, M. C., Levin, M., O'Reilly, F., Parsad, A., Roberston, A., & Warner, A. (2011). National assessment of IDEA overview IDEA national assessment implementation study executive summary and report. NCEE.

Bruininks, R. H., & Bruininks, B. D. (2005). *Bruininks-Oseretsky test of motor proficiency* (2nd ed.). Minneapolis, MN: NCS Pearson.

Case-Smith, J. (2002). Effectiveness of school-based occupational therapy intervention on handwriting. *The American Journal of Occupational Therapy, 56*, 17–25.

Colarusso, R. P., & Hammill, D. D. (2003). *Motor-free visual perception test* (3rd ed.). Torrance, CA: Western Psychological Services.

Coster, W., Deeney, T., Haltiwanger, J., & Haley, S. (1998). *School function assessment*. San Antonio, TX: The Psychological Corporation.

Dennison, P. E., & Dennison, G. E. (1994). *Brain gym*. Ventura, CA: Edu Kinesthetics.

Dunn, W. (1999). *Sensory profile, user's manual*. San Antonio, TX: The Psychological Corporation.

Dunn, W. (2006a). *Sensory profile school companion, user's manual*. Austin, TX: NCS Pearson.

Dunn, W. (2006b). *Sensory profile supplement, user's manual*. San Antonio, TX: Harcourt Assessment.

Folio, M. R., & Fewell, R. R. (2000). *Peabody developmental motor scales* (2nd ed.). Austin, TX: Pro-Ed.

Ford, A. N. (2003). *Write-on handwriting LLC*. Cambridge, MA: Educator's Publishing Service.

Frick, S. M., & Young, S. R. (2009). *Listening with the whole body: Clinical concepts and treatment guidelines for therapeutic listening*. Madison, WI: Vital Links.

Gerritsen, J. (2009). A review of research done on Tomatis Auditory Stimulation. www.mozartcenter.com/research

Gray, C. (2010). *The new social story book*. Arlington, TX: Future Horizons.

Hall, L., & Case-Smith, J. (2007). The effect of sound-based intervention on children with sensory processing disorders and visual-motor delays. *The American Journal of Occupational Therapy, 61*, 209–215.

Hammill, D. D., Pearson, N. A., & Voress, J. K. (1993). *Developmental test of visual perception-2*. San Antonio, TX: Pearson.

Inspiration® 9. (2011). Beaverton, OR: Inspiration Software.

Kidspiration® 3. (2008). Beaverton, OR: Inspiration Software.

Koenig, K. P., & Rudney, S. G. (2010). Performance challenges for children and adolescents with difficulty processing and integrating sensory information: A systematic review. *The American Journal of Occupational Therapy, 64*, 430–442.

Kranowitz, C. S. (2005). *The out of sync child: Recognizing and coping with sensory processing disorder*. New York: Berkley Publishing Group.

Martin, N. A. (2006a). *Test of visual motor skills*. Torrance, CA: Western Psychological Services.

Martin, N. A. (2006b). *Test of visual perception (non-motor)* (3rd ed.). Torrance, CA: Western Psychological Services.
Miller, L. J. (2006). *Miller function & participation scales*. San Antonio, TX: Pearson.
Miller, L. J., Nielsen, D. M., & Schoen, S. A. (2012). Attention deficit hyperactivity disorder and sensory modulation disorder: A comparison of behavior and physiology. *Research in Developmental Disabilities, 33*, 804–818.
Minson, R. (2007). *Integrated listening systems (iLs)*. San Diego, CA: Plural Publishing.
My School Day Enhanced CD. (2000). Leesburg, VA: Social Skill Builder.
Olsen, J. (2012). *Olsen's handwriting without tears*. Gaithersburg, MD. Publisher: Handwriting Without Years.
Parham, L. D., Ecker, C., Kuhaneck, H. M., Henry, D. A., & Glennon, T. J. (2007). *Sensory processing measure*. Torrance, CA: Western Psychological Services.
Schaaf, R. C., & Nightlinger, K. M. (2007). Occupational therapy using a sensory integrative approach: A case study of effectiveness. *The American Journal of Occupational Therapy, 61*, 239–246.
Stewart, K. (2007). *Helping a child with nonverbal learning disorder or Asperger's disorder* (2nd ed.). Oakland, CA: New Harbinger Publications.
Type to Learn® 4. (2010). Elgin, IL: Sunburst Digital.
Typing Instructor for Kids. (2009). Greensboro, NC: Carson-Dellosa.
Typing Quick & Easy 17. (2007). Pleasanton, CA: Individual Software.
UltraKey® 5. (2006). Buffalo, NY: Bytes of Learning.
Whitney, R. V. (2008). *Nonverbal learning disorder*. New York: Penguin Group.
Williams, M. S., & Shellenberger, S. (1996). *How does your engine run? Leader's guide to the Alert Program for Self Regulation*. Albuquerque, NM: Therapy Works, Inc.
Winner, M. (2005). *Think social! A social thinking curriculum for school-age students*. San Jose, CA: SCP Publisher.

Other Useful Resources Include

Ayres, A. J. (1991). *Sensory integration and learning disorders*. Los Angeles, CA: Western Psychological Services.
Bundy, A. C., Lane, S. J., & Murray, E. A. (2002). *Sensory integration: Theory and practice* (2nd ed.). Philadelphia, PA: F.A. Davis.
Levine, M. (2002). *A mind at a time*. New York: Simon & Schuster.

Chapter 4
Nonverbal Learning Disabilities: A Speech-Language Pathologist's Perspective

Joanne Volden

Consider Sam, an 8-year-old who, in the middle of a task about describing geometric shapes, asks "Did you know that a zebra is something like a horse?" Or Melissa, a 20-year-old in the same situation, who describes a striped triangle as "a unilateral triangle with a black dot running straight along the point from the apex to the base, lined with vertical stripes". Speakers like Sam and Melissa, whose communicative profile includes the production of fluent, grammatical sentences complete with sophisticated vocabulary, but who have difficulty in using language appropriately, are increasingly found on a speech-language pathologist's caseload. Some of these individuals may be diagnosed with a nonverbal learning disability (NVLD). The purpose of this chapter is to explore the communicative characteristics associated with NVLD, to examine areas of overlap with other diagnostic categories and to discuss implications for communicative assessment, intervention and future research.

As noted previously in this volume, Byron Rourke and his colleagues have argued since the late 1970s that subtypes of specific learning disability could be identified by their distinctive neuropsychological profiles (Rourke, 1989, 1995; Tsatsanis & Rourke, 2008). Nonverbal learning disability (NVLD), characterized by difficulties in processing nonverbal information, is one such subtype. Rourke (1989, 1995) proposed that NVLD arose out of primary deficits in tactile and visual perception which led to secondary difficulties in physical exploration of the environment and attention to visual or tactile stimuli. In turn, these secondary deficits resulted in flawed concept formation, problem solving and hypothesis testing. In the long run, linguistic, academic and psychosocial/adaptive skills were impaired as a result. Research to date, however, leaves many unanswered questions about the definition and characteristics of the NVLD syndrome, and the

J. Volden, Ph.D. (✉)
Faculty of Rehabilitation Medicine, University of Alberta,
3-48 Corbett Hall, Edmonton, AB T6G 2G4, Canada
e-mail: joanne.volden@ualberta.ca

J. Broitman and J.M. Davis (eds.), *Treating NVLD in Children: Professional Collaborations for Positive Outcomes*, DOI 10.1007/978-1-4614-6179-1_4,

degree to which it overlaps with other conditions. Because diagnostic criteria are not well established, it is difficult to describe a communicative profile that is specific to persons with NVLD, as there are very few studies that can reliably claim to have assessed children with NVLD who have no other condition. This chapter begins with a brief review of current issues in definition, before moving to an analysis of overlapping conditions and a critical examination of the literature on communication skills in NVLD. Areas in which research specific to NVLD is needed are specified throughout. The chapter concludes with suggestions for assessment and intervention.

Definition and Description

In Rourke's early descriptions of the NVLD syndrome, children with NVLD performed below age level on visual–perceptual, visual–spatial, motor (finger tapping, grip strength), psychomotor (e.g. timed measures for navigating through a maze) and tactile-kinesthetic (fingertip writing) skills but at age level or better on rote verbal and auditory perceptual measures, such as receptive vocabulary (Rourke & Finlayson, 1978; Rourke & Strang, 1978; Strang & Rourke, 1983). One of the early hallmarks of NVLD was a split between verbal IQ (VIQ) and performance IQ (PIQ) scores, with VIQ being significantly higher (Harnedek & Rourke, 1994).

In school, these children commonly experience difficulties in mathematics but display advanced skills in spelling and word recognition (Rourke, 1995). Children with NVLD are reported as being able to memorize math facts or theorems and repeat them, but they have difficulty in applying these same facts in problem solving. In later years, science courses that depend on such application, such as geometry or physics, become difficult (Tsatsanis & Rourke, 2008). Additional academic difficulties include problems in reading comprehension, so that these children are often unable to paraphrase or generate implications from a section of text (Tsatsanis & Rourke, 2008).

In terms of language, children with NVLD are described as highly verbal, fluent speakers, capable of using sophisticated vocabulary and appropriate sentence structure (Rourke, 1989). But despite being able to produce a large number of sophisticated words, these children often do not understand the full range of meanings that a word could represent (Rourke & Tsatsanis, 1996). As the child grows older and conversational interactions begin to demand the ability to employ contextual cues, the child's difficulties become more apparent. For example, they often have difficulty understanding inferences in conversation (Worling, Humphries, & Tannock, 1999) and they fail to understand figurative language, or humour (Rourke & Tsatsanis, 1996). Their discourse skills are also seriously impaired as shown by spoken language that is often inappropriate for the context and that is frequently disorganized and incoherent (Rourke & Tsatsanis, 1996).

This type of inappropriate discourse, coupled with their difficulty in interpreting nonverbal social cues such as facial expressions and gestures, led Rourke (1995) to suggest that children with NVLD would have difficulty in establishing friendships. In the long run, Rourke and his colleagues (Pelletier, Ahmad, & Rourke, 2001; Rourke, 1989; Rourke & Fuerst, 1992, 1995; Rourke, Young, & Leenaars, 1989) suggested that children with the NVLD profile were more likely to display "internalizing" psychopathologies (e.g. depression, withdrawal).

Rourke's conceptualization of the NVLD syndrome has evolved over time and NVLD is now described as a spectrum of disorders with varying degrees of expression. Tsatsanis and Rourke (2008) now emphasize that the *pattern* of performance, i.e. the gaps between an individual's neuropsychological assets and deficits rather than the level of any particular feature, is the most vital aspect of expression. For example, the presence of mathematical disability, which is the reason for referral of children in the initial studies by Rourke (1987) and long considered a necessary if not sufficient criterion (Rourke, 1993; Forrest, 2004), is now listed as occurring only in 72% (Forrest, 2004) to 86% of the NVLD population (Tsatsanis & Rourke, 2008). In addition, the considerable VIQ-PIQ split that was once considered a hallmark of NVLD (Harnedek & Rourke, 1994) has now been redefined as needing only to be a minimum of ten points, a gap that is not even statistically significant (Pelletier et al., 2001). Further, this discrepancy is now listed as the last feature in a ranked list and need not be present at all if other features are present (Tsatsanis & Rourke, 2008). Broadened diagnostic criteria have led many researchers and clinicians to question the utility of such a broadly inclusive diagnosis. In addition, evolving criteria have made Rourke's research results difficult to replicate and appropriate comparisons across research studies are often not possible.

Other models of NVLD also exist. Semrud-Clikeman (2007) proposed three broad areas of dysfunction as characteristic of NVLD: motor skills, visual–spatial organization and social functioning. In addition, Davis and Broitman (in this volume) suggest that NVLD is a spectrum disorder with core areas of deficit in visual–spatial skills and executive functioning. In some children, these deficits do not result in significant functional impairment while in others, social and/or academic problems are the result.

As an alternative to debating the relative merits of one diagnostic category over another, Rapin (2008) reminds us that classification of behaviourally defined syndromes is dimensional, not categorical. In other words, because we do not have a specific biological test that would unequivocally establish whether or not an individual has a condition, we place individuals in categories based on the behavioural dimensions that we observe. NVLD is one such condition and autism spectrum disorder (ASD) and pragmatic language impairment (PLI) are examples of others. Because these behaviourally defined, developmental disorders are believed to be multigenic as well as influenced by one's environment, behavioural presentations are variable. Thus, the margins separating one condition from another are inherently fuzzy and overlap among related syndromes is common. While this overlap is a liability in establishing the diagnostic validity of a condition like NVLD, this chapter takes the position that some insight into the communicative difficulties of children with NVLD can be gained by examining the research that has been done with children whose diagnoses represent overlapping conditions.

Overlap with Other Diagnostic Conditions

Asperger's Syndrome (AS), High-Functioning Autism (HFA), Autism Spectrum Syndrome and Pervasive Developmental Disorder-Not Otherwise Specified (PDD-NOS)

The NVLD profile of neuropsychological assets and deficits is strikingly similar to the symptoms displayed by individuals with Asperger's syndrome (AS) (Rapin, 2008). In fact, Rourke posits that the two conditions should not be dissociated (Rourke et al., 2002). If so, what is NVLD's relationship to HFA, which is a term that is sometimes applied to children who are diagnosed with ASD but whose nonverbal cognitive skills are within normal limits on standardized measures? Rourke et al. (2002) argued that AS and HFA are two separate conditions, and thus that NVLD would not be considered a part of the autism spectrum. On the other hand, the criteria for ASD in the proposed DSM-V (American Psychiatric Association, 2011) reflect the view that both AS and PDD-NOS are part of the autism spectrum (Happe, 2011) and that AS, HFA and PDD-NOS are indistinguishable (Ozonoff, 2008). Thus, NVLD, acknowledged as overlapping with AS, is a phenomenon that can be included at least on the "borderlands of autism" (Bishop, 1989). This debate remains unresolved, and a definitive conclusion awaits further research.

Developmental Coordination Disorder (DCD) and Developmental Attentional Motor Perceptual Disorder (DAMP)

Gillberg and Billstedt (2000) note that the lesser known disorders developmental coordination disorder (DCD), as it is called here in the United States, and developmental attentional motor perceptual (DAMP) disorder, as it is known in northern Europe, also overlap to a considerable degree with AS. Descriptions of DCD focus on motor incoordination in a child's development, but social sequelae and pragmatic language problems are also mentioned (Serra, Jackson, van Geert, & Minderaa, 1998). While NVLD has not been mentioned in the literature in regard to DCD or DAMP, its overlap with AS begs the question of whether these too are manifestations of NVLD or vice versa.

Pragmatic Language Impairment and Social Communication Disorder

In 2000, Bishop described children whose structural language was unimpaired but who displayed marked problems in appropriate language usage as having "pragmatic language impairment" (PLI; Bishop, 2000). The proposed DSM-V has introduced a new category, called social communication disorder (SCD), which appears congruent with PLI. SCD is defined as an impairment in pragmatics, diagnosed when a difficulty in the social uses of communication cannot be explained by low abilities in word structure, grammar or general cognitive ability (American Psychiatric Association, 2011). The relationship between PLI and ASD has also been a matter of considerable debate. Several investigators (Brook & Bowler, 1992; Gagnon, Mottron, & Joanette, 1997; Shields, Varley, Broks, & Simpson, 1996a, 1996b) have concluded that PLI is better thought of as a form of high-functioning autism. On the other hand, Bishop and Norbury (2002) suggested that children might display characteristics of pragmatic language impairment without displaying unusually restricted interests. Although it has not yet been systematically investigated, the same conclusion is likely to be true for the overlap of PLI or SCD and NVLD, i.e. children diagnosed with NVLD will display characteristics of PLI/SCD, but all children with PLI/SCD may not automatically be assumed to have NVLD. For example, there may be difficulties with spatial coordination that are present in NVLD but which would be irrelevant to the diagnosis of PLI. Nonetheless, the clinical description of symptoms in the *communicative* domain *appears* to be as appropriate for the population diagnosed with NVLD as it is for those diagnosed with HFA, AS, PDD-NOS or SCD.

As Volkmar and Klin (2001) point out, many investigators work only within their own disciplines and are therefore sometimes unaware of work in other areas. As a result, terms for children who display social disabilities have proliferated and the multiplicity of labels has added to the confusion about diagnostic categories. Careful research with clear diagnostic criteria will be needed to determine whether all of these conditions are essentially the same, overlap only in some dimensions (e.g. the social communicative domain) or are distinctly separate, with different causes, developmental courses and responses to treatment.

The Communication Profile

The communicative profile has largely been neglected in the research literature on NVLD (Rourke & Tsatsanis, 1996). There are several possible reasons for this neglect (Volden, 2004a). The first is the historical background of the disability. Efforts to isolate the NVLD syndrome arose from the attempt to establish subtypes of learning disability. Originally, labelling this phenomenon "nonverbal" was intended

(1) to establish the foundation of the disability as a deficit in nonverbal processing abilities and (2) to distinguish these nonverbal foundations from those associated with more traditional conceptions of learning disability where fundamental causes were language related (Rourke & Tsatsanis, 1996). The unfortunate by-product of this focus has been a reduced emphasis on systematic investigation of the communicative profile with clinicians and researchers alike ignoring the phenomenon because of a label that identifies the problem as "nonverbal" and therefore implies that difficulties lie outside the linguistic domain.

The second reason for some neglect in the literature is the behavioural presentation of the disorder. When a child displays an abundance of verbal output along with precocious vocabulary development and complex grammar, parents, clinicians, service providers and researchers are led to believe that language development is advanced. Although this conclusion is based on apparent rather than real language competence, identification of more subtle communication problems requires thoughtful, thorough and systematic investigation. To date, this has not been done in any comprehensive way.

A third reason is the difficulty with definitive diagnosis that was previously described. Diagnostic criteria for NVLD have evolved over time and definitive criteria that employ current and easily accessible diagnostic instruments have never achieved either stability or widespread acceptance (Semrud-Clikeman, Walkowiak, Wilkinson, & Christopher, 2010). A related issue is the difficulty of recruitment. Attempts to employ rigorous, conservative diagnostic criteria have resulted in small sample sizes even when recruitment was carried on for periods up to 3 years (Semrud-Clikeman et al., 2010).

In 2004, I reviewed the literature on communication in children identified with NVLD and found little empirical evidence to support the anecdotal and case history descriptions about communicative profile that are frequently found in the literature (Volden, 2004a). Regrettably, the situation has not changed substantially to date. This chapter presents a summary of those findings as well as recent pertinent findings from the research in ASD and PLI/SCD.

Language Form: Phonology, Morphology and Syntax

The most complete description of the communicative profile associated with NVLD continues to be provided by Rourke and Tsatsanis (1996) who divide their discussion into Bloom's (1988) domains of form, content and use. The domain of language form includes the dimensions of phonology, morphology and syntax. Phonology refers to the study of the sound system of language (Owens, 2007). Morphology involves the smallest units of meaning in a language (Owens, 2007). For example, a word like "cap" is a single morpheme. Grammatical affixes that change word meaning are also morphemes. Examples are suffixes like "s" to indicate pluralisation or "ed" to indicate past tense. While a word like "cap" is a single morpheme, the plural form "caps" is two. Syntax refers to rules that govern the way sentences are constructed (Owens, 2007). Rourke and Tsatsanis (1996) report that children with NVLD exhibit few difficulties in any of these three areas. In terms of phonology, they demonstrate advanced skills such as blending sounds together and segmenting words into component sounds (Rourke, 1989). Syntactic skills are also reported to be adequate, with grammatical morphology appropriately applied and a variety of sentence structures correctly produced (Rourke, 1989).

Data to support Rourke and Tsatsanis' (1996) description, however, are limited and their 1996 article does not rely on empirical support (Volden, 2004a). Examining the work in Rourke's laboratory that established the foundation for the NVLD diagnosis (Rourke, 1987, 1989, 1993, 1995; Rourke & Finlayson, 1978; Rourke & Fuerst, 1992, Strang & Rourke, 1983) revealed two subtests in their battery of neuropsychological measures that would provide evidence about phonological skill. In the auditory closure test (Kass, 1964, in Rourke & Finlayson, 1978), sound elements were presented via a tape recorder and the child was required to blend these sounds into words. Correct responding requires verbal memory skills and the ability to blend sounds together. The Speech Sound Perception Test (Reitan & Davison, 1974, in Rourke & Finlayson, 1978) required the child to listen to a series of speech sounds and to select the configuration of graphemes (i.e. letters) that matched the oral presentation. This test requires the ability to discriminate phonemes (i.e. speech sounds) and to match them to the appropriate letters. On these sub-tests, the children classified as NVLD performed at or above age level and well above the level achieved by children with the more traditionally acknowledged language learning disability (Rourke & Finlayson, 1978). Thus, these data provide some support for Rourke and Tsatsanis' description of phonological processing skills as an area of strength. Notably absent, however, from Rourke and Tsatsanis' account (1996) are any standardized measures of phonological or articulatory production, or any reports of systematic analysis of phonological competence as it could be observed in the speech used throughout the assessment. When Rourke and Tsatsanis (1996) report then that phonology is unaffected in the child with NVLD, the reader assumes that phonological production errors were not noted in conversation, but limited direct evidence of competence is actually reported.

With regard to the other dimensions of language form, none of the measures listed as part of the neuropsychological battery are designed to provide information about morphological or syntactic competence. Rourke and Tsatsanis (1996) appear to base their conclusions about integrity of these structural linguistic dimensions on clinical observation, and failed to note syntactic or morphological errors in the oral language used to complete various parts of the assessment. Systematic investigation of these dimensions using one or more standardized, comprehensive language assessments (see Paul, 2007 for an extensive list) and language sample analysis would begin to document and validate Rourke and Tsatsanis' (1996) observations.

In the population of persons with ASD, there is a long-standing consensus that phonology is relatively preserved and that morphology and syntax are not necessarily impaired relative to a person's cognitive level (Tager-Flusberg, Paul, & Lord, 2005). Nevertheless, Volden and Lord (1991) noted syntactic errors, that did not appear to be developmental in nature, in the language of some of their high-functioning participants with ASD. This possibility has also been raised in more recent papers by Rapin and Dunn (2003) and by Eigsti, Bennetto and Dadlani (2007). Overall, the consensus holds that syntax is not necessarily disordered in ASD, but it is possible that detailed analysis of sophisticated syntax may reveal disabilities in language structure that are present even in those whose scores on standardized language measures are within normal limits. Given the lack of precision in diagnosing differences between HFA and NVLD, subtle difficulties with sophisticated syntax may also be found in this population. While this area of investigation is not a pressing concern, a full description of the communicative profile in NVLD will require exploration of later-developing syntactic structures.

Semantics

In the domain of language semantics or content, Rourke and Tsatsanis (1996) describe children with NVLD as having large vocabularies but " relatively little in the way of meaningful content that is conveyed in their discourse" (Rourke & Tsatsanis, 1996, p. 37). These two observations may be reconciled by considering that, while they are often able to use a large number of sophisticated words, these children may not understand the complete meaning of the word or the full range of meanings that a particular term connotes. This lack can lead to words being used inappropriately. One example is a child who was describing the process of going to a grocery store. As part of the description he said "After you're finished then you go to the cashier. Then you go out the door. If it's at the *beginning* then you can go to the mall" (Volden, 2002). On questioning, it appeared that the child intended to describe the grocery store as at the *entrance* to a shopping mall, but chose the word "beginning" instead. While syntactic form was intact in this utterance, the selection of lexical items is unusual, and leads one to question the child's semantic skill.

Difficulties in comprehension become more apparent as the child grows older and conversational interactions begin to demand the ability to employ contextual cues. In addition, the appreciation of humour, irony, idioms or metaphor requires an adroit manipulation of literal and nonliteral meanings and is reported to be difficult for children with NVLD (Rourke & Tsatsanis, 1996). For example, children diagnosed with NVLD may have difficulty interpreting an utterance like "OK, time to wrap it up now" as an indication that an activity is finished or a sentence like "I just can't swallow that" as an expression of disbelief.

Turning to an examination of the evidence in support of these descriptions, the Peabody Picture Vocabulary Test (PPVT, Dunn, 1965) and the "verbal" subtests of the Wechsler Intelligence Scale for Children (WISC) (Wechsler, 1949, 1991) provide information about the content of language and were included in Rourke and Finlayson's (1978) original battery. The PPVT is a measure of receptive vocabulary that requires a participant to select one of four pictures that best represents the word spoken by the examiner. Multiple or less frequent word meanings are not assessed. The "verbal" subtests (information, similarities, vocabulary) of the WISC (Wechsler, 1949, 1991) tap basic semantic knowledge by assessing a child's understanding of words and the concepts they represent, as well as fundamental properties and relationships. On most of these measures, children classified as NVLD performed better than children with language-based learning disability but somewhat more poorly than chronological age peers. The only area in which children with NVLD were superior to test norms was in the area of word definitions. Unfortunately, none of these measures assessed sophisticated semantic skill such as the ability to understand extended discourse or figurative language (Volden, 2004a). Thus, most of Rourke and Tsatsanis' observations appear to have been based on their extensive clinical interactions rather than empirical data.

In order to evaluate some of the more subtle types of semantic comprehension difficulties, researchers have turned to an examination of the comprehension of narrative discourse. Narrative discourse involves recounting a sequence of events representing previous experience (McCabe, 1991). Beyond understanding individual words and sentences, a full understanding of discourse requires the ability to understand idea units, or propositions, and how they are related. It also depends upon the ability to make inferences based on one's world knowledge and on prior context. Despite verbal IQ scores that were comparable to chronological age (CA) peers, Worling et al. (1999) and Humphries, Cardy, Worling and Peets (2004) demonstrated that children with NVLD were worse at understanding the inferences contained in short stories than their CA-matched peers and were no better than children of the same age who exhibited verbal impairments. In addition, children with NVLD also showed similar difficulties to the children with verbal impairments in retelling the stories (Humphries et al., 2004). Dorfman (2000) found similar problems in inferencing, as well as in the ability to interpret ambiguous sentences and understand figurative language when she administered the Test of Language Competence—Expanded Edition (Wiig & Secord, 1989) to 19 children with NVLD and the same number of typically developing children matched on age, gender and verbal IQ.

These studies were limited by the lack of detailed investigation of the language status of the participants, with the only index of verbal functioning being the VIQ score. In addition, all of them cite small sample sizes as a limitation to widespread generalization of their results and all emphasize the need for replication with larger groups. Still, the inferential comprehension skills of children with NVLD were no better than those of children with verbal impairments, so the advantage that should have been conferred by measured age-appropriate levels of verbal abilities did not materialize. Overall, these findings provide empirical support for the semantic dysfunction reported anecdotally by Rourke and Tsatsanis (1996).

Comprehension of humour also presents an intriguing area of study with relevance to semantic communicative competence as understanding humour generally rests upon recognition of an inconsistency, often due to multiple word meanings, and subsequent resolution of the inconsistency by reassessment of the situation (Semrud-Clikeman & Glass, 2010). A single study on the comprehension of humour was found (Semrud-Clikeman & Glass, 2008). They found that children with NVLD who also had deficits in social perception were less able to select the humorous ending to a joke or a cartoon than age-matched children with a reading disability or typically developing controls. Unfortunately, detailed language data were not reported on these participants, so it is difficult to determine whether language status might also have had an impact on the comprehension of humour. More work is needed, in the population with NVLD, on examining sophisticated semantic communication skills such as abstract word meaning, communication where the information is implied rather than obvious and situations where an inconsistency has to be resolved such as jokes and the use of humour.

Pragmatics

Rourke and Tsatsanis (1996) report that the most deficient domain of language in children with NVLD is that of language use or pragmatics. Pragmatics refers to the appropriate social use of language across a number of social contexts (Berko-Gleason & Bernstein Ratner, 2009) and includes the ability to use language to accomplish a wide variety of social purposes (e.g. requesting objects, requesting information, commenting, greeting, etc.; Dore, 1974) as well as the ability to manage conversations successfully (e.g. initiating interactions and introducing topics, taking turns, maintaining and building on topics, recognizing and repairing conversational breakdowns and issues around politeness and formality) (Adams, 2005, Brinton & Fujiki, 1989; Klein & Moses, 1994). One can easily see that competence in the above skills requires more than the ability to formulate sentences. Competence in social communication requires social motivation and social knowledge, as well as knowing how to adjust language to fit the particular context and the ability to produce and understand a wide variety of linguistic forms (Adams, 2005).

Rourke and Tsatsanis (1996) describe the conversation of children with NVLD as seriously impaired, not only because so little content is expressed in their utterances but also because they appear to pay so little attention to how appropriate their language is within a particular situation. As a result their conversation is often inappropriate for the context, and frequently disorganized and incoherent (Rourke & Tsatsanis, 1996). As in the other language domains, empirical support is limited for Rourke and Tsatsanis' (1996) observations about pragmatic language skills. None of the measures of verbal ability reported throughout the literature on NVLD would yield conclusive evidence about the state of a child's pragmatic competence, especially in the sophisticated conversational skills that are reported as deficient.

In the population with ASD, pragmatic dysfunction has been documented in most areas of conversational management, including taking turns, initiating and maintaining topics, conversational repairs and adjusting language to fit a social situation (see Tager-Flusberg et al. (2005) for a review). Unfortunately though, the story is not entirely straightforward. While children and adolescents with ASD demonstrate weaknesses in these conversational skills as a group, there is also often great variability within the group. So, for example, some children may perform as well as their peers, even though the average performance of the group with ASD would be significantly lower than the norm (Young, Diehl, Morris, Hyman, & Bennetto, 2005). In addition, within a given individual, skills may be expressed under certain conditions but not under others, making it important to consider environmental variables before concluding that a particular ability is absent in the population with ASD (Volden, 2004b, Volden & Johnston, 1999, Volden, Magill-Evans, Goulden, & Clarke, 2007). For example, one would be tempted to conclude that children with ASD were unable to repair conversational breakdown if you only examined their spontaneous responses to a listener's request for a clarification (Paul & Cohen, 1984). When provided with multiple opportunities to repair the breakdown and prompts that were increasingly supportive, their performance improved (Volden, 2004b). These data were interpreted as indicating that the speakers with ASD were able to make repairs but were less efficient in deploying their repair strategies (Volden, 2004b). Given the apparent similarities between high-functioning children with ASD and children with NVLD, the same cautions should be applied in examining their performance. As is suggested for speakers with ASD, it is important to consider whether the relevant difficulty lies in linguistic performance (i.e. repairing the breakdown) or in executive control (i.e. deciding which repair strategy would be most useful at a particular time) (Volden et al., 2007).

Overall, anecdotal, clinical case descriptions of children with NVLD reveal a communicative profile that is characterized by significant pragmatic impairment in the presence of relatively preserved language form. While elementary semantic skills appear to be intact, the child with NVLD is likely to display deficits in semantic competence when situations demand deep rather than superficial comprehension and/or abstract or sophisticated semantic knowledge. Empirical evidence that would validate the clinical profile is limited. Research that would investigate the communicative parameters of NVLD is urgently needed.

Assessment

Very few of the above pragmatic dysfunctions are measured on traditional language assessment instruments because traditional tests focus mostly on linguistic structure and meaning rather than on pragmatic language use (Anderson, Lord, & Heinz, 2005; Bishop, 1998; Bishop & Baird, 2001; Young et al., 2005). Until recently, many of the assessment instruments that are commonly used by speech-language pathologists (SLPs) failed to test pragmatic skills at all (Adams, 2002; Russell & Grizzle, 2008). Thus, when a child demonstrated intelligence scores in the normal range and obtained scores within normal limits on traditional language measures, it was difficult for parents or professionals to document the need for intervention even though the child's dysfunctional social language skills were evident in conversation and placed him or her in jeopardy for full participation in school and community environments (Kamhi, 1998; Young et al., 2005).

Pragmatic language has proven difficult to assess for several reasons. First of all, pragmatics is defined as context-dependent behaviour, so the generally rigid structure of formal testing procedures fails to capture flexible adjustment to changing circumstances (Adams, 2002). In addition, children with pragmatic difficulties can often perform much better when given clear instructions in a concrete context, such as a standardized testing situation, than they do in a naturalistic setting (Bishop, 1998). Also, if a particular behaviour is not seen during the observation period, one is unsure whether it does not occur or whether it does occur but simply did not occur within the sample collected (Adams, 2002; Bishop, 1998).

Nevertheless, a number of formal measures have now been developed. Russell and Grizzle (2008) reviewed 24 pragmatic assessment tools to see if pragmatic language domains targeted on assessment could be reliably identified, and whether core domains emerged and were assessed across the range of instruments evaluated. They found that items from tests and parent questionnaires could be reliably categorized into 17 pragmatic language domains, but that tests varied widely in terms of what domains were assessed and for what ages they were appropriate. In addition, instruments varied in terms of the ages for which they were designed to be appropriate and whether they were norm referenced, criterion referenced or descriptive. Altogether, only seven of the measures were norm referenced, and of those only five were appropriate for ages spanning preschool to adolescent years. Of those five, only the Children's Communication Checklist—Second Edition (CCC-2; Bishop, 2003) sampled more than 10 of the 17 pragmatic domains that had been identified. As such, the CCC-2 appears to be an assessment instrument that would be appropriate and might be useful for identifying pragmatic impairment in the population with NVLD.

The CCC-2 (Bishop, 2006) is the US edition of the original CCC-2 that was published in the United Kingdom in 2003 (Bishop, 2003). The instrument is designed to screen for clinically significant communication problems of any type and to identify pragmatic language impairment, by obtaining judgements from parents or other adults who have regular contact with the child. Respondents are asked to rate the frequency with which the behaviour described in each item occurs. For example, one item asks the rater to judge how often (less than once a week or never, at least once a week but not every day, once or twice a day or several times a day or always) a child "talks about lists of things s/he has memorised such as the names of the capitals of the world". The checklist consists of 70 multiple-choice items divided into ten scales, with seven items each. Scales for speech, syntax, semantics and coherence assess aspects of articulation and phonology, language structure, vocabulary and discourse. Scales labelled initiation, scripted language, context and nonverbal communication address pragmatic aspects of communication that are not readily assessed by conventional language assessment. The remaining two scales, social relations and interests, focus on behaviours that are usually impaired in children with ASD.

The CCC-2 takes approximately 15 min of a parent's time to complete and another 15 min of an SLP's time to score and interpret. Two composite scores are derived,

(1) the General Communication Composite (GCC), expressed as a standard score with mean of 100 and standard deviation of 15, which may be used to identify children likely to have a clinically significant communication problem of any kind, and (2) the Social Interaction Difference Index (SIDI). The GCC is calculated by summing the scaled scores of the first eight subtests and converting that sum to a standard score. GCC scores less than 80 indicate a communicative impairment. The SIDI is calculated by subtracting total scaled scores of the subtests that measure initiation, nonverbal communication, social relationships and interests (i.e. pragmatic language and ASD-related behaviours) from the total scaled score of subtests measuring speech, syntax, semantics and coherence (i.e. structural language competence). When deficits in pragmatic skill are greater than deficits in structural language, a negative SIDI score results. Thus, a negative SIDI reflects disproportionate problems in pragmatic skill, i.e. pragmatic problems that exceed those expected given the child's general level of language competence. When the GCC score is less than 80, i.e. indicative of clinically significant communicative problems, an SIDI score below 0 indicates that while structural language problems may exist, there is also a disproportionate difficulty in pragmatic language use. In the event of an SIDI score below −15, Bishop (2003) suggests that pragmatic language impairment is present regardless of the GCC score. Recently, the Communication Checklist—Adults (CC-A; Whitehouse & Bishop, 2009) and a Communication Checklist—Self-Report (CC-SR; Bishop, Whitehouse, & Sharp, 2009), modelled on the CCC-2, have also been released in order to extend assessment of pragmatic skills to a broader population.

To my knowledge, the CCC-2 has never been evaluated with respect to the NVLD population, but in 2010, Volden and Phillips compared the effectiveness of the CCC-2 and the Test of Pragmatic Language (TOPL, Phelps-Terasaki & Phelps-Gunn, 1992) in terms of their ability to identify pragmatic language impairment in high-functioning children diagnosed with ASD. Sixteen 9-year-olds with ASD were matched to typically developing peers on chronological age, language age and on nonverbal IQ. Both groups exhibited age-appropriate levels of structural language competence, as measured by the Clinical Evaluation of Language Function—Version 4 (CELF-I 4; Semel, Wiig, & Secord, 2003), but children with ASD scored significantly worse than their matched controls on both language measures that included pragmatic language (i.e. the CCC-2 and the TOPL). The tests were not, however, equally effective at identifying individual children as having pragmatic language impairment. The TOPL identified 56% of the participants in this high-functioning group as pragmatically impaired while 81% were identified by the CCC-2 demonstrating a distinct advantage for the CCC-2 in detecting pragmatic language impairment in high-functioning speakers with ASD. Unfortunately, this comparison was done on the original version of the TOPL as the second version, the Test of Pragmatic Language—Version 2 (Phelps-Terasaki & Phelps-Gunn, 2007), was unavailable at the time data were collected. Whether the CCC-2 retains its advantage over the TOPL-2 is an open question. Nevertheless, our findings suggested that the CCC-2 would be useful for identifying children who might otherwise "slip through the cracks". Although the CCC-2 has not yet been investigated in children diagnosed with NVLD, the similarity of their communicative profile to that of the child with HFA suggests that the CCC-2 may prove a useful instrument to document the presence of pragmatic dysfunction in these children who have fluent and apparently sophisticated language.

Intervention

Definitive directions for effective intervention techniques are difficult to supply as so little research has been done. Some of the difficulties in conducting that research have already been outlined. An important early focus would be determining, at least in terms of communicative assets and liabilities, whether NVLD is simply another name for conditions that have been described with similar communicative symptoms (e.g. Asperger's syndrome, high-functioning autism, pragmatic language impairment, developmental coordination disorder). If these conditions are found to be essentially the same, research that has addressed language deficits in these other populations can be readily applied to children diagnosed with NVLD. If substantial and significant differences are found, the nature of those differences will have important implications for assessment and intervention with this population. In this chapter, I have taken the position that the communicative profile in NVLD does not differ substantially from the communicative profile of those with related diagnoses, but the research that would affirm or refute this position still remains to be done.

There is a much more extensive research literature on intervention in ASD, but many issues still remain unresolved. Intervention for the social communication deficit in ASD has been plagued by debates from a variety of theoretical perspectives (see Rogers, 2006 for a review), fuelled by small, often poorly controlled, studies and very few randomized clinical trials (RCTs) (Charman, 2011), which are considered the "gold standard" in experimental design for evaluating treatment effectiveness. An RCT is a study in which participants are allocated by chance to one of two or more treatments, and the outcomes from each treatment are then compared to determine which was the more effective. This rigorous methodology requires a large sample size; randomized assignment of participants; assessors who are unaware of the participant's treatment assignment; balance across treatment groups; a manualized (and therefore replicable) intervention procedure, including standards for ensuring that the procedure was followed reliably; as well as appropriate outcome measures (Spence & Thurm, 2010). Of the RCTs that have been published (e.g. Dawson et al., 2010; Green et al., 2010; Kasari, Freeman, & Paparella, 2006; Landa, Holman, O'Neill, & Stuart, 2011), each has focussed on a slightly different aspect of social communication impairment in young preschool children with ASD. Overall, these studies have shown that specific social communication behaviours that are the immediate focus of the intervention, such as parent and child synchrony in interaction and shared attention between child and carer, show improvement (Charman, 2011). Although these results are promising and indicate that social communication can be taught, much work still remains in terms of determining the cognitive mechanisms that underlie positive growth and in identifying which of the many components in a comprehensive intervention programme are "active" in promoting change and which are irrelevant (Charman, 2011; Spence & Thurm, 2010).

NVLD is more often associated with children of school age. In the population with ASD, I was unable to find published accounts of RCTs focussing specifically on social communication deficits in school-aged children, adolescents or adults with ASD. Often though, social communication skills are included, at least to some degree, in intervention programmes that target social skills in general. In addition, slightly less rigorous research designs, such as clinical trials using non-randomized groups or single-subject designs where an individual's performance is compared under different treatment conditions, have revealed some promising approaches. While these intervention methods would not yet have met the "gold standard", they may still prove useful. Some caution is, however, warranted. Until evidence from RCTs is available, parents, advocates and clinicians are cautioned that relying on research studies that employ simple pre- and post-treatment comparisons without using a control group is less reliable. In addition, one should only consider adopting a new or promising treatment if it is based on a convincing theoretical model and not comprised solely of an eclectic mix of methods (Prelock, Paul, & Allen, 2011).

In an effort to synthesize the results of a large body of intervention research, Reichow and Volkmar (2010) evaluated social skills interventions for individuals with ASD by examining research studies that had been published between 2001 and 2008 and which met criteria that they had established as constituting the "best evidence" (Reichow, Volkmar, & Cicchetti, 2008). Details of their criteria are available in Reichow et al. (2008), but essentially they only reviewed research that had been published in a peer-reviewed publication and that were rated methodologically "acceptable" or "strong". By restricting their review to these sources, Reichow and his colleagues (2008) were able to weed out weak evidence and concentrate only on those studies that demonstrated reliable and valid results.

In the school-aged population with ASD, Reichow and Volkmar reviewed 28 studies that met their criteria. A full report of their results is beyond the scope of this chapter, but they concluded that participation in social skills groups had amassed enough research evidence to be considered an "evidence-based practice" for school-aged children with ASD. Studies examining social skills groups were characterized by participants who were at least 10 years old with medium and higher levels of cognitive functioning. Thus, their level of cognitive skill would likely be comparable to children with NVLD. Effective social skills groups were held at least once per week for at least 12 weeks, and most of the studies examined groups that were held in clinical settings. More research is needed on curricula/best practices for social skills group instruction and on the feasibility and social validity of such groups delivered in school settings by special education teachers. Nevertheless, participation in a social skills group led by an experienced professional would seem a promising avenue for intervention for school-aged children with NVLD, given the overlap in social communication skills and deficits with HFA.

The use of video modelling met the criteria to be considered a "promising" intervention (Reichow & Volkmar, 2010). The technique involves watching a video vignette and practicing/evaluating targeted social skills. While some questions remain about whether "video modelling" alone was an effective intervention, and who (e.g. peer, adult, self) makes the most effective model for facilitating behavioural change, it is intuitively appealing as it targets skills in social judgement within specific contexts. It too may offer some hope for school-aged children with NVLD.

Summary and Conclusion

The communicative profile of speakers with NVLD bears striking similarities to those of speakers diagnosed with ASD. Fluent, sophisticated language may mislead conversational partners into assuming that the speaker with NVLD has equally sophisticated comprehension. Coupled with difficulties in taking appropriate conversational turns, repairing communicative breakdowns, maintaining conversational topics and navigating social situations, these children experience repeated failure and rejection in school and in the wider community. These children often "slip through the cracks" in terms of service provision. Much remains to be done to document the communicative profile, to establish its developmental course and to develop and test effective interventions. Until this evidence is available, this chapter has taken the position that guidance in terms of assessment and potentially effective intervention may cautiously be taken from the research evidence that has amassed around ASD. The CCC-2 is recommended as an assessment instrument that could be used to document the presence of pragmatic communication disorder in children for whom more traditional language assessments reveal no difficulties. Effective interventions, regrettably, lag behind.

References

Adams, C. (2002). Practitioner review: The assessment of language pragmatics. *Journal of Child Psychology and Psychiatry, 43*(8), 973–987.

Adams, C. (2005). Social communication intervention for school-age children: Rationale and intervention. *Seminars in Speech and Language, 26*(3), 181–188.

American Psychiatric Association, (2011). http://www.dsm5.org/proposedrevision/:ages?NeurodevelopmentalDisorders.aspx. Downloaded August 5, 2011.

Anderson, D., Lord, C., & Heinz S. J., (2005). Growth in language abilities over time among children with ASD and other developmental disabilities, International Meeting for Autism Research—poster presentation, Boston, May 2005.

Berko-Gleason, J., & Bernstein Ratner, N. (2009). *The development of language* (7th ed.). Boston, MA: Allyn & Bacon.

Bishop, D. (1989). Autism, Asperger's syndrome and semantic-pragmatic disorder: Where are the boundaries? *British Journal of Disorders of Communication, 24*, 107–121.

Bishop, D. (1998). Development of the children's communication checklist (CCC): A method for assessing qualitative aspects of communicative impairment in children. *Journal of Child Psychology and Psychiatry, and Allied Disciplines, 39*(6), 879–891.

Bishop, D. (2000). Pragmatic language impairment: A correlate of SLI, a distinct subgroup, or part of the autistic continuum? In D. Bishop & L. Leonard (Eds.), *Speech and language impairments in children: Causes, characteristics, intervention and outcome*. Hove, East Sussex, UK: Psychology Press.

Bishop, D. (2003). *The children's communication checklist, CCC-2 manual* (2nd ed.). London: The Psychological Corporation.

Bishop, D. (2006). *The children's communication checklist, CCC-2 manual (US edition)* (2nd ed.). San Antonio, TX: The Psychological Corporation.

Bishop, D., & Baird, B. (2001). Parent and teacher report of pragmatic aspects of communication: Use of the children's communication checklist in a clinical setting. *Developmental Medicine and Child Neurology, 43*, 809–818.

Bishop, D., & Norbury, C. (2002). Exploring the borderlands of autistic disorder and specific language impairment: A study using standardised diagnostic instruments. *Journal of Child Psychology and Psychiatry, 43*(7), 917–929.

Bishop, D., Whitehouse, A., & Sharp, H. (2009). *Communication checklist-self report (CC-SR)*. San Antonio, TX: The Psychological Corporation.

Bloom, L. (1988). What is language? In M. Lahey (Ed.), *Language disorders and language development*. New York, NY: Macmillan.

Brinton, B., & Fujiki, M. (1989). *Conversational management with language-impaired children: Pragmatic assessment and intervention*. Rockville, MD: Aspen.

Brook, S. L., & Bowler, D. M. (1992). Autism by another name: Semantic and pragmatic impairments in children. *Journal of Autism and Developmental Disorders, 22*, 61–81.

Charman, T. (2011). Commentary: Glass half full or half empty? Testing social communication interventions for young children with autism; reflections on Landa, Holman, O'Neill, and Stuart. *Journal of Child Psychology and Psychiatry, 52*(1), 22–23.

Dawson, G., Rogers, S., Munson, J., Smith, M., Winter, J., Greenson, J., et al. (2010). Randomized, controlled trial of an intervention for toddlers with autism: The early start Denver model. *Pediatrics, 125*, 17–23.

Dore, J. (1974). A pragmatic description of early language development. *Journal of Psycholinguistic Research, 4*, 343–350.

Dorfman, C. (2000). Social language and theory of mind in children with nonverbal learning disability. Unpublished doctoral dissertation, University of California, Berkeley.

Dunn, L. (1965). *Expanded manual for the Peabody picture vocabulary test*. Minneapolis, MN: American Guidance Service.

Eigsti, I., Bennetto, L., & Dadlani, M. (2007). Beyond pragmatics: Morphosyntactic development in autism. *Journal of Autism and Developmental Disorders, 37*, 1007–1023.

Forrest, B. (2004). The utility of math difficulties, internalized psychopathology, and visual-spatial deficits to identify children with the nonverbal learning disability syndrome: Evidence for a visualspatial disability. *Child Neuropsychology, 10*(2), 129–146.

Gagnon, L., Mottron, L., & Joanette, Y. (1997). Questioning the validity of the semantic-pragmatic syndrome diagnosis. *Autism, 1*, 37–55.

Gillberg, C., & Billstedt, E. (2000). Autism and Asperger syndrome: Co-existence with other clinical disorders. *Acta Psychiatrica Scandinavica, 102*, 321–330.

Green, J., Charman, T., McConachie, H., Aldred, C., Slonims, V., Howlin, P., et al., and the PACT Consortium. (2010). Parent mediated communication-focussed treatment in children with autism (PACT): A randomized controlled trial. The Lancet, 375, 2152–2160.

Happe, F. (2011). Criteria, categories and continua: Autism and related disorders in DSM-5. *Journal of the American Academy of Child and Adolescent Psychiatry, 50*, 540–542.

Harnedek, M., & Rourke, B. (1994). Principal identifying features of the syndrome of nonverbal learning disabilities in children. *Journal of Learning Disabilities, 27*(3), 144–154.

Humphries, T., Cardy, J., Worling, D., & Peets, K. (2004). Narrative comprehension and retelling abilities of children with nonverbal learning disabilities. *Brain and Cognition, 56*, 77–88.

Kamhi, A. (1998). Trying to make sense of developmental language disorders. *Language, Speech, and Hearing Services in Schools, 29*, 34–44.

Kasari, C., Freeman, S., & Paparella, T. (2006). Joint attention and symbolic play in young children with autism. A randomized controlled intervention study. *Journal of Child Psychology and Psychiatry, 47*, 611–620.

Klein, H., & Moses, N. (1994). *Intervention planning for children with communication disorders*. Englewood Cliffs, NJ: Prentice-Hall.

Landa, R., Holman, K., O'Neill, A., & Stuart, E. (2011). Intervention targeting development of socially synchronous engagement in toddlers with autism spectrum disorders: A randomized controlled trial. *Journal of Child Psychology and Psychiatry, 52*, 13–21.

McCabe, A. (1991). Preface: Structure as a way of understanding. In A. McCabe & C. Peterson (Eds.), *Developing narrative structure* (pp. ix–xvii). Hillsdale, NJ: Erlbaum.

Owens, R. (2007). *Language development: An introduction*. Boston, MA: Allyn & Bacon.

Ozonoff, S. (2008). Presentation to autism and the pervasive developmental disorders conference, February 3–5, 2008. http://www.dsm5.org/research/pages/autismandthepervasivedevelopmentaldisordersconference/february. Downloaded July 18, 2011.

Paul, R. (2007). *Language disorders from infancy through adolescence* (3rd ed.). St. Louis, MO: Mosby.

Paul, R., & Cohen, D. (1984). Responses to contingent queries in adults with mental retardation and pervasive developmental disorders. *Applied PsychoLinguistics, 5*, 349–357.

Pelletier, P., Ahmad, S., & Rourke, B. (2001). Classification rules for basic phonological processing disabilities and nonverbal learning disabilities: formulation and external validity. *Child Neuropsychology, 7*(2), 84–98.

Phelps-Terasaki, D., & Phelps-Gunn, T. (1992). *Test of pragmatic language*. Austin, TX: Pro-Ed.

Phelps-Terasaki, D., & Phelps-Gunn, T. (2007). *Test of pragmatic language-2*. Austin, TX: Pro-Ed.

Prelock, P., Paul, R., & Allen, E. (2011). Evidence-based treatment in communication for children with autism spectrum disorders. In F. Volkmar & B. Reichow (Eds.), *Evidence-based treatments for children with autism spectrum disorder* (pp. 93–170). New York, NY: Springer.

Rapin, I. (2008). Classification issues in the milder developmental disorders: Asperger syndrome, the syndrome of nonverbal learning disability and "Einstein children". In B. Shapiro & P. Accardo (Eds.), *Autism frontiers: Clinical issues and innovations* (pp. 29–47). Baltimore, MD: Paul H. Brookes.

Rapin, I., & Dunn, M. (2003). Update on the language disorder of individuals on the autism spectrum. *Brain & Development, 25*, 166–172.

Reichow, B., & Volkmar, F. (2010). Social skills interventions for individuals with autism: Evaluation for evidence-based practices within a best evidence synthesis framework. *Journal of Autism and Developmental Disorders, 40*, 149–166.

Reichow, B., Volkmar, F., & Cicchetti, D. (2008). Development of the evaluative method for evaluating and determining evidence-based practices in autism. *Journal of Autism and Developmental Disorders, 38*(7), 1311–1319.

Rogers, S. (2006). Evidence based interventions for language development in young children with autism. In T. Charman & W. Stone (Eds.), *Social & communication development in autism spectrum disorder*. New York, NY: Guildford Press.

Rourke, B. (1987). Syndrome of nonverbal learning disabilities: The final common pathway of white-matter disease/dysfunction? *The Clinical Neuropsychologist, 1*(3), 209–234.

Rourke, B. (1989). *Nonverbal learning disabilities: The syndrome and the model*. New York, NY: Guildford Press.

Rourke, B. (1993). Arithmetic disabilities, specific and otherwise: A neuropsychological perspective. *Journal of Learning Disabilities, 26*(4), 214–226.

Rourke, B. (Ed.). (1995). *Syndrome of nonverbal learning disabilities: Neurodevelopmental manifestations*. New York, NY: Guilford Press.

Rourke, B., Ahmad, S., Collins, D., Hayman-Abello, B., Sayman-Abello, S., & Warriner, E. (2002). Child clinical/pediatric neuropsychology: Some recent advances. *Annual Review of Psychology, 53*, 309–339.

Rourke, B., & Finlayson, M. A. (1978). Neuropsychological significance of variations in patterns of academic performance: Verbal and visual-spatial abilities. *Journal of Abnormal Child Psychology, 6*(1), 121–133.

Rourke, B., & Fuerst, D. (1992). Psychosocial dimensions of learning disability subtypes: Neuropsychological studies in the Windsor laboratory. *School Psychology Review, 21*(3), 361–375.

Rourke, B., & Fuerst, D. (1995). Cognitive processing, academic achievement, and psychosocial functioning: A neurodevelopmental perspective. In D. Cicchetti & D. Cohen (Eds.), *Developmental psychopathology* (Theory and methods, Vol. 1). New York, NY: John Wiley and Sons.

Rourke, B., & Strang, J. (1978). Neuropsychological significance of variations in patterns of academic performance: Motor, psychomotor and tactile-perceptual abilities. *Journal of Pediatric Psychology, 3*(2), 62–66.

Rourke, B., & Tsatsanis, K. (1996). Syndrome of nonverbal learning disabilities: Psycholinguistic assets and deficits. *Topics in Language Disorders, 16*(2), 30–44.

Rourke, B., Young, G., & Leenaars, A. (1989). A childhood learning disability that predisposes those afflicted to adolescent and adult depression and suicide risk. *Journal of Learning Disabilities, 21*, 169–175.

Russell, R., & Grizzle, K. (2008). Assessing child and adolescent pragmatic language competencies: Toward evidence-based assessments. *Clinical Child and Family Psychology Review, 11*, 59–73.

Semel, E., Wiig, E., & Secord, W. (2003). *Clinical evaluation of language fundamentals (CELF-4)* (4th ed.). San Antonio, TX: The Psychological Corporation.

Semrud-Clikeman, M. (2007) Social Competence in Children, New York: Springer.

Semrud-Clikeman, M., & Glass, K. (2008). Comprehension of humour in children with nonverbal learning disabilities, reading disabilities and without learning disabilities. *Annals of Dyslexia, 58*, 163–180.

Semrud-Clikeman, M., & Glass, K. (2010). The relation of humour and child development: Social, adaptive and emotional aspects. *Journal of Child Neurology, 25*, 1248–1260.

Semrud-Clikeman, M., Walkowiak, J., Wilkinson, A., & Christopher, G. (2010). Neuropsychological differences among children with Asperger syndrome, nonverbal learning disabilities, attention-deficit disorder and controls. *Developmental Neuropsychology, 35*(5), 582–600.

Serra, M., Jackson, A., van Geert, P., & Minderaa, R. (1998). Brief report: Interpretation of facial expressions, postures and gestures in children with a pervasive developmental disorder not otherwise specified. *Journal of Autism and Developmental Disorders, 28*(3), 257–263.

Shields, J., Varley, R., Broks, P., & Simpson, A. (1996a). Social cognition in developmental language disorders and high-level autism. *Developmental Medicine and Child Neurology, 38*, 487–495.

Shields, J., Varley, R., Broks, P., & Simpson, A. (1996b). Hemispheric function in developmental language disorders and high-level autism. *Developmental Medicine and Child Neurology, 38*, 473–486.

Spence, S., & Thurm, A. (2010). Testing autism interventions: Trials and tribulations. *The Lancet, 375*, 2124–2125.

Strang, J., & Rourke, B. (1983). Concept formation and non-verbal reasoning abilities of children who exhibit specific academic problems with arithmetic. *Journal of Clinical Child Psychology, 12*(1), 33–39.

Tager-Flusberg, H., Paul, R., & Lord, C. (2005). Language and communication in autism. In F. Volkmar, R. Paul, & A. Klin (Eds.), *Handbook on autism and pervasive developmental disorders* (3rd ed., pp. 335–364). New York, NY: John Wiley & Sons.

Tsatsanis, K., & Rourke, B. (2008). Syndrome of nonverbal learning disabilities in adults. In L. Wolf, H. Schreiber, & J. Wasserstein (Eds.), *Adult learning disorders contemporary issues*. New York, NY: Taylor & Francis.

Volden, J. (2002). Features leading to judgments of inappropriacy in the language of speakers with autism: A preliminary study. *Journal of Speech-Language Pathology and Audiology*, September, 26, 3, 138–146.

Volden, J. (2004a). Nonverbal learning disability: A tutorial for speech-language pathologists. *American Journal of Speech-Language Pathology, 13*, 128–141.

Volden, J. (2004b). Conversational repair in speakers with autism spectrum disorder. *International Journal of Language & Communication Disorders, 39*(2), 171–189.

Volden, J., & Johnston, J. (1999). Cognitive scripts in autistic children and adolescents. *Journal of Autism and Developmental Disorders, 29*(3), 203–212.

Volden, J., & Lord, C. (1991). Neologisms and idiosyncratic language in autistic speakers. *Journal of Autism and Developmental Disorders, 21*(2), 109–130.

Volden, J., Magill-Evans, J., Goulden, K., & Clarke, M. (2007). Varying language register according to listener needs in speakers with autism spectrum disorder. *Journal of Autism and Developmental Disorders, 37*(6), 1139–1154.

Volden, J., & Phillips, L. (2010). Measuring pragmatic language in speakers with autism spectrum disorder: Comparing the CCC-2 and the TOPL. *American Journal of Speech-Language Pathology, 19*(3), 204–212.

Volkmar, F., & Klin, A. (2001). Asperger's disorder and higher functioning autism: Same or different? *International Review of Research in Mental Retardation, 23*, 83–110.

Wechsler, D. (1949). *Wechsler intelligence scale for children*. New York, NY: The Psychological Corporation.

Wechsler, D. (1991). *Wechsler intelligence scale for children—III*. New York, NY: The Psychological Corporation.

Whitehouse, A., & Bishop, D. (2009). *Communication checklist—adult*. London: The Psychological Corporation.

Wiig, E., & Secord, W. (1989). *Test of language competence—expanded edition*. San Antonio, TX: The Psychological Corporation.

Worling, D., Humphries, T., & Tannock, R. (1999). Spatial and emotional aspects of language inferencing in nonverbal learning disabilities. *Brain and Language, 70*(2), 220–239.

Young, E., Diehl, J., Morris, D., Hyman, S., & Bennetto, L. (2005). The use of two language tests to identify pragmatic language problems in children with autism spectrum disorders. *Language, Speech, and Hearing Services in Schools, 36*, 62–72.

Chapter 5
Assessments for NVLD

John M. Davis and Jessica Broitman

How Do Psychologists Understand NVLD?

Capitalizing on Gerstmann's early work (1940), Johnson and Myklebust (1967) brought thinking about NVLD into the "modern age." In their book, *Learning Disabilities: Educational Principles and Practices* they described their version of the syndrome of nonverbal learning disorders. They observed fine motor difficulties, difficulties with math and writing, and difficulties in visual–spatial processing including something they called "social perception." They suggested that children with these issues had difficulties in the following areas: understanding gesture, nonverbal motor learning, body image, spatial orientation, right–left orientation, and social perception. Additionally, they also noted that children with NVLD also demonstrated distractibility, perseveration, and disinhibition. Later work has also found overlap with ADHD and executive function issues (Landau, Gross-Tsur, Auerbach, Van der Meer, & Shalev, 1999).

The next major advances in research and thinking about NVLD were made by Byron Rourke and his many colleagues. He is the leading proponent of the dominant model and/or definition of NVLD today. After decades of research and two seminal books, *Neuropsychology of Learning Disabilities: Essentials of Subtype Analysis* (1989) and *Syndrome of Nonverbal Learning Disabilities: Neurodevelopmental Manifestations* (1995), Rourke has left a significant mark on the field both by trying to establish a diagnostic set of criteria for NVLD and offering a theory for the cause of the disorder.

J.M. Davis, Ph.D. (✉)
California State University, East Bay, 25800 Carlos Bee Blvd, Hayward, CA 94542-3095, USA
e-mail: jack.davis@csueastbay.edu

J. Broitman, Ph.D.
San Francisco Psychotherapy Research Group, 9 Funston Street, San Francisco, CA 94129, USA
e-mail: drjess@comcast.net

J. Broitman and J.M. Davis (eds.), *Treating NVLD in Children: Professional Collaborations for Positive Outcomes*, DOI 10.1007/978-1-4614-6179-1_5,

Rourke's diagnostic criteria have remained fairly stable over time. Most recently, Rourke and his colleagues (Pelletier, Ahmad, & Rourke, 2001) have stated that the following criteria have to be met to determine NVLD:

1. Target test at least 1 SD below the mean.
2. No, or very minimal, simple tactile imperception and suppression versus very poor finger agnosia and/or finger dysgraphesthesia.
3. The highest scores on two subtests of the Verbal Scale of the Wechsler Intelligence Scale for Children-III (WISC-III): Vocabulary, Similarities, or Information.
4. Two of the subtests from the WISC-III nonverbal subtests of Block Design, Object Assembly, or Coding fall among the lowest scores of the Performance scale.
5. Wide Range Achievement Test—Revised (WRAT-R) standard score for Reading is at least 8 points higher than Arithmetic.
6. Tactual Performance Test, right, left, and both hand times, becomes progressively worse vis-à-vis the norms.
7. Normal to superior grip strength versus mildly to moderately impaired Grooved Pegboard.
8. WISC-III: VIQ exceeds PIQ by at least 10 points.

Rourke cites that the following criteria are needed for a "diagnosis" of NVLD:

- Children presenting with the first six criteria would definitely be diagnosed with NVLD.
- Seven or eight of the features present would constitute a positive diagnosis.
- Five or six criteria suggest probable NVLD.
- Three or four criteria suggest questionable NVLD.
- One or two criteria suggest low probability of NVLD.

However, more recent work is looking at NVLD somewhat differently, more as a disorder with subtypes than a monolithic structure (e.g., Grodzinsky, 2003; Grodzinsky, Forbes, & Bernstein, 2010; Mamen, 2006). Fine and Semrud-Clikeman (2010) have gone so far as to state that given the current empirical knowledge base for NVLD plus the lack of consensus for *what* NVLD is, evaluating for and diagnosing NVLD is problematic (see also Forrest, 2004). Also, consensus on core deficits has become less clear with new empirical data coming to light. There have also been questions regarding whether NVLD may share symptoms with both AS (Klin, Volkmar, Sparrow, & Cicchetti, 1996) and with ADHD (Hain, Hale, & Kendorski, 2009), which would then need to be *ruled out* to help establish an NVLD diagnosis.

Suffice it to say that currently we believe that a comprehensive psychoeducational or neuropsychological evaluation is needed to establish a diagnosis, as well as to identify the particular symptoms for a specific child. One must be able to explain and understand what a specific learner's strengths and weaknesses are in order to decide upon appropriate interveners and/or interventions, and to design accommodations and/or scaffolding to better enhance the learner's chance for success. In addition the test report should serve as a road map—a snapshot in time of the student's cognitive, socio-emotional, and academic functioning that can be used fluidly to navigate, guide, and inform future interventions. However, it should also be noted that currently no diagnostic nomenclature exists. In lieu of that we are offering a *heuristic* model which clinicians can utilize in order to best understand children who are suspected to have a NVLD. Details about how to accomplish this are presented below.

What Are Psychologists Using to Diagnose NVLD?

Referring back to Rourke's original criteria it can be seen that many of the tests recommended are outdated and/or no longer in use by many of today's practitioners. In order to update a system of assessment, Davis and Broitman (2011) developed a framework for assessment with some examples of tests in use today which may facilitate evaluations for NVLD. Table 5.1 is an overview of the model and Table 5.2 is the model with a variety of tests which could be used to measure those areas. Table 5.2 is not meant to be an exhaustive list, but a working list of clinically and psychometrically sound tests that are available. It is clear that other tests could be added and that newer tests will be developed which can be added at a later date.

How Might a Child with NVLD Look?

Let us consider how the student might present on the data accumulated by an assessment like that above. We will present the three areas of assessment that are most important to be considered in order to diagnose NVLD, cognitive/executive functions, social, and academic, and what the characteristic profiles might look like. We will then present a brief case study to provide an example of what a particular child did look like.

Cognitive/Executive Function

The one characteristic that has stood the test of time is that there are significant cognitive verbal strengths and cognitive weaknesses in the nonverbal areas, especially of intellectual ability (Fine & Semrud-Clikeman, 2010; Johnson & Myklebust, 1967; Rourke, 1989). In Carroll–Horn–Cattell nomenclature, verbal comprehension and reasoning is generally be referred to as crystallized intelligence (the breadth and depth of acquired knowledge) and the more nonverbal problem solving aspects of reasoning is generally referred to as fluid intelligence (cognitive processes used when confronted with a novel task) (Flanagan, Ortiz, & Alfonso, 2007). In Delis' Boston Processing model approach (Delis & Jacobson, 2000), children with NVLD

Table 5.1 Nine areas of essential cognitive functions

		Memory			Sensory motor	
IQ	Executive functioning and attention	Visual	Verbal	Vis/verb integration	Bilateral efficiency	Proprioceptive
Verbal or crystallized Fluid/pattern analysis Visuospatial quantitative	Attention/focus Initiation Working memory Planning/organizing internalized Planning/organizing externalized Self-monitoring Task completion	Real vs. abstract Recognition vs. retrieval Sequential vs. nonsequential Immediate vs. working vs. long-term memory	Contextual vs. decontextual Recognition vs. retrieval Sequential vs. nonsequential Immediate vs. working vs. long-term memory	Real vs. abstract Recognition vs. retrieval	Simple vs. complex Timed vs. untimed Sequential vs. nonsequential	Pencil grip
Graphomotor		Language			Visual processing	Affect and behavior
Timed	Untimed	Receptive	Expressive			
Grapho-symbol Non-symbol	Design drawing	Phonemic awareness Morphological awareness Syntax Sematics Pragmatics Receptive vocabulary	Rapid naming Expressive vocabulary Verbal fluency		Sequential vs. nonsequential Timed vs. untimed Orthographic processing	Depression Anxiety Thought problem Social problems Oppositional Conduct Self-esteem

Academic testing

Math	Reading	Writing
Math concepts	Basic word reading	Spelling
Math calculation	Non- or psuedoword Reading	Writing basics—punctuation, capitalization, grammar
Math application	Reading fluency	Writing fluency
Math fluency	Reading comprehension: literal and figurative/inferential	Sentence writing
		Paragraph composition
		Narrative
		Expository

Table 5.2 Davis–Broitman model assessment battery

IQ	Executive functioning and attention	Memory			Sensory motor	
		Visual	Verbal	Vis/verb integration	Bilateral efficiency	Proprioceptive
WISC-IV, DAS-II, KABC-II, Stanford–Binet-V	CPT-II NEPSY-II: Attention and Response Set Delis–Kaplan Executive Function System subtests BRIEF	WRAML-II: Design Memory and Finger Windows tasks Rey Complex Figure Test (RCFT) WISC-IV: Integrated Spatial Span task NEPSY-II: Memory for Designs task	WISC-IV: WMI tasks WRAML-II: Story Memory and Number–Letter tasks California Verbal Learning Test–Child Version (CVLT), WRAML-II: Verbal Learning subtest NEPSY-II: List Learning task	NEPSY-II: Memory for Names WRAML-I or II: Sound Symbol Learning tasks	WRAVMA: Pegboard NEPSY-II: Finger Tapping Other pegboard tasks	Observe pencil grip Observe amount of stress coming through on writing production

Graphomotor		Language		Visual Processing	Affect and behavior
Timed	Untimed	Receptive	Expressive	WISC-IV: Symbol Search,	Behavioral Assessment System for Children-2
WISC-IV: PSI	Beery-VMI-5	WISC-IV: Integrated—Similarities, Vocabulary, and Comprehension	WISC-IV: VCI	VMI–Visual	Conners Rating Scales-2
NEPSY-II: Visuomotor Precision	NEPSY-II: Design Copy	Peabody Picture Vocabulary Test	Test of Language Comprehension	NEPSY-II: Arrows task	Achenbach series
PAL-II: Alphabet Writing	WRAVMA: Drawing		Comprehensive Assessment of Spoken Language	Process Assessment of the Learner: Receptive and Expressive Coding	
			Expressive Vocabulary Test	Word Choice	
				Test of Orthographic Competence	

Academic testing

Math	Reading	Writing
Wechsler Individual Achievement Test-III (WIAT-III), the Key Math Test	WIAT-III, Gray Oral Reading Test Nelson–Denny Reading Test Test of Word Reading Efficiency	WIAT-III Oral and Written Language Scales, Test of Written Language-4

would generally be better at *local* reasoning (being able to see all the details of a situation) rather than *global* reasoning (being able to see the bigger picture of how all the details fit together). An apt metaphor one often hears is that these students have trouble seeing the forest for the trees (Foss, 1991).

Another potentially important contribution to understanding the thinking or processing styles of children with NVLD is Berninger and Richard's (2002) observation that *quantitative reasoning* also significantly contributes to math abilities. This may also contribute to a better understanding of the cognitive processing of students with NVLD, at least those that are experiencing arithmetic difficulties. That both *quantitative* and *spatial* reasoning can contribute to math abilities might help us to begin to explain why some students with NVLD may not be as impacted in math. Perhaps their strength in *quantitative reasoning* might help counter their weakness in constructional or spatial reasoning. Berninger's *Process Assessment of the Learner—Second Edition—Math* (2007), a test which assesses some of the important areas of functioning we describe above, may also be a valuable addition to our test battery to more fully understand students with NVLD processing difficulties. Hopefully future studies will shed light on these questions.

Upon psychological testing students with NVLD are often found to have visuo-constructional problems, often presenting with low scores on tasks such as the WISC-IV: Block Design or the DAS-II: Pattern Construction tests for example. On these tasks we often find they present with what Kaplan and her colleagues (Kramer, Kaplan, Blusewicz, & Preston, 1991; Kramer, Kaplan, Share, & Huckeba, 1999) have referred to as breaks in configuration. In essence this means being *captured* by the designs so that the overall *squareness* of the designs is forgotten, reducing the scores on these types of tests.

Another visual–spatial issue these students often have is difficulty with organizing a number of features into a whole, especially if the features are more complex and/or abstract and are more difficult to verbally encode. This is why the Rey Complex Figure Test (Meyers & Meyers, 1995) is widely used as part of a suspected NVLD case (Semrud-Clikeman, Fine, & Bledsoe, 2008). Here again what is often seen is that *pieces* of the RCFT are drawn while the overall gestalt of the design is lost. On this version of the RCFT, one also sees at times that the client performs better on the multiple choice/recognition part than on the free recall parts, since some of the *parts* of the design can be recalled better than the overall gestalt.

Another one of the better documented areas of difficulty for students with NVLD is visual working memory (Buchanan, Pavlovic, & Rovet, 1998; Cornoldi, Rigoni, Tressoldi, & Vio, 1999; Liddle & Rasmussen, 2005). The metaphor that we think captures this best is Baddeley's (1992) notion of the visuospatial sketch pad which he states is used to manipulate visual images. In this theory the central executive, which is assumed to be an attentional-controlling system, controls both the visuospatial sketch pad and what he refers to as its verbal counterpart, the phonological loop, which stores and rehearses speech-based information. When the visual–spatial sketch pad becomes overwhelmed or overloaded the student has trouble managing his or her workload and processing is impeded. This is often found with complex sequences of mental manipulation as are found in math (see Chap. 9).

Motor Skills

One of Rourke's (1989) initial concerns for children with NVLD was their motor development, both their gross and fine motor skills, describing these children as experiencing delays in motor development and difficulties with fine motor speed and gross motor skill acquisition. However, in his workshop presentations, Rourke often spoke of times when some of his clients would put a great deal of time and energy into task practicing, such as learning to ride a bike. They would often conquer their tasks; it would just take them longer. The issue of fine motor issues is less well documented. Whereas Rourke continues to use these criteria for helping to diagnose NVLD (Pelletier et al., 2001), others (Durand, Hulme, Larkin, & Snowling, 2005; Wilkinson & Semrud-Clikeman, 2008) have had differing results. One recent study (Semrud-Clikeman, Fine, & Bledsoe, 2010) may have helped clarify the issues. In this study they used the Delis–Kaplan Executive Function System (D-KEFS: Delis, Kaplan, & Kramer, 2001) Trail Making Test as the measure of fine motor/ graphomotor skills. They found that the children with NVLD did significantly more poorly on the more complex or demanding of executive functioning and spatial processing trials (Trails—Scanning, Number Sequencing, Letter Sequencing, and Number–Letter Switching tasks) than on the Fine Motor Speed task, which is a more *simple* connect-the-dots task.

Social

Socially, children with NVLD are often viewed as naïve, talkative, asking lots of questions, and engaging in parallel play longer than other children. One author (Davis) recalls a time when he was running a school for children with learning disorders watching a group of three elementary age boys with NVLD running around the playground. They were jumping and kicking in some sort of kung fu fashion. When queried about what they were doing, all said they were playing Ninja Turtles together, but without any interaction! Sweet, but with a context only they knew about, their play looked a bit odd and was essentially parallel play rather than interactive. Observing children's play is often an essential part of understanding and programming for the social aspects of their behavior. This school also tried to think systemically about children with these difficulties and how to program for their social needs (Davis, Nonverbal Learning Disabilities Conference presentation). Our post-evaluation team included a speech pathologist, social skills psychologist, classroom teacher, and playground supervisor. It was the job of the speech and language pathologist to draft the goals focusing on how to develop the student's pragmatic/social discourse. The speech pathologist chaired a meeting with the other experts so everyone was knowledgeable about what the goals were to be. The speech pathologist would then implement these in the one-to-one or one-to-two setting of the speech therapy. After a few sessions, or when the speech pathologist thought that the student(s) were ready, these students would start in a group of four to six students led by a psychologist focusing on the social skills already practiced. At the same time, the classroom teacher and playground aide would try to aid transfer and generalization of the skills being learned in the two therapeutic settings into the larger world of the classroom and school. Typically there would be 30–45 min team meetings every 6–8 weeks or as needed if the plan was not working well.

Mamen (2006) refers to a number of other social issues encountered by children with NVLD. These consist of things like difficulty with interpreting facial expressions and body language, difficulty with expressing emotions accurately through facial expressions and body language, overreacting to and misinterpreting other children's actions, none or few close friends, and difficulty with "unspoken" rules, pragmatics, and prosody. Due to these issues these children can also often find themselves bearing the brunt of bullying, teasing, and being made fun of (Little, 1993, 2002).

In terms of the assessment process, there are more psychometrically oriented instruments available for trying to capture aspects of social functioning. One of the more comprehensive approaches is the Social Skills Improvement System (SSIS) which consists of a series of rating scales (Gresham & Elliott, 2008), a classroom intervention program (Elliott & Gresham, 2007a, 2007b), and an intervention guide (Elliott & Gresham, 2007a) all of which can be used to assess and guide interventions for the youth(s) of interest. It is one of the most comprehensive assessment programs focusing on social skills. There are also certain scales on adaptive behavior measures, like the Vineland-II (Sparrow, Cicchetti, & Balla, 2004) and the Adaptive Behavior Assessment System-II (ABAS-II: Harrison & Oakland, 2003) that are very useful in identifying strengths and weaknesses in social and communication areas.

Other possible tests have been mentioned. One of the older tests, the Draw-A-Person test, was advocated by Johnson and Myklebust (1967), not necessarily to be scored in any way with psychometric properties, but in a more intuitive approach. In our experience, however, many children with NVLD feel very anxious about trying to draw. Projective techniques have sometimes been used, but we believe that these have to be utilized with the utmost care, or perhaps not at all. The Rorschach in particular, given the issues students with NVLD face, is highly suspect in terms of the results they produce. Apperception tests, like the Robert's-2 (2001), may have some clinical validity; however with the paucity of normative data for students with NVLD, using the scoring guidelines should be done with a great deal of caution if at all. See Chap. 10 for additional information on social skills.

Educational

Math: Trouble with mathematics, especially arithmetic calculation, has always been noted as the hallmark for NVLD from Gerstmann (1940). And trouble with mathematics continues to be thought of as a deficit for children with NVLD by ourselves

(Davis & Broitman, 2011) and others (Fine & Semrud-Clikeman, 2010; Forrest, 2004; Gross-Tsur, Shalev, Manor, & Amir, 1995; Shalev, 2004). Forrest's (2004) research supports the notion that it may be that math calculation is more impacted than math reasoning, but clearly more research is necessary in this area. Anecdotally, it has also been reported that students with NVLD can also struggle with the abstract concept formation often associated with math. Due to visual–spatial deficits they may struggle more with geometry then other types of math, and have difficulty being able to utilize graphs and diagrams.

Since math abilities and processes vary for each student with NVLD, we suggest that all primary areas of math functioning should be assessed. These include the areas of math calculation, math reasoning, math fluency, and in some cases applied math skills, especially as part of the transition planning from high school to young adulthood. Most of the standard academic measures, like the Wechsler Individualized Achievement Test-III (WIAT-III: 200×) and the Woodcock–Johnson-III (WJ-III: Woodcock, McGrew, & Mather, 2001), have subtests that can be used for these purposes. Two other tests that we have found useful for some of our clients are the Test of Early Mathematics Ability (TEMA: Connolly, 2007) for children 3 years to 8 years, 11 months for those children who are experiencing difficulties early enough to use this test, and the Key Math-3 (Connolly, 2007) for a more in-depth assessment of math abilities when needed to better understand and/or program for a particular students intervention plan.

Reading: Reading, or at least basic decoding, has typically been reported as a relative strength for students with NVLD. However, Rourke (1985) and others, i.e., Thompson (1997), have pointed out that the very beginning of reading skills can sometimes be a concern. It is believed that this is likely to be a struggle with the orthographic aspects of reading at the kindergarten and first-grade levels until the graphemes/letters are over learned and connected with their appropriate phonemes/morphemes/words. More typically the concerns that have been reported in the area of reading are in the advanced reading comprehension areas, especially those more demanding of inferential rather than literal comprehension (Foss, 1991; Thompson, 1997). Unfortunately there aren't any reading tests that have a formal scoring for picking up these differences, but the WIAT-III (Psychological Corporation, 2010) and the Nelson–Denny (Brown, Fishco, & Hanna, 1993) allow you to get the raw scores for the specific question in each category that the student has gotten incorrect. This is sometimes interesting because some of the students with NVLD have been found to do somewhat better on the more detail/literal comprehension questions than the more inferential types of reading comprehension questions. Students who present in this way might be referred to a speech pathologist for a more comprehensive language assessment. Such results are also useful to the educational therapist or special education teachers who are designing intervention plans for them.

Written language: As noted above, fine motor issues have always been somewhat of a concern, although now the data is less consistent about the role of fine motor issues in NVLD. But for those students who do struggle with penmanship it clearly interferes with writing production abilities (Berninger, 1999). Other descriptions of writing difficulties often refer to difficulty with topic sentences, getting caught up in detail, and trouble with some of the organizational aspects of writing (Tanguay, 2002; Thompson, 1997). Again, the basic achievement tests assess some of the important areas; however in terms of samples produced we believe that the WIAT-III task is more demanding of the kinds of weaknesses which might emerge for students with NVLD than the WJ-III which requires less production and organization. If a more in-depth assessment is needed, the Test of Written Language—fourth edition (Hammill & Larsen, 2009) is a very useful instrument although takes much longer to administer. Sometimes administering some of the subtests, such as Contextual Conventions or Story Composition, may be all that is needed.

The Case of Katie

We present the case of Katie to illustrate a few of the critical issues relevant to our discussion of the assessment of NVLD. Katie came into the ninth grade from an East Coast private school. Early birth and developmental histories were unremarkable. Early school history was positive for some beginning reading issues which seemed to resolve themselves with some brief private tutoring, and some math issues that began around fifth grade. There were no significant social or behavioral issues reported, but Katie was described as somewhat shy, generally good with adults, and had a couple of close girlfriends. By the sixth grade parental concerns persisted and they had Katie evaluated by a learning specialist recommended by the school. As you can see below, the evaluator used the Woodcock–Johnson-R cognitive and academic batteries.

	Standard scores
WJ-R (1999)—Cognitive	
Fluid Reasoning	124
Long-Term Retrieval	100
Short-Term Memory	91
Processing speed	94
Visual processing	91
Verbal comp./vocab.	106
Auditory processing	81
WJ-R (1999)—Academic	
Basic reading	107
Passage comprehension	118
Calculation	95
Applied problems	92
Dictation	96
Proofing	101

Auditory processing data seemed to be problematic for Katie, but Katie appeared to have a relative strength found on the cognitive battery in Fluid Reasoning. The report suggested that there may have been some attentional or memory issues but she did not exhibit eligibility criteria for a specific learning disability. And, given her weaknesses in auditory processing, it was interesting that they did not seem to be negatively impacting her reading skills the way we would have presumed they should. Recommendations from this report consisted primarily of subject matter tutoring as needed. Unfortunately, Katie's difficulties did not stop there. She continued to struggle in school and things seemed to become relatively more difficult in math and science somewhat. Katie's parents continued to be concerned and decided to have her reevaluated by another learning specialist. These were the results obtained at the second testing.

	Standard scores
WJ-III (2001)—Cognitive	
Fluid Reasoning	96
Long-Term Retrieval	107
Short-Term Memory	106
Processing speed	93
Visual processing	91
Verbal comp./vocab.	109
Auditory processing	73
WJ-III (2001)—Academic	
Basic reading	100
Passage comprehension	109
Calculation	116
Applied problems	104

Again, Katie appeared to struggle with auditory processing. This time no particular strengths emerged, she still did not meet the criteria for a specific learning disability, and again there were no apparent academic weaknesses. Katie performed significantly more poorly on the Fluid Reasoning tasks on this testing while all other scores are within predicted limits. This difference was more or less accepted and left unexplained in the report. However, this time her parents decided to follow up with Fast Forward Language, which they believed was helpful for the perceived auditory processing.

Katie began ninth grade in her neighborhood public high school. The transition from the East Coast to her new West Coast public school was not easy for her. In ninth grade her parents reported that Katie was working hard, making some acquaintances, but struggling to make closer friends. School was "ok," but she was having some difficulty keeping all the major projects and study schedules organized and would need extra parental support when feeling overwhelmed. From the fifth grade, math and science had been a bit harder, so she had some tutorial support for both subjects. Her parents reported that they were afraid that Katie would "burn out" if she had to continue to work so hard, but she managed a 3.2 GPA for the year. Then tenth grade began. Within the first few weeks Katie was overwhelmed by her geometry class and her confidence was significantly shaken. Katie's parents were more concerned than ever that Katie's self-esteem and motivation would be impacted, and again sought the help of an evaluation to see if there was anything that could be done to provide additional support for her in the school.

As the evaluator, Davis met with Katie's parents, read the previous reports, and presented them with what we would try to assess. A comprehensive evaluation, similar to the one above, was agreed upon. The following are the results:

Cognitive Results

• Wechsler Intelligence Scale for Children-III (1989)	
Index scores	Standard scores
Verbal comprehension index	108
Perceptual organization index	67
Freedom from distraction index	98
Processing speed index	122
• Differential Ability Scale (1990)	
Subtests T-scores	
– Matrices	58
– Sequential and quantitative	49
Index scores	Standard scores
Nonverbal/fluid	104

Wide Range Assessment of Memory and Learning-II		
Subtests	*Subscale scores*	
Story memory	8	
SM recall	8	
SM recognition	13	
Verbal learning	6	
VL recall	6	
VL recognition	10	
Picture memory	8	
Finger windows	11	
Rey Complex Figure Test		
Subtests	T-Scores	Percentiles
Copy		>16
Time to copy		<1
Immediate recall	40	16
Delayed recall	38	12
Recognition total correct	39	14

Comprehensive Test of Phonological Processing	
Subtests	*Subscale scores*
Elision	8
Blending words	7
Memory for digits	12
Nonword repetition	5
Rapid digit naming	10
Rapid letter naming	11
Wide Range Assessment of Visual Motor Abilities	
Subtests	*Standard scores*
Drawing	100
Pegboard-dominant (R)	92
Non-dominant	93
Delis–Kaplan Executive Function System	
Subtests	*Subscale scores*
Trail making tests	
Visual scanning	13
Number sequencing	9
Letter sequencing	10
Number-Letter switching	6
Motor speed	12
Verbal fluency	
Letter fluency	8
Category fluency	12

Child Behavior Checklist—all scales within normal limits

Teacher Report Form—not administered as parents thought that none of her teachers knew her well enough

Youth Self-Report—all scales within normal limits

Connors' Continuous Performance Test II—results more like the non-ADHD group.

Academic Results

Wechsler Individual Achievement Test-II	
Subtests	*Standard scores*
Listening comprehension	111
Oral expression	115
Word reading	106
Reading comprehension	109
Pseudoword reading	95
Spelling	111

(continued)

(continued)

Wechsler Individual Achievement Test-II	
Written expression	100
Numerical operations	118
Mathematics reasoning	101
Nelson–Denny Reading Test, 1993	
Subtests	*Standard scores*
Comprehension	111
Rate	100
Test of Word Reading Efficiency	
Subtests	*Standard scores*
Sight word	100
Phonemic decoding	88
Woodcock–Johnson-III	
Subtests	*Standard scores*
Writing fluency	112
Math fluency	108

Brief Overview and Interpretation of Results

At the time, Katie was a 15-year-old student who was experiencing some intra-individual differences in her cognitive development. She exhibited relative strengths in the areas of verbal comprehension and reasoning, immediate "incremental" short-term memory, and adequate social skills and athletic abilities. Relative weaknesses are apparent in three primary areas. The first area continues to be in auditory processing, or what would be called phonological blending issues. It would seem from these data that the Fast Forward Language program did not transfer to the skills needed for this type of assessment; however her parents believed that Fast Forward helped in the "real world" in some unknown way. This aspect of her processing was also observed in her previous two assessments. The next two areas were not.

Her second area of difficulty was in visuoconstructional/spatial reasoning. This is likely the area that would be most responsible for her significant struggles with geometry. It is an area that was noted in the former evaluations as her visual processing scores were in the low average range, but Katie did not seem as impacted as she does here. This became most apparent on the WISC-III and RCFT data. And, as discussed below this may be likely because of the increased memory, complexity, and/or spatial/organizational demands relative to the less complex tasks of the WJ-III in the previous testing or here on the WISC-III: PSI (93rd percentile). Interestingly, given her adequate fluid/quantitative reasoning skills on this testing, and on a lot of the math presented to her on the academic testing, she was able to perform in the average range. However, an item analysis on the math sections of the WIAT-II revealed that Katie was able to solve many of the basic math and algebraic equations, but she was not successful in using basic geometry. Unfortunately most academic diagnostic tests do not try to separate these areas out in any useful kind of format.

Katie's third area of difficulty was in verbal and visual memory. Katie could become overwhelmed when the memory tasks were *not* incremental and therefore required more simultaneous organization and encoding. Here Katie could become overwhelmed without context (see WRAML-II: Verbal Learning, RCFT, D-KEFS: Verbal Fluency). But she could *produce* better in a recognition format which reduces some of the organizational demands of information retrieval. Likewise this sort of overwhelm could also be seen on some of the reading tasks. While she scored in the average range for reading comprehension, on the Nelson–Denny Katie was able to finish 34 of the 38 questions within the allotted time, and 26 were answered correctly. It is of interest that of the eight items missed, only one was of the literal type while seven were of the inferential or interpretive type, which some believe would be consistent with nonverbal learning disorders (Rourke & Tsatsanis, 1996; Worling, Humphries, & Tannock, 1999).

Summary

This case study points out that NVLD is both complex and often coexists with other disorders. Katie showed some of the classical signs of a verbal learning disorder created by an underlying auditory processing or phonological processing disorder. Given Rourke's (Pelletier et al., 2001) criteria, this should have been an area of strength for a child with NVLD. However, when a more comprehensive battery was administered it became clearer that not only was there a persistent and somewhat treatment-resistant phonological processing disorder, but also that Katie was experiencing processing issues consistent with a nonverbal or spatial processing disorder. Further, some of the academic weaknesses like geometry and inferentially oriented reading comprehension skills were actually more consistent with NVLD than auditory processing difficulties.

Recommendations were consistent with her processing issues. The more important had to do with some direct instruction in organization and study skills: having content-oriented tutoring in the geometrically oriented math and sciences with a tutor who understands that verbal mediation and discussion will be essential to the tutorial process, and should reading comprehension become more problematic, a structured approach to reading comprehension strategies. More specifically for literature, the use of study guides or Cliffs Notes was suggested to help Katie understand some of the broader issues and themes in the material she read, to help her to better organize and understand the material.

Finally, Katie's results highlight how important it is to consider which test measures will be used. The WJ-III was able, at least for Katie, to pick up her auditory processing difficulties, but it was not very good at picking up her spatial processing issues and was also unable to pick up the kinds of memory tasks that were more problematic for her.

NVLD is not always an easy disorder to diagnose. It is often more difficult to find in younger children than older children given the nature of the academic tasks they are forced to face, and it can be hidden when cognitive strengths, motivation, and family support provide coping strategies to help the student maintain in school.

There are numerous recommendations that can be useful additions to help guide the professions who will be using the child's assessment report. We close with a list of some of those we have found most beneficial to children with NVLD. Of course the areas of strength and weakness for a particular child will determine its inclusion in a particular report. We have grouped these recommendations into four categories: general approaches, approaches for visual–spatial/executive function, approaches meeting the student's socio-emotional needs, and approaches for academic support. Please note that not all recommendations will be needed for all students with NVLD. This isn't an exhaustive list of all that can be done, but rather examples of things that may be useful with particular guidelines about how they might help.

General Approaches/Attitudes Toward Students with Nonverbal Learning Disorders

1. Avoid figures of speech, and be literal. Children with NVLD often have trouble interpreting metaphors and may grow emotional in response to them. At minimum, they tend not to admit that they have not understood the figurative language.
2. When working with students with NVLD, if they exhibit a behavior that you do not want/like, do not assume that this is a "character flaw" or "bad behavior." It will be more helpful to assume that it is likely a misunderstanding or miscommunication and then approach the child with that mindset.
3. Assume their "Why …" questions are *literal* questions. Answer them literally before continuing to respond as you would to a child without NVLD.
4. As Russell Barkley (2005) has stressed for children with ADHD, every day is a new day. Holding grudges and creating resentment over the long term is likely to interfere with the relationship. Instead help lay out causes and effects, especially but not limited to the social ones. Mistakes made yesterday don't necessarily lead to progress tomorrow if one cannot understand the effects of one's actions, on self or on others.
5. Children with NVLD have more difficulty than average with constructing sequences. For example, there are at least 50 steps involved in getting to his or her next appointment on time: hear bell in class, put books away, remember to take backpack, leave class, turn left, go downstairs, go to the bus stop, find the right bus, remember to pick up backpack, find seat, put backpack down, get off at the right stop (*with* backpack!), enter building, and find the correct room.
6. Observe the child's behavior closely, especially in novel or complex situations. We believe that the child's actual behavior should be our guide to understanding

his or her struggles. It is generally understood that the new or novel situations will most likely generate the greatest problems for the child with NVLD. Directly observing the child will allow the professional to develop an intervention plan that focuses more specifically on the needed skills.

Visual–Spatial/Executive Functions (Core Deficits)

1. It is important for teachers and treatment professionals to recognize that there may sometimes be limitations in the child's/adolescent's visual, perceptual, and/or sensory processing modalities. He or she may be less "in sync" whenever material is presented in a purely visual modality.
2. Instructions with visual tasks should be verbally broken down in a logical step-by-step fashion. When something is presented in a visual or multimodal format, it should be accompanied by verbal cues and/or explanations. Keep in mind that the child will likely appreciate and benefit from, not tire of, lengthy, concrete verbal instructions and/or examples.
3. The child/adolescent may have difficulty "seeing the big picture" or the context from which details are extracted. While most people take a whole-part-whole approach to learning novel material, children and adolescents with these issues tend to take a part-whole approach whereby he or she can become easily stuck in the details. These children/adolescents tend to benefit from assistance in "stringing" the details together to form the whole, which should be facilitated by the integration of step-by-step verbal instructions. Teach the child to utilize verbal mediation for problem solving.
4. Try to make cause-and-effect relationships verbally explicit whenever possible.
5. Try to demonstrate how details are part of a larger whole and/or how details can be grouped together as part of a whole, e.g., words may be grouped into categories within a larger list.
6. The child can be overwhelmed by large amounts of materials; thus information should be presented in small "chunks" whenever possible. Large amounts of material, information, and homework assignments that have not been structured for him or her may be counterproductive given that he or she could become overwhelmed and distractible when challenged thusly.
7. Teach the child/adolescent to use his/her verbal strengths to mediate his/her experiences. Verbal mediation is a powerful tool for these youngsters.
8. Rely on his/her verbal strengths to teach decision making, goal setting, and making action plans to achieve goals and evaluate results.
9. Try to make the demands for performance as reasonable as possible, i.e., make sure demands are not overwhelming.
10. Teach and practice organizational skills. Utilize structure, routine, and rote or "scripted" rules when necessary to help the child/adolescent better manage situations.

11. Teach the child/adolescent to self-monitor his/her own understanding of situations/instructions and to ask clarifying questions when necessary.
12. Teach the child to make better use of his or her visual–perceptual–organizational. We caution professionals to help the child to exercise and develop his or her less-developed skills to work toward achieving the highest level possible through age-appropriate remedial exercises.
13. Teach the child to use age-appropriate aids to reach a specific goal. These may include digital watches, calculators, laptops, and various forms of assistive technologies which could be utilized to help improve the child's performance.

Social/Emotional

1. Many people with NLD tend to see only extremes as choices, and miss the "gray zone." Therefore, helping them to slow down enough to consider gray areas can be very helpful, esp. in social situations where the options generally are quite a bit more complex than "fight or surrender," "win or lose."
2. The child's/adolescent's tendency to get stuck in the details of social events can be anxiety provoking, and once started this cycle may tend to escalate. The best way to deal with escalating frustration is to utilize relaxation techniques that can be used immediately when the frustration cycle begins. These techniques should be practiced often and in non-anxiety provoking situations as well. Once the child/adolescent masters this technique, it can be applied to numerous situations that cause him/her anxiety or distress. Further, once relaxed, one can better learn to switch strategies and take an alternative strategy to a novel situation.
3. The child's/adolescent's nonverbal weaknesses can cause social difficulties and possible misperceptions. He or she may have trouble reading nonverbal cues, especially when they are subtle, and may have difficulty knowing how to respond in novel social situations. It is important to understand that the child may not accurately perceive the "gestalt" in social situations as well and might require assistance in the same step-by-step manner. He/she will likely do better in more highly structured social situations, but social skills training can help to better adapt to less structured situations.
4. Help the child develop insight into situations that are easy for him or her and those that are particularly troublesome. Here we stress the importance for the child [or adult] to understand his or her own cognitive functioning over time with the goal of developing a realistic understanding of his or her capacities. Once achieved, this understanding can help guide the child to get assistance when needed, and help him or her avoid situations that may be more likely to end in failure. It is also the cornerstone of self-advocacy.
5. Anticipate the situations where he/she might have difficulty with transitions or novelty and provide advanced practice and support for how to deal with them.

6. Teach the child/adolescent to attend to and interpret facial expressions, gestures, prosody, vocal inflections, and other nonverbal aspects of communication.
7. Teach the child to interpret visual information when there is competing auditory information.
8. Teach the child to refine and use appropriately his or her verbal skills. The child with NVLD needs to be taught what to say, how to say it, and when to say it. Considerable time should be spent training and retraining the child to stop, look, listen, and weigh alternatives even in the most mundane circumstances. Failure to do so leaves the child subject to negatively reinforcing consequences which can promote a withdrawal and avoidance.
9. There is a need to teach appropriate nonverbal behavior. Pragmatic skills should be thought of as both receptive and expressive. So there is a need to work with the student on how to read nonverbal behavior and how to present nonverbal behavior consistent with how the child actually feels and for what the child is actually trying to transmit.
10. Clinicians must facilitate structured peer interactions. If needed, start with individual instruction in social skills but do not assume transfer and generalization. Provide social group instruction for repetition and practice and generalization. Let teachers and aids also know what skills are being taught so that they can scaffold within the classroom and/or playground.
11. Be cognizant of the professional's role in preparing the child with NVLD for adult life. Professionals have a unique and crucial role in helping the child plan for and achieve success. Our domain is as vast as all of life, since the child with NVLD needs help accruing all life's social and survival skills.
12. Encourage the child to describe in detail important events that are transpiring in his or her life. We have found that engaging in a detailed discussion of an event can allow the child to hear the discrepancies between his or her perception and the perception of others. Using a technique of reteaching can allow the professional to check what the child has analyzed and integrated. It also allows the child to develop a verbal "context" within which to more easily store information.

Pre-academic and Academic

1. Promote, encourage, and monitor systematic explorative activities. This is especially true at younger ages when students with NVLD are less likely to move around their environment to explore and experience the sort of things Piaget talks about during his sensory motor phase.
2. Go slowly and ensure understanding when working with visual material. Recognize that the geometric maths and sciences will be particularly difficult.
3. Teachers and clinicians must adopt realistic attitudes. The professional must use his or her refined understanding of the child's strengths and weakness to plan for success. If there is no way for a school to accommodate the child's

deficits, alternative programs must be found. In cases where this is not possible the family should be helped to avoid the situation.

4. Teachers should permit the use of laptops and calculators in the maths and sciences as needed. For some students, independent studies of the particular subject may be required. Students should be allowed longer test time in a distraction-free environment for in-class and standardized testing.
5. For in-class or standardized testing utilizing bubble or Scantron methodologies, a recorder should be provided or the answers should be allowed to be left in the test pamphlet, especially high stakes testing.
6. Revise spacing on homework and tests when needed. For instance provide math problems not 30 to a page but perhaps 5–10 per page. Also, consider that the homework not be about the number of problems completed, but rather achieving mastery.
7. If physical education is problematic, having other exercises or activities may be needed.
8. On longer homework or class assignments, allow the student to dictate or record, especially if handwriting and keyboarding are slow.
9. Lecture notes should be made available before class to reduce the note taking demands and to allow the student to prep for the lecture and create a context for new material to aid in retention.
10. Get school personnel to make modifications of assignments involving visual–spatial skills such as graphs and/or charts.

References

Baddeley, A. (1992). Working memory. *Science, 255*(5044), 556–559.

Barkley, R. A. (2005). *Attention-deficit hyperactivity disorder: A handbook for diagnosis and treatment* (3rd ed.). New York: Guilford Press.

Berninger, V. W. (1999). Coordinating transcription and text generation in working memory during composing: Automatized and constructive processes. *Learning Disability Quarterly, 22*, 99–112.

Berninger, V. W. (2007). *Process assessment of the learner- Math* (2nd ed.). San Antonio, TX: Pearson Education.

Berninger, V. W., & Richards, T. L. (2002). *Brain literacy for educators and psychologists*. New York: Academic Press.

Brown, J. A., Fishco, V. V., & Hanna, G. (1993). *Nelson-Denny reading test: Manual for scoring and interpretation, forms G & H*. Rolling Meadows, IL: Riverside Publishing.

Buchanan, L., Pavlovic, J., & Rovet, J. (1998). A reexamination of the visuospatial deficit in Turner syndrome: Contributions of working memory. *Developmental Neuropsychology, 14*, 341–367.

Connolly, A. J. (2007). *Key math-3*. San Antonio, TX: Pearson Education.

Cornoldi, C., Rigoni, F., Tressoldi, P. E., & Vio, C. (1999). Imagery deficits in nonverbal learning disabilities. *Journal of Learning Disabilities, 32*, 48–57.

Corporation, P. (2010). *Wechsler individual achievement test III*. San Antonio, TX: Psychological Corporation.

Davis, J. M., & Broitman, J. (2011). *Nonverbal learning disabilities in children: Bridging the gap between science and practice*. New York: Springer.

Delis, D. C., & Jacobson, M. (2000). *Neuropsychological testing. Encyclopedia of psychology.* New York: Oxford University Press.

Delis, D. C., Kaplan, E., & Kramer, J. H. (2001). *The Delis-Kaplan executive function system.* San Antonio, TX: The Psychological Corporation.

Durand, M. D., Hulme, C., Larkin, R., & Snowling, M. (2005). The cognitive foundations of reading and arithmetic skills in 7 to 10 year olds. *Journal of Experimental Child Psychology, 91*, 113–136.

Elliott, S. N., & Gresham, F. M. (2007a). *SSIS classwide intervention program teacher's guide.* Minneapolis, MN: NCS Pearson.

Elliott, S. N., & Gresham, F. M. (2007b). *SSIS performance screening guide.* Minneapolis, MN: NCS Pearson.

Fine, J. G., & Semrud-Clikeman, M. (2010). Nonverbal learning disabilities: Assessment and intervention. In A. S. Davis (Ed.), *Handbook of pediatric neuropsychology.* Cambridge, UK: Cambridge University Press.

Flanagan, D. P., Ortiz, S. O., & Alfonso, V. C. (2007). *Essentials of cross-battery assessment* (2nd ed.). Hoboken, NJ: Wiley.

Forrest, B. (2004). The utility of math difficulties, internalized psychopathology, and visual-spatial deficits to identify children with the nonverbal learning disability syndrome: Evidence for a visuospatial disability. *Child Neuropsychology, 10*(2), 129–146.

Foss, J. (1991). Nonverbal learning disabilities and remedial interventions. *Annals of Dyslexia, 41*, 128–140.

Gerstmann, J. (1940). Syndrome of finger agnosia, disorientation for right and left, agraphia and acalculia. *Archives of Neurology and Psychiatry, 44*, 389.

Gresham, F. M., & Elliott, S. N. (2008). *SSIS rating scales.* Minneapolis, MN: NCS Pearson.

Grodzinsky, G.M. (2003). *Subtypes of nonverbal learning disability: A neuropsychological analysis.* Presented at the 13th Annual Nelson Butters' West Coast Neuropsychology Conference, March 20–23, San Diego, CA.

Grodzinsky, G. M., Forbes, P. W., & Bernstein, J. H. (2010). A practice-based approach to group identification in nonverbal learning disorders. *Child Neuropsychology, 16*(5), 433–460.

Gross-Tsur, V., Shalev, R. S., Manor, O., & Amir, N. (1995). Developmental right-hemisphere syndrome: Clinical spectrum of the nonverbal learning disability. *Journal of Learning Disabilities, 28*(2), 80.

Hain, L. A., Hale, J. B., & Kendorski, J. G. (2009). The comorbidity of psychopathology in cognitive and academic SLD subtypes. In S. G. Feifer & G. Rattan (Eds.), *Emotional disorders: A neuropsychological, psychopharmacological, and educational perspective* (pp. 199–225). Middletown, MD: School Neuropsych Press.

Hammill, D., & Larsen, S. C. (2009). *Test of written language* (4th ed.). Austin, TX: PRO-ED.

Harrison, P. L., & Oakland, T. (2003). *Adaptive behavior assessment system* (2nd ed.). San Antonio, TX: Harcourt Assessment.

Johnson, D. J., & Myklebust, H. R. (1967). *Learning disabilities: Educational principles and practices.* New York: Grune & Stratton.

Klin, A., Volkmar, F. R., Sparrow, S. S., & Cicchetti, B. P. (1996). Validity and neuropsychological characterization of Asperger Syndrome: Convergence with nonverbal learning disabilities syndrome. *Journal of Child Psychology and Psychiatry, and Allied Disciplines, 36*, 241–259.

Kramer, J. H., Kaplan, E., Blusewicz, M. J., & Preston, K. A. (1991). Visual hierarchical analysis of block design configural errors. *Journal of Clinical and Experimental Neuropsychology, 13*(4), 455–465.

Kramer, J. H., Kaplan, E., Share, L., & Huckeba, W. (1999). Configural errors on WISC-III block design. *Journal of the International Neuropsychological Society, 5*, 518–524.

Landau, Y., Gross-Tsur, V., Auerbach, J., Van der Meer, J., & Shalev, R. (1999). Attention-deficit hyperactivity disorder and developmental right-hemi-sphere syndrome: Congruence and incongruence of cognitive and behavioral aspects of attention. *Journal of Child Neurology, 14*, 209–230.

Liddle, G. A., & Rasmussen, C. (2005). Memory profile of children with nonverbal learning disability. *Learning Disabilities Research and Practice, 20*, 137–141.

Little, S. S. (1993). Nonverbal learning disabilities and socioemotional functioning: A review of recent literature. *Journal of Learning Disabilities, 26*, 653–665.

Little, S. S. (2002). Middle-class mothers' perceptions of peer victimization of children with Asperger's syndrome and nonverbal learning disorders. *Issues in Comprehensive Pediatric Nursing, 25*, 43–57.

Mamen, M. (2006). *Nonverbal learning disabilities and their clinical subtypes: A handbook for parents and professionals—New edition*. Ottawa, ON: Centrepointe Professional Services.

Meyers, J. E., & Meyers, K. R. (1995). *Rey complex figure test and recognition trial (RCFT)*. Odessa, FL: Psychological Assessment Resources.

Pelletier, P. M., Ahmad, S. A., & Rourke, B. P. (2001). Classification rules for basic phonological processing disabilities and nonverbal learning disorders. *Child Neuropsychology, 7*, 84–98.

Roberts, G. (2001). *Roberts apperception test for children and adolescents* (2nd ed.). Los Angeles, CA: Western Psychological Services.

Rourke, B. P. (Ed.). (1985). *Neuropsychology of learning disabilities: Essentials of subtype analysis*. New York: Guilford Publications.

Rourke, B. P. (1989). *Nonverbal learning disabilities: The syndrome and the model*. New York: Guilford Press.

Rourke, B. P. (1995). The NLD syndrome and the white matter model. In B. P. Rourke (Ed.), *Syndrome of nonverbal learning disabilities: Neurodevelopmental manifestations*. New York: Guilford Press.

Rourke, B. P., & Tsatsanis, K. D. (1996). Syndrome of nonverbal learning disabilities: Psycholinguistic assets and deficits. *Topics in Language Disorders, 16*(2), 30–44.

Semrud-Clikeman, M., Fine, J. G., & Bledsoe, J. (2008). Meta-analysis of Empirical Research in Assessment and Diagnosis in NVLD. Paper presented at the International Neuropsychological Association. Honolulu, Hawaii

Semrud-Clikeman, M., Fine, J. G., & Bledsoe, J. (2010). Executive functioning in children with Asperger's Disorder, nonverbal learning disabilities, and typically developing children. *Journal of Abnormal Psychology, 38*, 509–519.

Shalev, R. S. (2004). Developmental dyscalculia: Review. *Journal of Child Neurology, 19*, 765–771.

Sparrow, S. S., Cicchetti, D. V., & Balla, P. A. (2004). *Vineland adaptive behavior scales* (2nd ed.). Bloomington, MN: Pearson Assessment.

Tanguay, P. B. (2002). *Nonverbal learning disabilities at school*. London, England: Jessica Kingsley.

Thompson, S. (1997). *The source for nonverbal learning disorders*. East Moline, IL: Linguisystems.

Wechsler, D. (1989). Wechsler Intelligence Scale for Children- Third Edition. The Psychological Corporation. San Antonio, TX.

Wilkinson, A., & Semrud-Clikeman, M. (2008). *Motor speed in children and adolescents with nonverbal learning disabilities*. Paper presented at the International Neuropsychological Society. Honolulu, Hawaii

Woodcock, R. W., McGrew, K. S., & Mather, N. (2001). *Woodcock-Johnson III tests of achievement*. Itasca, IL: Riverside.

Worling, D. E., Humphries, T., & Tannock, R. (1999). Spatial and emotional aspects of language inferencing in nonverbal learning disabilities. *Brain and Language, 70*, 220–239.

Chapter 6
The Physician's Role in Treating NVLD

Meryl E. Lipton

Introduction

Children with nonverbal learning disabilities (NVLD) present a complex, varied set of characteristics. This chapter provides a framework to help better understand these children and the role that physicians can have in providing these children, adolescents, and young adults excellent care.

Some parents take their child to a physician only for medication to treat the ADHD, anxiety, or the depression that may be a part of their child's clinical picture. Other parents come to a physician for diagnosis, intervention suggestions, or case management. When the physician can provide the services required, it is a good match. When the physician is fully aware of the social and neurocognitive elements of NVLD, it can be a great match.

The chapter addresses the following seven questions, which are essential when planning how to work with children who have these difficulties:

1. What are the NVLD characteristics that prompt a referral to a physician?
2. What are the developmental NVLD milestones families and professionals should know about?
3. What types of physician specialists are most likely to be skilled in caring for individuals with NVLD?
4. Why aren't some physicians able to provide services needed by children with NVLD?
5. How can parents and professionals partner with physicians to create the best outcomes?

M.E. Lipton, M.D., Ph.D. (✉)
Rush University Medical Center, Medical Director Rush Neurobehavioral Center, 1653 West Congress Parkway, Chicago, IL 60612, USA
e-mail: meryl_lipton@rush.edu

J. Broitman and J.M. Davis (eds.), *Treating NVLD in Children: Professional Collaborations for Positive Outcomes*, DOI 10.1007/978-1-4614-6179-1_6,

6. What medications might be useful for which symptoms?
7. What is a clinical model of physician as case manager? Case histories are included that will highlight important issues including the role of medication in treatment.

NVLD Symptoms that Might Prompt a Referral to a Physician

For infants and toddlers who are later diagnosed with NVLD, the initial concerns are most often problems with sensory and motor processing. These behaviors (sensitivity to light or loud noises, difficulty with fine and gross motor skills, etc.) are not specific to NVLD. They are found in many children with neurobehavioral disorders such as ADHD, Autism Spectrum Disorders, and Learning Disorders.

Children with NVLD have a cognitive pattern characterized by strong verbal language and weak processing of visual information which include faces, spaces, and places (Denckla, 2000, personal communication). In addition, these children frequently have difficulties with attention regulation (ADHD) and organizational challenges. During the early years in school, some children with NVLD are able to perform at an academically acceptable rate and are not especially loud and/or boisterous enough to call attention to their behavior. As a result, their neurobehavioral problems may not be identified. As they develop—and the demands of school, family, and social life increase—challenges may become apparent. As the school years progress, difficulties with reading comprehension, math, attention, and organization often surface. Social, emotional, and behavioral difficulties become more pronounced and referrals are made to physicians such as general pediatricians, behavioral pediatricians, child and adolescent psychiatrists, and pediatric neurologists.

Children with NVLD have a variety of characteristics that prompt being seen by a physician. By definition, this population of children typically has social difficulties with making and maintaining friendships. These children want to have friends yet find it hard to initiate and sustain reciprocal interactions with age mates. They often have trouble knowing how to enter into a conversation or where to stand in a small group of peers. Their challenges reading nonverbal cues in a 1:1 situation amplify when participating in a group. Integrating and interpreting all the simultaneous messages can be frustrating for them. Hence they are frequently left alone. Children with NVLD have social interest but frequently lack social know-how. These social challenges often lead to secondary problems with self-esteem, anxiety, and problems with mood that prompt a referral.

A common clinical presenting complaint is inattention. Usually the teacher at school notices inattention and communicates this concern to the family. Another important referral is for secondary symptoms such as poor self-esteem, anxiety, and sadness which can lead to depression. Children who experience social failure are at risk for developing poor self-esteem, anxiety, and depression. When social failure is linked with academic difficulties in the school environment, those risks are increased.

Some family situations may be a safe haven for these children, but other family situations may independently facilitate the development of poor self-esteem, anxiety, and/or depression.

Anxiety is a frequent presenting complaint for children with NVLD. Children who have significant problems reading the visual/nonverbal cues which make up 75% of communication (Mehrabian, 1971) often have a hard time making sense of what is happening in their environment. Anxiety can be a natural response to living in a confusing place where you understand neither what is happening nor what may happen.

The next section provides some of the specific developmental content/expertise that a physician should have if s/he is going to have an increased probability of success recognizing and treating an NVLD patient.

Essential Developmental Aspects of NVLD

NVLD is characterized by delay in the emergence of developmental social–emotional behaviors. Therefore it is important that families and professionals know the social–emotional developmental symptoms that children with NVLD may manifest. Like other neurobehavioral problems, NVLD comes in small, medium, and large. Integrating the continuum of severity with a child's social–emotional development helps create a deeper understanding which will inform a more focused set of interventions.

Clinically observed relevant behaviors of children with NVLD include:

- Infant behaviors: generally quiet, slow to explore the environment, content watching others rather than being interactive.
- Preschool: avoidance of fine and gross motor activities, poorly developed daily living skills, observe others play but rarely interact, continued parallel play.
- Elementary school: initial period of difficulty with letter and number recognition followed by improvement, reading words and spelling are easy, motor difficulty when writing, interested in books with facts rather than relationship-based stories, problems with reading comprehension, inattention, difficulty with organizational strategies for writing, struggles with numeral writing and calculations, limited peer interactions.
- Middle and high school: academic problems with math, writing (motor and organizational), and reading comprehension; organizational challenges; social difficulties; anxiety; and depression.
- College and beyond: some adolescents with mild to moderate NVLD are successful in college. Their academic, organization, and social problems provide challenges but they are able, often with support, to complete a course of study. Others find independent living, coupled with the academic and social demands, to be overwhelming. Anxiety and depression can be the result of these life challenges.

In some children these behavioral descriptions provide enough information a professional to begin to recognize symptoms of NVLD. Other circumstances are better served with specific research tools based on specific behaviors. In Charts 6.1 and 6.2 (Lipton & Evans-Smith, 2006), research-based social–emotional learning milestones are broken out across both age and by where those behaviors fit within a framework known as the SELF (social–emotional learning framework) (Lipton & Nowicki, 2009). The SELF integrates information about social–emotional processing from multiple academic areas: neuroscience, education, and psychology (Lipton & Nowicki, 2009). In an attempt to provide a conceptual structure for social–emotional learning skills, the SELF separates abilities to take in social emotion information, comprehension, abilities to engage in social–emotional behaviors, and execution. The SELF's comprehension begins with awareness—decoding nonverbal signals of emotion. It is followed by meaning—integrating verbal and nonverbal cues within the social context. Reasoning is the last aspect of comprehension and refers to social problem solving. Expression includes connect (behaviors that demonstrate an association with others in the environment) and interact (behaviors that support reciprocal social interactions and deepen behaviors associated with evolving and maturing reciprocal relationships).

Additional information about the SELF is found in Chart 6.3.

On Charts 6.1 and 6.2, bar lines indicate when a specific social–emotional learning skill appears. As an example, during the initial 2 years of life, babies learn to recognize basic emotions such as happy, sad, angry, and fearful (Browne, Rosenfield, & Horowitz, 1977; Labarbera, Izard, Vietze, & Paris, 1976; Nelson, Morse, & Leavitt, 1979). During years 2–9, they learn more complex emotions, known as social emotions, including pride, embarrassment, and envy (Brody & Harrison, 1987; Michaelson & Lewis, 1985).

These social developmental milestones might be helpful to professionals who work with young children as it is well accepted that the earlier the intervention takes place, the more opportunity there is for gains to occur.

Finding the right physician for a child with NVLD is an important and sometimes difficult undertaking. Getting references from satisfied parents and professionals in the field is a good starting place. The next section offers information that may help in that process.

Physician Specialists Most Likely to Be Skilled in NVLD

There is wide variation in training, experience, and commitment among physicians who provide care for individuals with NVLD. Multiple factors will influence the parent's choice of practitioner such as the physician's knowledge of and experience with children's brain-based social, academic, behavioral, and learning issues such as NVLD. Although beyond the scope of this chapter, the family's finances, insurance coverage, access to subspecialists, and available time will be additional factors that influence the choice of physician. The initial inquiry should be for locally based pediatricians with a special interest in NVLD, behavioral/developmental pediatricians, child and adolescent

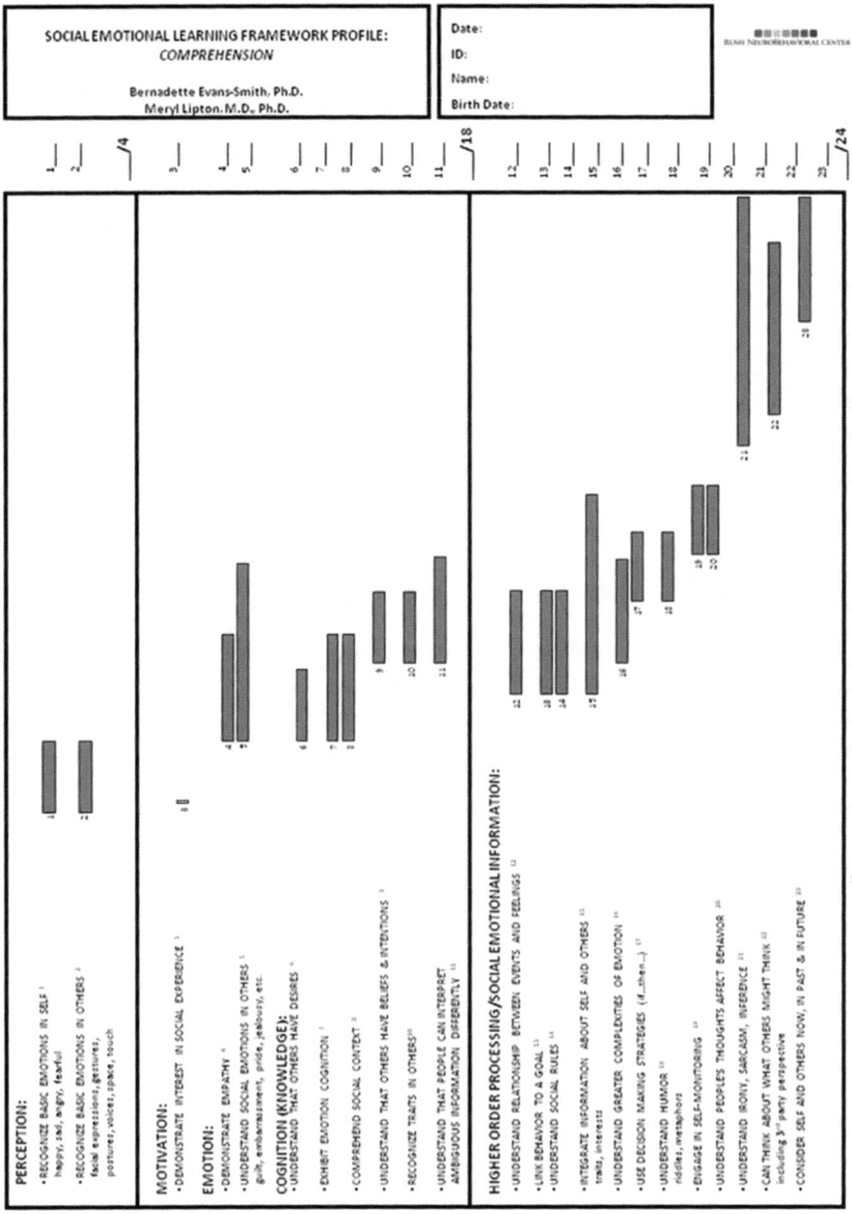

Chart 6.1 SELF: Comprehension. Developmentally arranged aspects of social emotional comprehension

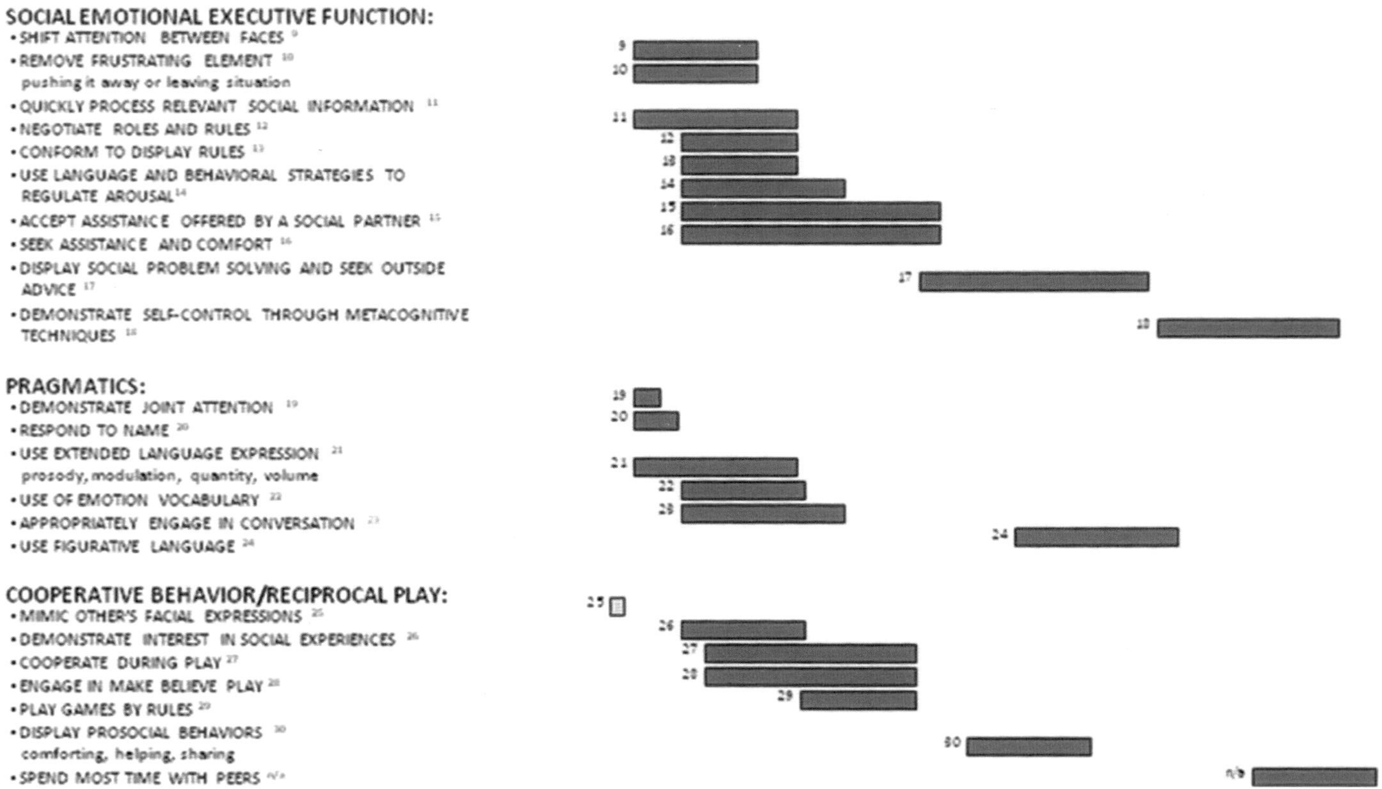

Chart 6.2 SELF: Execution. Developmentally arranged aspects of social emotional execution

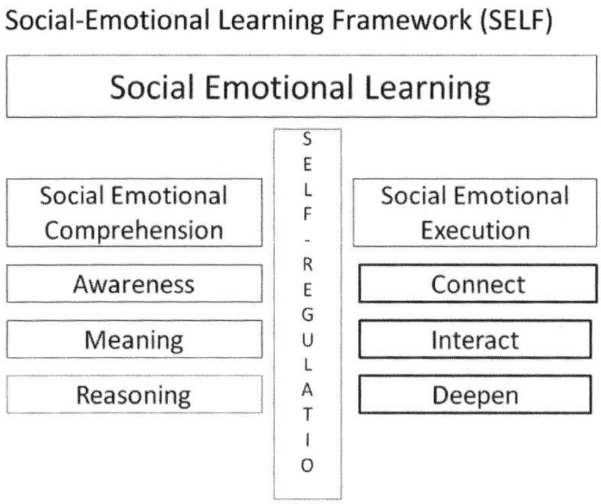

Chart 6.3 SELF Overview of major divisions of social emotional learning

psychiatrists, and/or pediatric neurologists. Rather than searching for a specific type of physician, such as a psychiatrist, neurologist, etc., the search should be focused on finding a physician who has experience with and an interest in this population.

Begin the search by talking to parents and professionals in schools and the community who have first-hand experience with children who have NVLD. Find out who is comfortable and knowledgeable about diagnosing NVLD. Some physicians are known in schools and the community as being particularly skilled in managing medications.

When a professional or parent recommends a doctor, ask first about the physician's strengths and weaknesses. Then ask if the doctor was the first choice that they made or if they tried someone else before they found someone they were satisfied with. If possible, never take one person's recommendation. Their advice may be sound, but having 2–3 people recommend the same physician will enable you to make a wiser selection. If possible, interview two physicians. Some important aspects of choosing a physician go beyond expertise and background. They include such things as "fit" with the personality and communication styles of the child and her or his parents. These qualitative factors are best judged in-person.

Finding the physician who fits the needs of the NVLD child is a difficult but important process. Understanding some of the reasons that many physicians are unable to fit the role of a physician for children NVLD youngsters is discussed in the section below.

Some Physicians Can't Provide Services Needed by Children with NVLD

There are various types of physicians that can help care for children with NVLD. Often the child's pediatrician is the first physician to evaluate a child with NVLD. The child with NVLD may initially present and even be treated for attention problems by the primary care physician while the child's other neurobehavioral issues go undiagnosed. Finding a pediatrician who initially understands and or considers the possibility of a diagnosis of NVLD is unfortunately unusual.

Prior to 1997 there was no requirement for pediatricians in training to have behavioral pediatrics as part of their education. Given that at least 25% of children's problems fall into the behavioral/developmental category, a change in pediatric training requirements was created. Since 1997, pediatric trainees have a minimum of a 1 month developmental/behavioral rotation (Boreman, Thomasgard, Fernandez, & Coury, 2007). Pediatricians in training currently receive structured experiences in the broad area of learning problems. However, there is another barrier. Nonverbal learning disabilities are not a medically accepted diagnosis nor is it a term seen frequently in the medical literature. Thus, NVLD is unlikely to be part of many pediatricians' training curriculum. Exemplifying this is that in a literature search limited to medical rather than psychological journals, it was rare to find a reference dedicated to the subject of NVLD. In a PubMed review covering years 1988–2011, there were eight articles in pediatric medical journals where NVLD was mentioned and none of the articles were dedicated to the topic of NVLD: Agarwal, Agarwal, Upadhyay, and Singh (1991); Bishop and Baird (2001); Christianson, Chesler, and Kromberg (1994); Ekstrom, Hakenas-Plate, Tulinius, and Wentz (2009); Elbert and Seale (1998); Graham, Bashir, Stark, Silbert, and Walzer (1998); Lingman et al. (2010); and Turgay, Binder, Snyder, and Fisman (2002).

Given this lack of specific knowledge about NVLD, pediatricians will often refer children with learning/behavioral problems to a subspecialist such as a child psychiatrist, developmental/behavioral pediatrician, or a pediatric neurologist. Even at this level of specialization, many well-trained physicians are not well versed in NVLD and may not recognize, diagnose, and treat this disorder. Therefore the search for a physician who understands NVLD and can help children with it requires more effort on the part of parents and professionals who are seeking medical help.

Another barrier that deserves attention is the role health care insurance companies' play in effecting diagnosis and interventions. Even if physicians want to take on these cases, many are pressured by insurance companies to keep visits short, so even if they can be helpful, doctors, especially in pediatrics and family practice, often don't have the time to observe and recognize the behavioral components of NVLD. In addition, because NVLD is not an accepted medical diagnosis, many insurance companies will not pay for physicians to diagnose or treat NVLD—though they may pay for the treatment of other associated problems such as Attention Deficit Hyperactivity Disorder (ADHD), anxiety, and mood disorder. Physicians with pharmacologic expertise can be very helpful for children with NVLD as some of the co-associated symptoms respond to medications.

Whatever role the physician plays in caring for the child with NVLD, optimizing the ***relationship*** *will lead to better outcomes. The next section offers some suggestions on enhancing the relationship of the family and professionals with the physician.*

Parents and Professionals Partnering with Their Physicians to Create the Best Outcomes

Physicians are best able to serve children with NVLD when they work in a constructive partnership with the child, the parents, and other professionals who provide interventions to the patient.

Planning the first physician visit will benefit everyone. Parents should be encouraged to bring all of the relevant materials about the child to the initial meeting. When possible it can be helpful to organize and edit them. Unfortunately physicians (like all professionals) often have limited time and they can be much more helpful if lengthy school reports are summarized, grades are presented in a way that they can be easily reviewed, and professional tests are presented in a thoughtful order that shows progress over time.

Parent can be invited to address two helpful questions: *What are the child's problems? What is his or her story?* They should be coached to succinctly tell the physician what the child's problems are as you see them. It may be helpful for them to make notes prior to the meeting to help assure all the information you think is important will be addressed. Next, help them answer the question: *What do you hope to get from the doctor?* What can the physician do that would make you feel that the child has received excellent care?

As parents plan for the visit and consider these questions, it can be helpful to remember that there are a variety of roles that physicians can play. In terms of time and involvement, they are quite separate, but each of them is important, such as:

1. The physician can diagnose and administer medication. If the physician is managing medications it is important to know what information the physician will need about dose and side effects, and how often that information should be provided. No changes in the amount or timing of the medication should be made without consulting the physician. If the physician is playing a role on a team, then it's important for all of the team members to agree on how they are going to proceed and to set up a communication system that takes as little time as possible but keeps everyone up to date.
2. The physician can act as a referral source for other professionals who are expert in speech and language, neuropsychological testing, social–emotional groups, etc. If the physician is referring the patient to other professionals, it is wise to ask why the professional she or he recommends was selected. What are their professional strengths and weaknesses?
3. In the most integrated scenario, the physician can become a member of the team that some children with NVLD require. This means that the doctor would come to team meetings with other professionals and/or join professionals at the child's school to develop and then monitor an academic and care plan.

No one of these roles is better or less valuable than another; they are just different. Depending on which alternative has been agreed upon, the role of the parents is also different.

- Parents (or referring professionals) can ask the physician about similar cases and related training and case load. There are many ingredients, but it is prudent to ask the doctor about their training in NVLD and how many children with this disorder s/he regularly treats. NVLD is not a frequent diagnosis, and on balance, it would be better to work with a physician who has treated many children rather than a few.
- Discuss costs and insurance coverage. It is important to have a frank conversation with the physician about what she or he charges (including for reading reports) and what is or isn't covered by health insurance. This should happen in advance of making decisions that cost money. That way there will be no surprises, and if resources are limited, strategic decisions can be made that will maximize the benefit from the coverage that is available.

Choosing and monitoring medications used for neurobehavioral problems such as ADHD, anxiety, and *mood disorders is the physician's role. Care is optimized when the family, the child (when age appropriate), and the professionals understand the roles of the various medications that may be used.*

Medications that Might Be Useful for Specific Symptoms

Medication may be one aspect of a well-developed intervention plan. The medications used for children and adolescents with NVLD are targeted to the associated conditions rather than to the primary problem of sociability and visual spatial motor functioning. Many children with NVLD have difficulty with attention regulation (ADHD) and benefit from stimulant medication (Ritalin, Concerta, Focalin, Adderall, Vyvanse, etc.), antihypertensives (Intuniv, Kapvay, Tenex, clonidine), or other non-stimulant ADHD medication such as Strattera or bupropion (Wellbutrin). Others have anxiety and mood disorders that may be treated with selective serotonin reuptake inhibitors (SSRI's) such as Prozac, Zoloft, Lexapro, etc. Children with more complex psychological and behavioral issues are sometimes treated with combinations of medication which may include atypical antipsychotics (Risperdal, Abilify, etc.). See Chart 6.4 below.

There are many pieces to the puzzle of organizing the diagnosis and treatment of a child with NVLD. How does it all get done? There are many models that can be used. One option is having the physician as case manager. Below you will find the description of such a model as well as some cases that illustrate various aspects of the process.

A Clinical Model of a Physician as Case Manager. To be effective for patients with NVLD (or other neurobehavioral issues) the role of the physician expands as it varies with each situation. Some parents take their child to the physician only for medication to treat the ADHD, anxiety, or depression that may be a part of their child's clinical picture. Other parents come to the physician for diagnosis, intervention suggestions, or case management.

Medications for NVLD and Associated Disorders		
Associated Disorders:		Medications:
ADHD	Stimulants:	Ritalin, Ritalin LA, Concerta, Focalin, Focalin XR, Metadate CD, Adderall, Adderall XR, Vyvanse, Daytrana Patch
	Non-Stimulants:	Strattera, Clonidine, KapVey, Tenex, Intuniv, Wellbutrin, Provigil
Anxiety	Selective Serotonin Reuptake Inhibitors:	Zoloft, Celexa, Lexapro, Prozac, Paxil
	Benzodiazpines:	Klonipin, Ativan, Xanax
Mood	Selective Serotonin Reuptake Inhibitors:	Zoloft, Celexa, Lexapro, Prozac, Paxil
	Atypical Anti-Depresant	Wellbutrin, Effexor, Cymbalta
	Atypical Anti-Psychotics	Risperdal, Zyprexa, Abilify, Seroquel

Chart 6.4 Overview of neuro-emotional disorders found in children, adolescents and young adults with NLD and helpful medication classes

The most comprehensive role for the physician is as the case manager. This requires the physician to understand the child's neurobehavioral strengths and challenges and the effects of this profile on the child, the family, peers, and school performance. All of this information is used to inform a comprehensive, individualized intervention plan. The child with NVLD often has a team of interventionists, including school personnel, with whom communication is very important. Regular follow-up with the patient and parents is an important aspect of expanded medical care.

The process utilized with great success at the Rush Neurobehavioral Center to develop an understanding of the child with NVLD, provide support to parents, and help develop and monitor an intervention plan.[1] Parts of this model overlap the general

[1] This chapter is written from the point of view of physician who, before going to medical school, was a special education teacher and then earned a doctorate in educational psychology and then became a behavioral pediatric neurologist. That background and my having created a practice with extended time with patients. That is not an option for many of my peers, but the framework that is laid out here can help parents and professionals when they are interviewing physicians to care for NVLD children. From it, both sides can more meaningfully discuss what can and can't be provided towards the child's care.

approach detailed above. Other sections are different. The point is to adapt the best of both to fit the local situation.

Initial contact with the physician is usually an in-depth meeting with parents who are seen without the child present. This allows parents to speak freely about their concerns. For children in preschool or elementary school, whenever possible, a school visit consisting of an observation of the child in a structured setting with academic content (when age appropriate) and an unstructured free time setting is the next step. For preschool children, observing during free play time can be very useful. A meeting with the school team is included. This allows for the consulting physician to develop insights into the school team, learning where the team is in the process of understanding the child, what interventions have been tried, how successful they feel about their work with the child, etc. At this point in the process of getting to know the child, she/he hasn't yet met the physician so they can freely observe social skills, self-regulation, play, attention regulation, facility with nonverbal and verbal language, and general behavior during structured and unstructured aspects of the school day. The school visit is also an opportunity to promote a good working relationship with the school. For middle school and older children, school observation is generally not conducted as it is not as productive as for the younger children.

Following the school visit, the physician will see the child to conduct a neurobehavioral evaluation. If some areas of functioning have not been well evaluated, and the information is pertinent, further evaluation is solicited. At this point, information from the parent visit, school observation, child visit, a neuropsychological evaluation (if available), and any other evaluations that have been done (occupational therapy, speech and language, etc.) are integrated into a neurobehavioral framework.

A neurobehavioral framework for diagnostic integration is then utilized. This includes noting strengths and weaknesses in the following domains: sensory, motor, cognitive (processing and academics), regulation (attention, behavior, anxiety, executive functions, tics, and repetitive behaviors), social interest and abilities, as well as emotional status (mood, anxiety, obsessive-compulsive behavior, etc.). From this neurobehavioral framework, a diagnostic understanding is developed and transformed into suggested interventions for the individual child, the family, and the school. While standard diagnoses are utilized for the school, insurance, etc., this more nuanced diagnostic understanding allows for more meaningful treatment plans.

Following the diagnostic process, feedback sessions with the parents, school personnel, and with the child (when age appropriate) are conducted. At the school session, up-to-date information is integrated with the school's experience, knowledge, and observations. The school meeting is an excellent opportunity to develop goals and measurement criteria, interventions, and future communication plans in a cooperative manner.

While a child with NVLD may have many potential interventionists (tutor, therapist, family therapist, OT, speech and language pathologist, social skills group leader, etc.) it is important not to overdo the hours a child spends getting help outside of school. Choosing the highest priority items to target for therapy allows the child downtime, alone time, and time with the family. For the interventions chosen, it is optimum to have measureable goals and a time table developed with the interventionist. Quarterly team communication through conference calls or e-mails can keep everyone focused and coordinated. The frequency of physician follow-up visits with the patient and family is defined on an individual basis.

This clinical model has been used with many hundreds of patients over the last two decades. Below you will find a sequence of case histories that highlight a series of lessons learned through clinical practice.

Case 1: A Path Toward the Diagnosis of NVLD in Children

Johnny exemplifies how complicated the diagnostic path can be for children with NVLD. He is a middle schooler whose symptoms of NVLD were clearly present at the age of 7, yet he was not diagnosed with NVLD until the age of 11. Parents and teachers became worried about Johnny in the second grade. At that time, his teachers noted that he tried to make friends but wasn't able to develop relationships with the other children. He would walk over to a group of children who were looking serious as they spoke to each other with a big smile and inappropriately ask if anyone wanted to play a computer game with him. No one wanted to play with him or sit near him. His fine motor skills were lacking, and he had an especially hard time copying from the whiteboard.

Now that Johnny is in sixth grade, he appears very sad. He is easily overwhelmed at lunch, during transitions, and in gym. Johnny still has no friends. His parents are concerned because he no longer even wants to participate in activities he loved to do like reading his books, walking to the ice cream store, and playing with his dog.

When Johnny was seen at 7 years of age he had social issues, motor coordination problems, and visual processing issues. At the time, with increasing concern about the rise in the numbers of children with Autism Spectrum Disorder, the school psychologist declared Johnny was "ok" because he passed the diagnostic tests for autism. Johnny's pediatrician was relieved and a wait-and-watch approach was taken.

Now that Johnny is 11 years old, the waiting has stopped as he appears depressed to his pediatrician who sends him to a counselor for therapy. After 6 months of therapy and little change, he is sent to a psychiatrist who suggests medication for his depression. A second opinion was requested and the developmental pediatrician asked for a neuropsychological evaluation which revealed social problems and a neurocognitive profile consistent with NVLD. Johnny started on Zoloft to relieve his anxiety and depression while school accommodations were put in place for his NVLD. His counselor, who now understood more about Johnny's cognitive and emotional function, became more effective. As Johnny's depression started to lift and his anxiety decreased, his desire for social experiences emerged and he joined a social development group.

Unfortunately, this is a typical path for the discovery that a child has NVLD. When we do a better job teaching physicians about the developmental signs of NVLD, early identification and treatment might well prevent Johnny's world from becoming anxious and depressed.

The next case is an example of early intervention.

Case 2: Successful Outcome Can Follow Early Intervention

Maya is an 8-year-old girl who was initially seen when she was an almost 5-year-old preschooler. Her parents brought her to a behavioral pediatric neurologist for a second opinion regarding her social problems. Maya's parent's initial concern began because the teacher had questions about her social behavior. The teacher mentioned that Maya demonstrated no interest in other children except for watching them. Her mother said, "I rarely see Maya with other kids in her neighborhood." Maya's parents were afraid she was autistic. A psychologist had ruled out autism, but her parents wanted a "medical opinion."

Maya was described as a quiet baby who preferred to sit rather than explore. She loved being read to and listening to music. She had no interest in blocks, coloring, playing with clay, etc. She had a trying time in busy, noisy, and new environments. There was no history of repetitive behaviors or special interests.

During trips to the supermarket, she covered her ears and clung to her father. Her language development was advanced. When her class was doing a Thanksgiving-related craft activity she declined to join and said, "My fingers just don't work so well." During free play at school she was usually on her own. Occasionally she was seen watching others. When working in small groups in school she was unable to use her words to connect with the children. Without noticing, she might stand too close making the other students feel uncomfortable. Maya was an only child, and her parents had small families who did not live nearby. They rarely saw Maya in social settings with peers and were not aware of any social issues. If the teacher hadn't raised an issue about Maya's social behavior, her parents would not have been concerned as both parents were also not particularly social.

Maya's neurobehavioral examination revealed a nervous 4-year 9-month-old girl who took an extended amount of time to calm. She had hyper-responsiveness to sensory stimuli. Her fine and gross motor coordination difficulties were moderate in nature. Her eye contact with the examiner was limited but seemed to vary with her anxiousness. She had difficulties identifying affect on pictures of children's faces. When shown pictures of children who were engaged in activities, she would describe the activity (girl on a swing) rather than the two girls talking near the swing. When talking to her parents or about things she likes, her language was excellent. Maya went on to have an occupational therapy evaluation that demonstrated sensory-motor problems.

Case Summary and Discussion

Maya was a bright, almost 5-year-old child with social impairments, sensory and motor dysfunction, expressive and receptive language strengths, and pragmatic language difficulties. There were no apparent attention issues. Language was well developed, while visual spatial motor processing was an area of deficit. She struggled with anxiety seemingly related to environmental situations that are difficult for her to process, perhaps related to both her sensory–motor issues, visual–spatial deficits, and her social impairment. Her clinical social–emotional learning skill assessment revealed impairment in emotion recognition, social problem solving, and processing speed.

Maya appeared to have a neurocognitive and social–emotional learning pattern suggestive of NVLD of a mild to moderate nature. Focused intervention and close follow-up were started. She received occupational therapy from a therapist who is trained in the developmental individual difference relationship method (DIR) developed by Dr. Alan Greenspan (Greenspan & Wieder, 2005). To enhance her social behavior, once a week she worked with another child and the DIR therapist. Teacher and parents worked on preparing Maya verbally for new situations using the auditory/language modality for presentation of information and using a variety of activities for encoding and interpreting emotion in themselves, in Maya, and in other people in the social context.

For the classroom, the school social worker incorporated a social–emotional learning (SEL) curriculum that she developed. Maya was previewed the class SEL lesson in a 1:1 setting the day before the class had the lesson. This worked well for her. A small social skills lunch group was formed and took place twice a week. One of the girls in the group went on to have play dates with Maya.

Maya is now in third grade. She is achieving beyond grade level in language-based academics. For the past 3 years, she has had a tutor for math which has served her well. She has support at school for organization, math, and reading comprehension. She continues to work on her individual social learning skills and takes part in an ongoing social development group during the academic year. Maya has two friends she enjoys. Her anxiety is not currently a problem.

Transitioning to the independence of adulthood has many challenges for adolescents and young adults with NVLD. Next is a case that demonstrates some of those issues.

Case 3: Transition to Independence

Eric is a 21-year-old business student at an excellent Midwestern university. He was initially seen when he was 15 years of age for attention issues. Eric's attention problems became apparent in high school when there was so much academic work to do that his usual style of getting by on his very high verbal IQ no longer worked for him. Eric's neuropsychological evaluation revealed a significant discrepancy with verbal IQ in the 99th % and performance IQ in the 70th %. His visual spatial and visual motor scores were highly discrepant with his language scores and these cognitive measures were reflected in his academic performance. Eric was a loner from preschool on. He had three brothers and the family was socially self-sufficient. In school and at home, Eric was accepted for the nonsocial boy he was.

Eric and his parents sought pharmacologic treatment of his inattentive ADHD. He was successfully treated with a stimulant. We talked about his neurocognitive strengths and issues and his social abilities. Eric was glad to know "what I am made of" but had no desire to work on social skills. Life was good for him. School was going well, and the family was his social world.

Eric went off to college at a school that provided high-quality support for students with learning issues. He availed himself of the services and made a good transition. Some executive function problems emerged but the learning center at the school provided support. In his junior year, Eric called in a panic. He reported that "it has all caught up with me. I have two big problems." The biggest is that he finds himself lacking in the ability to communicate with girls, something that is now very important to him. The second problem was that in a number of his classes, the students needed to work in teams, and he had a hard time keeping up with what was going on in the group situation. Eric wanted help with his social skills but being at a school in a very small Midwestern town, there were no social skills specialists there. So, a theater teacher was found who was willing to work with Eric on emotion reading and expression. Eric gained enough social ability to work in a team and have some successful dates.

With the current popularity of medications for neurobehavioral disorders like ADHD, anxiety, etc., many parents hope that their child's NVLD can be helped with a pharmacologic treatment.

Case 4: Medication for NVLD?

Like many patients whose children have NVLD, Mark's parents came for a consultation regarding medication for "his NVLD." Mark was a third grader who had behavioral difficulties at home and school; he had social interest but lacked social know-how, his academic strengths were in language and reading and his academic difficulties were in math. Organization was a challenge. In unstructured settings he found a quiet corner to sit in. In the busy lunch room he sat alone. At home he kept to himself. Mark's parents needed to remind him to do his chores. He refused to go to big family events like the circus and similar noisy, busy activities. Mark had been in the same school since kindergarten and had a buddy who he played with for years when the play dates were arranged by parents. But now that the children choose who they wanted to play with, he would rarely see his friend. Mark was becoming more isolated and recently had "lost his spark."

His parents took Mark to a neuropsychologist who evaluated him and diagnosed him with NVLD, and his parents came to me for medication for the NVLD. After reviewing with Mark's parents what NVLD was, I had to tell them there was no medication for his NVLD. Medications don't improve social skills or the neurocognitive aspects of NVLD. I was able to make suggestions for intervention that could help Mark and that was the path we took.

Case Summary and Discussion

NVLD is a pattern of combined deficits in the social, cognitive, and academic domains which are not helped with medication. There are, however, co-occurring neurobehavioral disorders that are improved with pharmacologic treatment. We often see ADHD, anxiety, depression, tics, mood dysregulation, and obsessive-compulsive behavioral traits co-associated with NVLD. These are the disorders that are possible targets of medication.

Intervention planning varies for each patient. While medications don't directly treat the basic neurocognitive features of NVLD, they can be very helpful in treating some of the associated conditions as you will see in Case 5.

Case 5: Behavioral Issues in NVLD and Their Treatment

Mandy, a second grader, was brought in for a consultation because of her difficult behavior. She was adopted, and said to be a "handful" since the day she arrived. Her infancy was characterized by poor sleep and constant crying. An early occupational therapy evaluation diagnosed sensory-motor difficulties and she received occupational therapy that focused on her sensory-motor dysfunction since she was 3 years old. As a toddler she knew no behavioral boundaries. She did what she wanted and rarely did what parents wanted. Family therapy was started and there was some improvement, but Mandy still was easily frustrated and had frequent meltdowns.

In preschool Mandy showed interest in other children, but when she approached them with her vivacious energy they would scatter. If two girls were taking turns on the swing, Mandy would go over and announce that she was next. She seemed to have a difficult time reading social context. She was frequently in trouble for "bothering other students." Mandy didn't understand social space and would go nose to nose just to ask a question of a schoolmate. And when the other child went away Mandy would get angry and sometimes she would express her anger physically.

Her mother told an interesting story about Mandy. When Mandy was 5, she was sitting with mom while she was on the phone. Mom got some bad news about her father's health. Mom put down the phone and was visibly upset. Mandy wanted her mom to take her outside. Mom told Mandy that she just found out that her father was ill and in the hospital so she felt upset. Mandy said "you look happy … this is what it looks like when you are upset," and Mandy proceeded to act out her meltdown behavior.

Once the academics of kindergarten and first grade became a challenge for Mandy, she would often refuse to go to school. Every morning was a battle. She got anxious at the thought of going to school. Sunday nights were filled with anxiety and meltdowns.

Mandy's neuropsychology evaluation described a cognitive and social pattern of NVLD with inattentive ADHD, anxiety, and the presence of sensory–motor problems. The school instituted many accommodations that were helpful and Mandy did a little better but there were significant behavioral problems both at home and school. Mother reported that at home she needed to be with Mandy all the time to be sure she was doing what she was supposed to.

Mandy's parents were looking for a pharmacologic treatment. Given Mandy's behavioral issues and neuropsychological evaluation, the targets of the pharmacologic treatment were anxiety and attention. We successfully worked over the next 4 months on finding a medication that was well tolerated and helpful for Mandy's inattention. Unable to tolerate stimulants, Intuniv was tried and Mandy's attention and anxiety were better controlled. Behavior at home and school improved. Mandy was now able to profit from a cognitive behavioral approach to her anxiety.

Case Summary and Discussion

Children like Mandy who have NVLD and behavioral problems require an insightful perspective. Their behavioral problems are often secondary to their sensory–motor and neurocognitive weaknesses. We ask these children to function in a world with complex behavioral, emotional, and cognitive stimuli that they have a difficult time encoding and interpreting. What does it feel like when you don't understand what is going on around you and when you are asked to do things that don't make sense?

While medication can be helpful with the inattention, anxiety, and depression we find in children with NVLD, it is only one part of the treatment plan. Medications make the child more available for accommodated learning situations and well-targeted interventions. However, medications alone are not an optimum treatment plan.

Summary

NVLD is a complex pattern that has social and cognitive elements. Each person with NVLD has a unique set of strengths and challenges that need to be evaluated and understood. The key to being a successful physician for children or adults with NVLD is first to understand the social, motor, sensory, regulatory, neurocognitive, and emotional strengths and problems that each patient experiences; transform that information into an individual intervention plan for the patient, family, and school; and then help support them in managing the plan over time. One must join the family on the path they are taking as they learn to parent a child with NVLD.

References

Agarwal, K. N., Agarwal, D. K., Upadhyay, S. K., & Singh, M. (1991). Learning disability in rural primary school children. *The Indian Journal of Medical Research, 94*, 89–95.

Bishop, D. V., & Baird, G. (2001). Parent and teacher report of pragmatic aspects of communication: Use of the children's communication checklist in a clinical setting. *Developmental Medicine and Child Neurology, 43*(12), 809–818. Erratum in Developmental Medicine and Child Neurology 47(4), 287.

Boreman, C. D., Thomasgard, M. C., Fernandez, S. A., & Coury, D. L. (2007). Resident training in developmental/behavioral pediatrics: Where do we stand? *Clinical Pediatrics, 46*, 135–145.

Brody, L. R., & Harrison, R. H. (1987). Developmental changes in children's abilities to match and label emotionally laden situations. *Motivation and Emotion, 11*, 347–365.

Browne, G. Y., Rosenfield, H. M., & Horowitz, F. D. (1977). Infant discrimination of facial expressions. *Child Development, 48*, 555–562.

Christianson, A. L., Chesler, N., & Kromberg, J. G. (1994). Fetal valproate syndrome: Clinical and neuro-developmental features in two sibling pairs. *Developmental Medical Child Neurology, 36*(4), 361–369.

Ekstrom, A. B., Hakenas-Plate, L., Tulinius, M., & Wentz, E. (2009). Cognition and adaptive skills in myotonic dystrophy type 1: A study of 55 individuals with congenital and childhood forms. *Developmental Medical Child Neurology, 51*(12), 982–990.

Elbert, J. C., & Seale, T. W. (1998). Complexity of the cognitive phenotype of an inherited form of learning disability. *Developmental Medical Child Neurology, 30*(2), 181–189.

Graham, J. M., Jr., Bashir, A. S., Stark, R. E., Silbert, A., & Walzer, S. (1998). Oral and written language abilities of XXY boys: Implications for anticipatory guidance. *Pediatrics, 81*(6), 795–806.

Greenspan, S., & Wieder, S. (2005). *Infant and early childhood mental health: A comprehensive, developmental approach to assessment and intervention*. Washington, DC: American Psychiatric.

Labarbera, J. D., Izard, C. E., Vietze, P., & Paris, S. A. (1976). Four- and six-month old infants' visual responses to joy, anger, and neutral expressions. *Child Development, 47*, 535–538.

Lingman, R., Golding, J., Jongmans, M. J., Hunt, L. P., Ellis, M., & Emond, A. (2010). The association between developmental coordination disorder and other developmental traits. *Pediatrics, 126*(5), 1109–1118.

Lipton, M., & Evans-Smith, B. (2006, August). Social emotional learning framework (SELF): Conceptual, clinical, and research aspects. The Summer Institute on Neurodevelopmental Disorders, MIND Institute, University of California, Davis, CA.

Lipton, M., & Nowicki, S. (2009). The social emotional learning framework (SELF): A guide for understanding brain-based social emotional learning impairments. *The Journal of Developmental Processes, 4*(2), 99–115.

Mehrabian, A. (1971). *Silent Messages*. Belmont, CA: Wadsworth.

Michaelson, L., & Lewis, M. (1985). What do children know about emotions and when do they know it? In M. Lewis & C. Saarni (Eds.), *The socialization of emotions* (pp. 117–139). New York: Plenum.

Nelson, C. A., Morse, P. A., & Leavitt, L. A. (1979). Recognition of facial expressions by seven-month-old infants. *Child Development, 50*, 1239–1242.

Turgay, A., Binder, C., Snyder, R., & Fisman, S. (2002). Long-term safety and efficacy of risperidone for the treatment of disruptive behavior disorders in children with sub average IQ's. *Pediatrics, 110*, e34.

Chapter 7
Coaching: Addressing the Psychosocial and Executive Functioning Challenges of NVLD in K–12 and the Transition to Adulthood

Catherine M. Brown and Bridget Leary

The educational process that children with nonverbal learning disabilities (NVLD) experience can differ significantly from children without disabilities. Furthermore, many parents discover that the psychological, social (psychosocial), and executive functioning challenges that children with NVLD face can delay attaining typical developmental milestones (Epstein, Saltzman-Benaiah, O'Hare, Goll, & Tuck, 2008). Although individuals with NVLD may possess many strengths, such as a robust vocabulary, strong reading skills, aptitude for technology, specialized interests, atypical or unique associations, sustained attention, attention to detail, or memorization, compared to neurotypical individuals (Bedrossian & Pennamon, 2007; Price & Fisher, 2010; Stothers & Cardy, 2012), it is critical for parents and educators to understand the subtypes of NVLD and their functional impact on related domains (Davis & Broitman, 2011; Franz, 2000). This chapter will explore an emerging type of support available to individuals with NVLD referred to as "coaching."

The Individuals with Disabilities Act (2004) mandates parent participation in the special education process and in the development of the child's Individualized Education Plan (IEP). Typical recommendations in the IEP, such as modifications to course content, assistive technology, waivers for testing, and occupational or speech therapy, address academic progress of children with learning disabilities. Consequently, it is necessary for parents to be intensely involved in educational decision-making, maintain frequent communication with school personnel, and provide daily assistance in homework for children with NVLD (Bennis, 2011; Brown, 2005; Case, 2001; Starr, Foy, Cramer, & Singh, 2006).

C.M. Brown, Ph.D. (✉) • B. Leary
Accessibility Services, California State University, East Bay,
25800 Carlos Bee Blvd, Hayward, CA 94542-3095, USA
e-mail: katie.brown@csueastbay.edu

J. Broitman and J.M. Davis (eds.), *Treating NVLD in Children: Professional Collaborations for Positive Outcomes*, DOI 10.1007/978-1-4614-6179-1_7,

Most often, the IEP designed for each child in the special education system will only address concerns that significantly impact the learning process. However, many children with NVLD or children with similar diagnoses require significant support with the development of their psychosocial and executive functioning skills, in addition to their academic skills. Best practices call for attention to these areas (Bravo, 2001; Gutstein & Sheely, 2002; Krsti , 2001; Lyle, 1998), yet in practice, these concerns do not receive significant attention from special education professionals (Braaten, 2011; Franz, 2000; Ris & Nortz, 2008; Wright, 2008). The IEP may not address these nonacademic behavioral and emotional issues unless they have a substantial impact on the individual's educational progress. In these cases, a behavior support plan or counseling is warranted (Etscheidt, 2006; Raines, 2006; Schwenn, 1991). When behavioral interventions are mandated by the IEP, some school districts employ support personnel with varying degrees of training (Cook et al., 2007; Quinn, Gable, & Fox, 2001; The Behavior Analyst Certification Board, 1998).

Non-mandated Special Education Needs

Regardless of what the identified needs are in the IEP, many parents of children with NVLD are routinely developing strategies to accommodate the child's learning disability and related challenges. Monitoring schoolwork, encouraging the development of social skills, and adjusting to the child's unique sensitivities to sensory input can become a daily strain between the child and parent, thereby increasing the frequency and intensity of involvement with their child's entire K–12 educational and developmental process (Christenson, 2005; McKinney & Hocutt, 1982; Otterbourg, 1996). The issues with executive functioning such as attention, organization, and time management require rigorous supervision of the youth's education and acquisition of independent skills. To prepare children to attain appropriate developmental milestones and future aspirations for college or career will likely require parents to provide supports to their children into adulthood (Casey, Rourke, & Picard, 1991; Galway & Metsala, 2011; Little, 2003; Rourke, Young, & Leenaars, 1989). Moreover, research in the field indicates that addressing the associated psychosocial issues of children with NVLD early will result in positive outcomes maintained over the lifespan (Evans, Shultz, & Sadler, 2008; Vogel, Hruby, & Adelman, 1993).

Disproportionate Parental Accommodation and Involvement

It is important to note that aside from family members or friends, no other support exists to address these non-mandated psychosocial and executive functioning needs for the individual with NVLD. Therefore, parents or other family members allocate a disproportionate amount of time supervising their educational, domestic, and social activities. Monitoring schoolwork for children with NVLD often requires that parents breakdown homework assignments into multiple concrete steps for easy completion. Even a child with stronger organizational skills may have attention problems that require multiple prompts after school from parents to decrease procrastination of homework completion. Once on task, children may become easily distracted and require frequent reminders until completion. Difficulties with executive functioning do not end with academics. Organization and time management can be equally frustrating in the independent living, emotional, and social skills domains. Some children with NVLD require numerous prompts for dressing, mealtimes, hygiene, and bedtime routines to accomplish these activities. Even during leisure time, parents may prompt children to participate in social activities with peers, as well as monitor friendships to encourage appropriate social interactions (Wiener, 1998). For children with more emotional issues parents may also need to maintain an awareness of fluctuating emotional thresholds to elicit the best outcomes. Parents may find themselves becoming apprehensive when they become familiar with their child's triggers, such as noise level, unexpected changes, unstructured activities, new environments, or social settings that may contribute to undesired behaviors (Baker & McCal, 1995; Margalit & Heiman, 1986).

The frequency and intensity of support that some children with NVLD need can be impractical for overall household functioning (Antshel & Joseph, 2006), especially if other children or responsibilities require attention. Parents may experience a level of monitoring that can become fatiguing for them and stressful for the child.

Furthermore, parents that attempt to ameliorate all social, academic, or risks can unwittingly increase feelings of dependency on family supports and can be counterproductive to increasing independent living skills (Little, 2003; Little, & Clark, 2006; Martin, 2007; Shessel & Reiff, 1999; Smith, English, & Vasek, 2002; Speckman, Goldberg, & Herman, 1992). Providing assistance without decreasing the levels of support over time can lead to behaviors, such as learned helplessness, negative self-concept, and a lack of initiative in employment settings (Sanders, 2006; Valås, 2001). Although it may seem counterintuitive, students with disabilities should have an equal opportunity for success and failure, just as students without disabilities may fail or succeed (Forrest, 2003).

For most neurotypical children, independence can be expected within typical age-appropriate, developmental timelines. In this sense, neurotypical children inherently possess social capital that many children with NVLD lack (Riddell, Baron, & Wilson, 1999; Stanton-Salazar, 2011). For parents of children with NVLD, disproportionate parent involvement is generated by perceived functional necessity rather than a conscious decision to tirelessly monitor these activities. Over time, parents may choose to augment their parenting roles or transition parent involvement in the education system with support from others to increase social capital and address issues that are not mandated by the IEP.

Coaching Support

Coaching is not a new concept and the definition of coaching depends on the individual and the environment where coaching takes place (Fletcher, 2007). This chapter will review evidence-based strategies that coaches can implement to go beyond the mandated requirements of special education programs in public schools to assist in other developmental areas where many otherwise bright and talented youth with NVLD find obstacles to progress. These strategies can be implemented with elementary, secondary, and postsecondary settings or if needed in the workplace. Coach support can be provided in the home or academic settings, to increase positive outcomes throughout the formative educational years and beyond (Marti, 2004). The goal is to increase independence in decision-making, behavior, independent living, and social skills (Kouwenhoven, 2011). College students with learning disabilities who used coaches for assistance with organizational and time management challenges have described this type of coaching as "…a personalized, self-directed service that promoted their self-determination" (Parker & Boutelle, 2009, p. 208).

Coaching has also been referred to in the literature as "mentoring," "tutoring," "counseling" or as a "life coach," "personal coach," or an "executive coach" (Dansinger, 2000; Fletcher, 2007; Marti, 2004). Coaches can develop rapport with the client and, with permission, coaches have an opportunity to work in collaboration with instructors or other school personnel for a more comprehensive type of support. Therefore, coaches differ from tutors since tutoring is typically conducted over brief periods of time to address subject-specific work or assist with academic remediation (Nesselrodt & Alger, 2005; Ratey, 2002). Similarly, coaches build rapport with the youth with NVLD and can work in any domain needed in addition to assisting with more rigorous academic demands. Coaches can be similar to life coaches since life coaches work with individuals with disabilities to assist with the transition from high school to vocational school or work. Typically life coaches for people with disabilities assist with financial transactions, living arrangements, employment, overall health, and social life (Landmark, 2011). Coaches also differ from personal coaches since personal coaches are more similar to counselors and may use psychological strategies, insight, or "talk" therapy (Kouwenhoven, 2011; Lewis, 2008; Ratey, 2002).

Anyone can benefit from working with a coach, and there are many types of coaching services available for all age groups and objectives. Coaches do not only work with people with disabilities. Other coaching services such as academic coaching differ from the type of coaching discussed in this chapter because it is specifically designed to assist individuals with the admission process for competitive colleges by developing personal essays and test-taking strategies (Academic Coaching Services, 2010; Kenny & Faunce, 2004) or establishing goals that are based on individual strengths (Hardy, 2001; Robinson & Gahagan, 2010). Finally, executive coaches focus on the transition process to leadership positions in employment settings (Smith Glasgow, Weinstock, Lachman, Suplee, & Dreher, 2009). An individual's level of independent functioning, life goals, or specific challenges will determine the type of coaching services that will be required.

Qualifications

Coaches can be used in professional, educational, home, or community settings. Choosing the right kind of coach will depend largely upon the goals of the youth and family. Any individual who implements strategies to achieve specific developmental objectives can be considered a coach, regardless of the person's educational level or professional experience (BiswasDiener, 2009). However, some institutions are beginning to offer specialized certificate programs for "coaching" (Coach Training Alliance, 2001; International Coaching Federation, 2011; The Behavior Analyst Certification Board, 1998). Therefore, individuals with a professional interest in working with this population can formally attain this skill set. The need for this type of training will depend on many factors, such as the family's personal preference, age of the child, severity of challenges, and requirements of certain educational settings. Coaching can lead to more positive outcomes for individuals with NVLD as well as improved overall family functioning (Goldberg, Higgins, Raskind, & Herman, 2003; Speckman et al., 1992; Truesdale-Kennedy, McConkey, Ferguson, & Roberts, 2006).

Characteristics

The coaching literature indicates some general qualities that would benefit most age groups and educational goals. For example, one of the strongest assets is establishing rapport between the coach and the individual. Trust and mutual respect is important (Herrera, Sipe, McClanahan, Arbreton, & Pepper, 2000). In the beginning stages, coaching contact should be frequent. Daily check-ins will allow the coach and student to establish appropriate goals and expectations for this collaborative relationship. The number of coaching hours needed will depend on the course load, grade level, and individual skill level of the client (Robinson & Gahagan, 2010). In addition, students and families should anticipate that the need for coaching hours will likely increase when the individual with NVLD is transitioning to a new schedule or environment. Even for college students, the more frequent the contact with the coach in the first years, the more likely the student will experience benefits such as higher GPA and a likelihood to complete school programs (Troiano, Liefeld, & Trachtenberg, 2010).

The best success will occur with long-term relationships between the client and the coach. Depending on the family's need and resources, it may be best to make arrangements for more than one coach to work with the client to provide stability when a coach is unavailable due to illness, vacations, or other commitments. The greatest potential benefit is the client's increasing independence and decreasing need for support from others. Coaches working closely with the client and family may have more opportunities to determine if the youth with NVLD has learned to generalize skills to new situations. A coach that is closer in age to the client may hold a stronger belief than the parents are able to perceive that independence is attainable. Sometimes coaches can offer a more objective observation of the client's level of functioning than the parents' perceptions (Espiner & Guild, 2011; Williams, 2010). Therefore, clients that can offer incentives for meritorious coaches to commit to at least a year or more would likely experience the best outcomes.

Further, a coach should not act as an authority figure that substitutes for the parent, a supervisor, or a teacher nor does the coach attempt to control the individual's choices (Ratey, 2002). The coach may guide the individual to make the best choices based on the individual's own education, independent living, or social goals, as well as careful monitoring of the progress towards those goals. Coaches need to understand what intrinsically motivates the individual in an organic and dynamic setting with varied types of opportunities for learning. This type of learning is not available in more formal settings, such as the classroom or structured groups.

The characteristics of a coach will depend on the specific needs of the individual. Hiring a coach can be an additional cost to the family but this is not necessary if the coach is willing to work for other forms of payment, such as room and board, educational experience, familial reciprocity, or community service projects. There are also ways to use one coach for a group of students, rather than one-on-one to reduce the out-of-pocket cost for coach services. For example, one coach in a group setting can move from student to student and prompt students to organize or initiate homework, set educational goals, monitor progress towards homework completion, and guide students towards areas of interests and strengths to make schoolwork more enjoyable.

Coach Relationships with Parents, Youth, and Educators

Coach–Parent Relationship

Specialized trainings or publications that focus on strategies to address a child's distinct psychosocial and organizational challenges are available (Martin, 2007; Stewart, 2007). Some research using collaborative techniques with parents indicated increased gains in independent living skills (Panerai, Ferrante, & Zingale, 2002). Cognitive coaching techniques have been shown to significantly improve skills in cognitive performance in younger children when parents are involved in the individualized treatment plans, regardless of type of treatment implemented in the home (Ozonoff & Cathcart, 1998). However, research on parent effectiveness in implementing specific interventions for children with LD is inconclusive (Mikami, Lerner, Griggs, McGrath, & Calhoun, 2010; Speckman et al., 1992). For coaches working with younger children, educating parents to use the same techniques reinforces learning (Ozonoff & Cathcart, 1998). Although, positive outcomes may have more to do with the child's preexisting skills than with type of support from trained service providers and parents (Sallows & Graupner, 2005).

In the academic domain, the coach can work with the parent on homework routines that promote the student's ability to self-regulate, prompts to maintain organization of schoolwork, and to use daily planners or electronic devices to complete tasks or assignments. For any behavior intervention, it is important for all those involved to agree on the method, rationale, and consistency of the youth's developing daily living skills. For example, some behaviors at home will not improve if the parent and coach do not use established prompts and sequences of domestic routines designed to improve these skills. Socially, parents and coaches will need to come to an agreement on appropriate social skills goals, modeling consistent expected behaviors, and using strategies for thinking through consequences and perspective taking.

Coach–Student Relationship

Individuals with NVLD should be able to work collaboratively with the coach (and parents, depending on age of individual) to identify goals and view the coaching session as a positive experience. The individual must be prepared to explore strategies with the coach until they find a system that works for the specific individual and be willing to follow the coach's recommendations. However, hiring a coach is not a guarantee that the individual will be successful. If the client does not follow through with a plan or fails to collaborate, the client will likely be unsuccessful (Evans Getzel, McManus, & Briel, 2004; Ratey, 2002).

Coaches must also maintain a healthy rapport with their clients and be mindful of developing the youth's skills in order to consistently increase independence. It is easy for a coach to perpetuate dependence on the coach if the coach loses an ability to be objective about the youth's potential. The coach may fear a loss of rapport with the youth as the youth gains independence and has a decreased need for coaching services. Due to the independent nature of the role of the coach and potentially increasing responsibilities, the coach must also be careful to regularly examine their practices by consulting with other professionals and literature in the field. The coach and parent should regularly self-reflect on actions that may be assisting the youth to increase or decrease dependence on familial or coach support.

Coaching adults with NVLD is very different from coaching youth. However, it is important to consider the developmental stage of the client. Although young adults may be entering college and transitioning to an adult setting, students with NVLD with social challenges can be at one age intellectually but at quite another emotionally. Each client is unique and in order for a coach to make informed choices on strategies a coach must value the knowledge base and acquired experiences of an adult individual with NVLD. Whether the student is attending a 2-year or a 4-year college, the role of the coach is to decrease dependence on such supports. By examining outcomes a coach can tell if the intervention worked, but more importantly, the coach will need to focus on the eventual fading of the intervention supports.

Strategies to increase independence include cognitive behavioral training skills, such as reviewing steps to problem solving, linking effort to outcome, decreasing negative self-talk, and comprehending the purpose of the assignment (Butler, 1998). Self-advocacy skills are also very important. However, it is important not to continually overemphasize the individual's identity as a person with a disability. To do so can perpetuate the stigma, dependency on others, and instill a sense of need for support, rather than increasing independence (Wang & Dovidio, 2011). A good practice in coaching students with disabilities is to guide them to discuss specific needs that are based on themselves as a person, rather than a person with a disability. For example, rather than repeating, "I have a NVLD that affects my ability to prioritize and organize my work," a more positive self-affirming statement could be "I prefer structure, so I would like to write these steps down." In this way, the individual is still advocating for themselves to mitigate specific challenges, reinforcing feelings of competency, and promoting positive self-concept.

Coach–Educator Collaboration

While the youth with NVLD is a minor, an educator's communication with parents is essential and required by law. However, the educators are not able to communicate with anyone other than the youth's legal guardian. Therefore, the student and parent will need to grant special permission to allow this communication with a coach. In addition, parameters about the nature of the communications will need to be specified. Educational progress is a specific type of communication. Behavior and emotional issues are another issue that may require communication with the school counselor or psychologist. Again, these types of communications will need to be agreed upon in writing. In the initial stages, the coach and instructor will need to clarify responsibilities of the student, coach, and instructor (Troiano, Liefeld, & Trachtenberg, 2010). In addition, "shadowing" the student in class or other school activities can be a valuable assessment tool. This requires full collaboration from instructors. The coach must be familiar with the typical and specific characteristics of individuals with NVLD in order to be effective (BiswasDiener, 2009; Ratey, 2002). A coach differs from other types of support because the coach can be involved in a full range of environments and employ various strategies to ensure generalization of learned skills in different settings. With the support of the individual, the coach can also interact with key people in the youth's expanding ecological domains. This also allows a coach to observe how personal factors will affect outcomes (Dansinger, 2000; Ratey, 2002).

A child with behavioral, emotional, or organizational issues can affect the entire culture of the classroom (Dodge, Dishion, & Lansford, 2006; Evertson & Weinstein, 2006; Walbeck, Menlove, Garff, Menlove, & Harris, 2003). Although many special education teachers have successfully mastered the behavior modification skills needed to deliver academic content and maintain the functioning of the classroom, these efforts can also be time consuming depending on the individual and the significance of the behaviors.

Once an individual with a disability graduates from high school, the laws differ significantly and special education instructors and small class sizes are not mandated. Typically the coach or parent will not have access to communication with educational staff in a higher education setting due to the adult status of the student. The student's written permission and consent is required prior to any communications about educational progress or behavioral issues. However, if the student is in agreement, this communication and consent is preferable and will greatly enhance the work the coach can do with the student in numerous domains. It is important to check with the college the student is attending for policies and procedures that are particular to each campus.

Support for Parents

To increase independence in children with NLVD, it may take many years to address issues as they occur throughout the child's development. Therefore, even with the support of coaches, parents may want to consider finding support for themselves throughout this process. There are many nonprofit organizations or support groups designed for parents and other family members who care for a child with a disability.

Support groups can offer validation to emotional feelings and provide informational resources when a child transitions to a new school or has new responsibilities (Graziosi, 2010; Heiman & Berger, 2008). Some organizations can also match parents to other caregivers with children with similar disabilities or concerns (Santelli, 2002). These services are often offered at no cost to families.

Diagnostic Tools

Initial assessments may not point to a diagnosis of NVLD. Educational and school psychologists use a battery of psychoeducational tools to diagnose an individual with a learning disability (LD). However, currently a diagnostic tool specific to identifying NVLD is not available. Therefore, one of the most meaningful indicators of an NVLD is a significant discrepancy between verbal and performance domains on standardized cognitive assessments, such as the commonly used Wechsler Intelligence Scale for Children (WISC), the Wechsler Adult Intelligence Scale (WAIS), Woodcock–Johnson III, (WJ III), Wide-Range Assessment of Memory and Learning (WRAML), and neuropsychological assessments such as the NEPSY-II or the Cognitive Assessment System (CAS). These tools also provide insight to the related subtypes of each individual youth with NVLD (for more information see the Assessment Chap. 5).

Professionals can determine the specific executive functioning and psychosocial supports that are needed with additional diagnostic tools. Organization and attention issues are diagnosed with instruments, such as the Behavior Rating Inventory of Executive Functioning, BRIEF or BRIEF-A for adults, and Child Behavior Checklist (CBCL). Social and emotional issues can be identified with tools, such as Behavior Assessment System for Children II (BASC-II) and Social Skills Rating System (SSRS), to name a few (Sosna & Mastergeorge, 2005). The Adaptive Behavior Assessment System, 2nd edition (ABAS-II) (Harrison & Oakland, 2002), diagnostic tool or other independent living skills checklists are helpful for determining when typically developing same-age peers begin to develop these skills (i.e., self-responsibility for meeting daily personal needs, simple meals, use of appliances, safety, transportation, and purchasing items). These tools will provide guidance to target areas of supports for coaches.

Similar Strengths and Challenges of NVLD and Other Disabilities

Children with a diagnosis of Asperger Syndrome (AS), autism spectrum disorder (ASD), pervasive developmental disorder, obsessive–compulsive disorder, bipolar, anxiety, ADD/ADHD, anxiety, depression, or oppositional defiant disorder also share related psychosocial and organizational issues with NVLD. Some youth lack friends in school, perceive literal versus figurative interpretations in communication, or experience social anxiety. Attention deficit or difficulties with transitions are also common symptoms. For these reasons differentiating between several possible diagnoses can be confusing (Fitzgerald, 1999; Leplow, Murphy, & Nutzinger, 2002; Packer & Pruitt, 2010). Some experts believe that NVLD and Asperger syndrome diagnoses may be on the same spectrum (Ambery, Russell, Perry, Morris, & Murphy, 2006; Gunter, Ghaziuddin, & Ellis, 2002), while other experts differentiate between these two diagnoses (Davis & Broitman, 2011; Nydén et al., 2010; Ryburn, Anderson, & Wales, 2009; Semrud-Clikeman, Walkowiak, Wilkinson, & Christopher, 2010). Children diagnosed with autism typically receive supports to mitigate challenges such as visual–spatial, executive functioning, comprehension, social, motor, sensory, behavioral, and emotional issues.

Interestingly, a diagnosis of ASD, which is characterized by challenges with social interaction, communication, and executive functioning, presents more significant concerns than a diagnosis of NVLD does and requires additional supports in the home and in school with a one-on-one "coach" or "behavior interventionist" to address these issues. It is common for children on the ASD spectrum to receive up to 40 hours a week of this type of coach support service at the age of diagnosis and similar individualized support in the educational setting as early as preschool (Autism Speaks, 2005; Magiati, Moss, Charman, & Howlin, 2011; Smith, 2010). It is the school district's responsibility to pay for these extra services. However, the IEP will typically not address similar challenges for youth with a more mild diagnosis of NVLD (Little, 2003).

Although many authors have identified significant differences between NVLD and Asperger's or autism, such as the lack of restricted interests and repetitive sensory behaviors, both populations still share some similar characteristics (Ambery et al., 2006; Lewis, 2008). Therefore, the coaching strategies mentioned in this chapter to assist individuals with NVLD are also appropriate for individuals with AS or ASD (Adreon & Durocher, 2007). Likewise, coaching programs targeted to the ASD population may be a good match for students with NVLD. Research on using coaches for children and young adults with disabilities is limited, and even more limited on the topic of NVLD and coaching. Regardless, the research-based strategies mentioned in this chapter can be implanted by individuals with coaching responsibilities apart from whether the coach is a professional or paraprofessional. Some struggles that youth with NVLD may have are discussed below together with evidence-based strategies.

Evidence-Based Strategies

There is limited literature on evidence-based strategies that is specific to individuals with NVLD. However, research on strategies for other diagnoses that share similar challenges to individuals with NVLD (i.e., executive functioning, cognitive processes, emotional regulation, and sensory issues) is more prevalent and included in this review.

Visual Memory and Visual–Spatial Organization

Poor visual recall can manifest in a variety of ways. Therefore, unique interventions specific to the individual will be necessary. Some individuals, depending on their age and experience, will have difficulty recalling faces which can interfere with social interactions (Dimitrovsky, Spector, Levy-Shiff, & Vakil, 1998; Petti, Voelker, Shore, & Hayman-Abello, 2003; Vallabha, 2003). Others may have difficulty remembering where they last saw personal items or where to find information or directions. One strategy is using a static image to refer back to such as photos of key people to remember at school or take a picture of how a task is supposed to look when completed correctly. This way, the individual does not have to rely on visual memory. A coach can assist in determining what type of visual recall issues are preventing growth and assist with creating visual prompts or taking photos. Interestingly, improvements in visual–spatial working memory and processing have been associated with both fine and gross motor skills interventions (Alloway & Warner, 2008; Wilson & McKenzie, 1998). Therefore a coach may consider having the individual with NVLD create the visual prompts which may increase engagement in learning and allow the client to develop fine motor skills in the process.

However, visual–spatial organization may be a more common challenge. This can manifest as difficulties finding classrooms or navigating a route to school. Teaching individuals to talk through the problem step-by-step out loud to oneself initially, then decreasing external verbal problem solving, and transition to internal verbal problem solving is a type of cognitive behavioral approach with promise (Williams, Richmond, & Yarbrough, 1992). Schematic visualization can more easily illustrate relationships such as when solving math equations, a visual representation of how concepts are connected to each other by using diagrams and lines connected to pictures can be effective (van Garderen, 2006).

Further, it can be difficult for some individuals with NVLD to make sense of tables and charts in texts which are not accompanied by explicit instructions on how to read these graphic organizers. This type of visual–spatial challenge will need concrete verbal or visual instructions. Coaches can assist with how to organize information with various strategies to minimize visual distractions for reading or math. Coaches can create simplified visual organizers with charts, colors, photos, and lists, to prompt individuals with NVLD through consecutive steps in problem solving for academic, residential, or work settings.

Executive Functioning

While academic deficits may be mild, the absence of organizational and time-management skills may appreciably inhibit the youth's ability to demonstrate academic competency. Executive functioning includes skills, such as organization, time management, attention, and prioritizing that affect successful outcomes in differing environments (Panerai, Ferrante, & Zingale, 2002). To increase the child's independence in this area, structure, routines, and consistency will help with maintaining learned skills. The coach should also teach the youth (as developmentally appropriate) to use a planner, calendar, or electronic device and teach methods or steps to assist the individual to operate independently (Parker & Boutelle, 2009; Ratey, 2002). Individuals with NVLD may need to visually picture what the day or week looks like. Children who want to "do homework later" can look at the daily time slots in a planner to see where they will have time to complete work. However, children with organizational challenges are often not realistic about the amount of time a project will take. Therefore, part of the coach's responsibility is to walk through the steps of a task and determine realistic timeframes. A coach can assess the amount of actual time taken on each type of task, and then provide an ongoing list of tasks with the estimated amount of time to complete the task, so that youth with time management issues can refer to the chart and can make independent choices about how to meet their goals.

Coaches can address executive functioning issues by assessing task complexity to determine how to break the task down into concrete steps or how to "chunk" instructions. Guided notes, such as creating an outline from the text and then comparing this outline with an outline prepared by the coach or the instructor, has been shown to be an effective strategy to increase student academic performance (Lazarus, 1993). Using writing prompts can assist the individual to generate ideas and get them down on paper. College students with attention problems report less ability to self-monitor daily activities and take longer to respond to certain types of stimuli depending on the complexity of the activity (Chang, Davies, & Gavin, 2009). Therefore, the coach working with an adult with NVLD and executive functioning challenges will spend a significant amount of time building organizational systems for the individual (Ratey, 2002; Ratey & Sleeper-Triplett, 2011). Challenges with attention and organization may result in overlooking smaller details. The individual with NVLD may not notice changes in formatting that provide contextual clues, read written instructions thoroughly, or attend to verbal instructions. Such an individual may not have any difficulty completing an assignment, but may forget to turn in the assignment for grading, or forget identifying information such a name or title of an assignment. Misplacing the assignment or the instructions to complete a task is also common for individuals with attention problems. Attention and organization problems also presents as an unorganized school binder, backpack, room, or workplace. Not all interventions for executive functioning are guaranteed to exhibit the same effectiveness with all individuals. Successful strategies can depend on the differing diagnoses, as well as the unique difference of the individual with this type of deficit (Semrud-Clikeman, Walkowiak, Wilkinson, & Christopher, 2010).

Independent Living Skills

Increasing the individual's independent living skills has to be a conscious choice. It is important to establish a healthy balance between family involvement and the youths' own developing independence. A parent that remains overly involved can unknowingly delay development of social and independent living skills (Smith, English, & Vasek, 2002), especially in the area of the child's safety. Literal interpretations of social interactions or lack of attention to surroundings may become potentially hazardous situations. For example, interpersonal problems arise when a child does not "read" a situation well, such as noticing subtle humor, sarcasm, anger, or "tones" of a conversation. The individual may need concrete instructions for situations involving traffic, crowds, strangers, bullying, and peer pressure.

Some youth with NVLD have intense needs. It is easy for parents to continue in their role of assisting children beyond the child's developmental need for this assistance by continuing to prepare simple food, cleaning up after meals, picking out clothes, gathering needed school materials in the backpack, prompting to care for hygiene, minding morning and evening routines, or completing chores around the home. This can be due to several factors. First, it can be a timesaving strategy. For example, parents or siblings without NVLD can often complete these tasks much quicker than an individual with attention challenges can. Second, it is practical for parents, since they can ensure that children get to school with the needed materials to prevent parent trips to the school to bring forgotten items at home. Third, parents who perform tasks for their children can affect some measure of control over unique sensory and emotional needs that daily living skills responsibilities can exacerbate, especially when under the pressure of time. Parents who assist with these responsibilities can often avoid negative outcomes, such behavior or emotional problems, and anxiety (Albert, Maia, Saracco, Brunatto, & Mataix-Cols, 2010). Therefore, it is possible for parents to inadvertently increase their child's dependence on them by performing tasks themselves rather than teaching children mastery of these tasks.

To avoid lingering dependence on parents, coaches can provide objective observations of developmentally appropriate goals for independent living skills. In addition, a coach can help in the child's (and the parent's) transition process from dependence to independence. A coach can create visual structure and meaningful prompts to the child that parents can continue to use at home when a coach is not present. Coaches can teach independent living skills in structured settings individually or in groups. Coaches can implement many strategies at home or at school. For example, coaches working with students who live at home or on campus can teach cooking skills in a structured setting, similar to home economic classes, or in a more naturalistic setting, such as when the individual is intrinsically motivated to prepare a snack at home or in college housing, to demonstrate how to do the dishes, laundry, clean a room, or organize, by providing schematic representations of these tasks for reference.

Cognitive Processing, Reading Comprehension, and Written Expression

Some individuals with NVLD have cognitive processing challenges that affect their understanding of how concepts are connected to each other. Additionally, individuals with NVLD have difficulty solving problems in novel situations, as they may not generalize what they learn and apply one problem-solving technique to a different type of problem (Schiff, Bauminger, & Toledo, 2009). Other strategies include meta-cognitive learning approaches to create learning objectives in reading materials and teaching emotional regulation during learning (Paris & Oka, 1989).

Coaches should also be familiar with assistive technology. Research supports the use of text-to-speech technology to increase reading comprehension (Izzo, Yurick, & McArrell, 2009). Other promising strategies that coaches can use include priming the student to recognize text structure and subject-specific text features, such as titles, vocabulary, diagrams, and maps (Kelley & Clausen-Grace, 2010), and to cue the reader to look for specific ideas, such as main ideas, and compare and contrast text (Gaddy, Bakken, & Fulk, 2008). Self-advocacy skills are critical to assist with reading and writing, especially in the transition from high school to college. The professors, coaches, and family members need to understand the importance of student self-advocacy so that extra time may be awarded to students with NVLD to process information and to adjust to the lack of special educators proficient in teaching students with LD that they once had in high school (Hadley, 2006; Izzo et al., 2009).

After-school tutoring programs that assist students with writing skills may not provide enough staff scheduling consistency to become familiar with the individual learning style of the student with NVLD. Similarly, students with LD find that the typical tutoring offered in college is not helpful because most tutors are not trained to work with students with LD (Hadley, 2006). Collaboration between tutors and coaches can help reduce frustration and educate tutors on how to work with the student more effectively.

Social Understanding

It is important for coaches to teach students meta-cognitive methods for social skills development. Using "Social Thinking" (Crooke, Hendriz, & Rachman, 2008; Winner & Crooke, 2011) strategies to teach individuals why we do specific behaviors, such as eye contact and perspective taking, is an effective means of facilitating a learned behavior to a novel setting. Coaches can also be integral in implementing many of these strategies, such as using Social Stories that model social norms in various interpersonal or community situations (Kalyva & Agaliotis, 2009; Kokina & Kern, 2010; More, 2008). Due to the time involved to individualize this strategy (Gray, 2000; Whitehead, 2007), find resources, or create unique materials the coach seems to be the best choice for this targeted activity. There are software products on the market that simplify this concept, such as books and digital support (Gray, 2011; Smith, 2003), but time involved to facilitate the individual's appropriate engagement with the software, monitor effectiveness, and continually incorporate new skills can be a daunting project. Older individuals that receive socials skills training may increase their skills in initiating social activities, responding to emotional situations appropriately, and in conflict resolution. However, these skills may not necessarily translate into improved relationships with fellow peers with similar challenges (Schechtman & Katz, 2007).

Coaches can assist in social understanding in creative ways. Coaching activities can be enhanced through movies, cartoons, video games, and stories, and can be used for discussion on appropriate social interactions. Common situations that can occur in school, such as lunchtime interactions, making authentic friends, bullying, and school dances, are good topics for review. Discussions between a coach and a client pertaining to humor, social nuances, customs, etiquette, and other behaviors can occur naturally during or after a movie. Certainly, a movie or other entertainment chosen by the individual will hold attention and place "the lesson" in context.

Social Skills

Delayed development of social skills may manifest due to several factors, such as a preference for activities that do not require the participation of others, for instance, reading or video games. Consequently, some youth with NVLD lack peer friendships. Certain subtypes of NVLD that experience problems with social skills do not inherently understand common social customs, such as not interrupting when someone else is talking, perceiving that peers lack interest in the subject of the conversation, naturally occurring segues that end conversations, or how to transition to other topics. Lack of social awareness can present challenges with peer collaboration in the classroom, developing authentic friendships, or confusion about romantic relationships for individuals with NVLD. Children without friends in school can lead to a feeling of disconnect to the community. Further isolation from the mainstream may encourage affiliations with fringe groups that perceive rejection from peers or family members, leading to involvement in risk-taking behaviors (Farmer et al., 2011; McNamara & Willoughby, 2010).

Professionals often recommend facilitated social groups for children with certain subtypes of NVLD that are designed to teach skills that children without disabilities inherently learn from their social interactions with peers, such as turn taking, sharing, and verbal and nonverbal social cues in communication (Marti, 2004). Social coaching can facilitate appropriate behaviors such as increasing opportunities for communication with others by teaching how to initiate a conversation or engaging in activities with others with mutual interests; although training may influence outcomes in social skills more than the rapport between group members (La Greca & Mesibov, 1979; Schechtman & Katz, 2007; Tanguay, 2000).

Initially social skills can be taught to youth with NVLD one-on-one with the coach, such as turn taking, interrupting, transitioning, listening, and social comprehension. In a naturalistic or organically occurring setting, a coach can prompt the use of these skills. This can occur in the playground with prompts from the coach or in a social skills group with a facilitator of an activity acting as the coach. Other children's activities, such as playing a team sport, attending a child's birthday party, or playing with siblings, are situations that can become naturalistic learning opportunities. The coach needs to be available to make social adjustments and provide prompts along the way until the skill is internalized and mastered.

Social Support

It is not enough for coaches and parents simply to provide social support for individuals with NVLD. It is important that individuals concretely comprehend that this social support is present and reliable. Without this understanding, they risk suffering from anxiety, depression, low self-esteem, peer rejection, isolation, or even suicidal thoughts (Winterowd, Street, & Boswell, 1998). In the social self-concept domain, it is important to understand the potential for vulnerability in this population, address self-concept at an early age, and establish a supportive classroom culture (Elbaum & Vaughn, 2003; Givon & Court, 2010). Not all students with NVLD possess low self-esteem or academic self-concept. However continued and developmentally appropriate social support is recommended at home and at school.

Emotional Regulation

It is very common for students with NVLD to experience depression, anxiety, low self-esteem, stress, and concentration problems. Without support, individuals will likely lack necessary coping skills. A coach can play an important role in helping the individual to identify negative self-talk patterns and emotions related to living with a disability and address how these patterns may affect motivation to complete goals (Ratey, 2002). Family members report that extra transition time is needed from one activity to the next. An individual that experiences difficulty with transitioning may exhibit increasing anxiety over seemingly simple tasks or interpersonal exchanges. This can result in frequent emotional outbursts. This continuous effort to mitigate these issues can increase the amount of stress, affecting the entire family dynamic (Epstein et al., 2008; Risdall & Singer, 2004).

Once educational accommodations have been established, often other manifestations of the NVLD need to be managed. A coach can assist with daily check-ins to monitor the clients. Coaches can also provide daily structure and reminders about what coping strategies to use before tests to minimize test anxiety, how to plan for breaks throughout the school day, and how to reduce sensory overload, and remind the student about cognitive behavioral strategies. Even if school personnel in the educational setting have the time to regularly address these issues, a coach with a unique rapport with the student would be able to provide guidance on the kinds of issues to share with counselors, instructors, or peers. Coaches can help the individual with NVLD to systematically discern when it is appropriate or necessary to share personal information.

Anxiety

In general, anxiety can be experienced as excessive fear or worrying of internal or external events. It can manifest in a variety of academic and psychosocial domains. For some individuals with NVLD, difficulties with executive functioning or social situations can have a negative effect on one's self-confidence. It is important for individuals with NVLD to take ownership of their strengths and cognitively rehearse these strengths when self-doubt sets in. Narrative therapy is a process that can assist with reframing negative perceptions of past experiences into neutral or positive perceptions of self in the present and future. This can assist with perceptions of control over irrational fears (Foster & Banes, 2009; Young, 2008). It is also helpful to write out or picture the new narrative to help make concepts more concrete for individuals who possess more visual than verbal strengths (Cashin, 2008). Strategies also exist regarding specific types of anxieties.

Test Anxiety. It is common for individuals with NVLD to experience test anxiety. Coaches can teach the individual test-taking strategies, with multiple choice exams, to perceive some control over anxiety by choosing the order of questions to answer (Holzer, Madaus, Bray, & Kehle, 2009). This tactic is something a coach can work on with the youth for various subjects to help with mastery and generalization of skills to novel test-taking environments. Coaches can also teach and encourage the student to use relaxation techniques before exams to reduce stress (Broota & Sanghvi, 1994; Cheek, Bradley, Reynolds, & Coy, 2002; Purcell, 1999).

Math Anxiety. For certain subtypes of NVLD, it behooves a psychologist to differentiate between an individual who has a disability related to applying math concepts to problems and an individual who is unable to do math due to math anxiety. In other words, it is important to discern between a cognitive challenge and an emotional factor that is affecting academic performance. A coach may need to focus on strategies to address the anxiety first before attempting required math courses (Prevatt, Welles, Li, & Proctor, 2010). See Chap. 9 for more detail.

Obsessive–Compulsive Disorder. Obsessive–compulsive disorder (OCD) is a type of anxiety disorder. Cognitive behavioral therapy, when used consistently and collaboratively within the individual's varied ecological settings, has demonstrated beneficial results for obsessive–compulsive challenges (Barrett, Farrell, Pina, Peris, & Piacentini, 2008). However, most likely, parents and some coaches will require training and professional feedback prior to the implementation of this technique. Coaches and parents will need to understand that some individuals with NVLD may lack insight into how specific OCD behaviors have a negative impact on their quality of life and on others (Ruta, D'Arrigo, Vitiello, & Mazzone, 2010). Mindfulness strategies teach the individual not to judge themselves or the intrusive thoughts, but rather to examine the rationale of the thoughts, decide on their practicality, and perceive some control over behaviors (Fairfax & Barfield, 2010).

Depression

Clinical depression can result when effective academic or social interventions have not been applied over the typical milestones of a child's development (Marti, 2004; Roman, 1998). If depression reaches significant levels, it can lead to very severe consequences, such as suicide (Rourke & Leenaars, 1989). Some researchers believe that increased suicidal tendencies may also be related to the subtype of NVLD that also experiences impulsivity (Bender, Rosenkrans, & Crane, 1999). Coaches working with a client long term can provide an objective perspective on symptoms of depression that family members may not perceive, especially if they have received training in this area. In addition, the rapport between a coach and the individual can provide anecdotal information regarding correlations between types of events and episodes of depression such as before or after specific academic or social experiences. Families that receive respite support for children with similar disabilities have been correlated with decreased hospitalizations (Mandell et al., 2012). Therefore using a coach can support the family as well as the client.

Self-Esteem and Self-Understanding

Self-esteem can be a critical factor in the developmental lifespan of children with NVLD. The individual's self-perception of whether or not the LD limits them academically or socially is affected by parents, peers, teachers, and the child's surrounding environment (Cosden, Brown, & Elliott, 2002). Academically, if individuals with LD have negative self-perceptions of their achievement abilities, this can contributew to their overall educational aspirations (Lackaye & Margalit, 2006). Research indicates that children who understand that their LD is domain specific and not a global deficit have higher self-esteem or a more positive academic self-concept (Cosden, Brown, & Elliott, 2002; Cosden, Elliott, Noble, & Kelemen, 1999; Rothman & Cosden, 1995). Social comparisons with peers and perceptions of teacher evaluations of schoolwork also contribute to the child's academic self-concept (Bear, Minke, Griffin, & Deemer, 1998). On the college campus coaches can model successful study habits to increase the perceived value of a college education. (Zwart & Kallemeyn, 2001) See the Social Skills chapter 10 for more detail.

Motor Skills

A child with fine motor challenges will demonstrate difficulty with handwriting. Many informal and fun fine motor activities can ultimately assist with handwriting, such as building models, art projects, or playing computer games that require keyboard strokes, a steady hand, and hand-to-eye coordination. In addition, internal self-talk or internal rehearsing has been shown to increase fine motor coordination in older children with NVLD (Tuller, Olvera, & Scott Kelso, 2007).

Parents and teachers of children with NVLD will notice that poor gross motor skills can affect balance, athletic ability, gait, timing of movements, and awareness of surroundings. This can also cause the individual to frequently bump into people, or knock over objects. Although this may not be a primary concern for parents compared to learning problems, some research indicates that the greater the deficits in this area, the lower the academic achievement in reading and math (Westendorp, Hartman, Houwen, Smith, & Visscher, 2011). Very young children will benefit by encouraging them to engage in general playground-type activities (Kamps, 2001; van der Mars & Butterfield, 1987). To intensify the opportunities for gross motor activities, the family may want to consider identifying a "coach" on the playground such as an older peer or hiring a coach playmate (Caldwell & Heller, 2003; Moon et al., 1992; Shumaker, 2008). As with other types of interventions, naturally occurring opportunities and the child's involvement in determining the type of activity or goal will have the best effect (Missiuna & Pollock, 2000).

When motor skills significantly differ from peers, it may draw negative attention, teasing, bullying, or isolation from peers in play or athletic settings (Bejerot, Edgar, & Humble, 2011). However, motor tasks that require collaboration and interaction with others have also been shown to increase adaptive and social skills (Legoff & Sherman, 2006). Furthermore, some researchers suggest that rather than focusing on motor skill development to prevent rejection by peers, it is more advantageous to focus on improving self-concept and cultural acceptance of differences (Lingam, Coad, Novak, & Emond, 2011). Coaches can provide support to encourage motor activities, self-understanding, self-advocacy, and social interaction to assist with development in this area.

Sensory

Some individuals may experience excess or diminished sensitivity in visual, auditory, touch, taste, or smell compared with peers without NVLD. It is important to know if children are seeking sensory input or are attempting to avoid it (Schaaf, 2011). See the Occupational Therapy chapter 3 for more detail. Previous success with exposure and sensory integration strategies over time and the individual's particular developmental stage affects sensitivity. Coaches that have a strong rapport with the student can play an integral role in educational settings by providing input for instructors and students in class activities, course selection, special projects, or extracurricular events that have the potential to demonstrate strength challenges. Children seeking such stimulation will not respond well to rote routines that are void of novel sensory experiences. On the other hand some students may require modification for activities that generate particular odors, physical contact, or coordination or require changes in routines such as field trips or fire drills. Even when some environments seem relatively innocuous and routine, some individuals sense things that others may not. For example, the fluorescent lighting commonly used in educational or work settings can "buzz" or appear to blink for individuals with hypersensitivity to auditory or visual input.

It is necessary to have personal knowledge about the youth with sensory issues such as how to use physical movements to know when it is necessary to increase or to reduce stimuli in order to elicit the best performance or compliance with educational activities (Murray, Baker, Murray-Slutsky, & Paris, 2009). Coaches can intervene with prompts to the student to self-advocate appropriately to modify external stimuli in the environment when appropriate (i.e., turn off one light, reduce volume of an activity) to decrease issues with sensory input. Coaches can help the individual to think of ways to adapt to the environment individually, such as taking a break from stimuli, using earplugs, wearing sun glasses, or moving to an area with reduced visual distractions, such as seating in a cubicle when available (Cheng & Boggett-Carsjens, 2005).

Behavioral Issues

For a child with NVLD, transitions and adherence to preestablished routines can be one of the most challenging aspects for a coach or parent. Youth that have difficulty with transitions are likely to experience initial problems in academic or social settings. Preparing the individual for the next activity can make the difference in a successful outcome. Likewise lack of individual preparation can be an obstacle to progress. It is important to be proactive and teach the client how to cope and self-soothe to aid in transitions, or new situations that could be stressful (Cheng & Boggett-Carsjens, 2005). The coach can practice taking the client to a location the day before an activity or review the expected procedures. Prior to entering a specific type of community setting such as store or restaurant, using public transportation, or engaging in certain social activities, the coach can prepare the youth with reminders of what will occur, what behaviors are expected, and of how to help themselves feel better when anxious. Videos, stories, and pictures can be helpful to depict potentially troublesome situations and appropriate behavior (Crooke et al., 2008; O'Conner, 2009; Winner & Crooke, 2011), but it is also important to remind the individual that colors, sights, sounds, and sequence of activities can vary and of how to adapt to changes.

Medication

Though medication specific to treating NVLD or similar diagnoses are not available (Marek, 2004; Teeter, 2009), some psychiatrists may recommend medication that can address specific symptoms that individuals with NVLD experience. Research on the typical comorbid issues of NVLD such as managing their attention, depression, or anxiety (Cuijpers, van Straten, Hollon, & Andersson, 2010; Shireman, Reichard, & Rigler, 2005; Tanguay, 2000) or compulsive behaviors is more common. (For example, for a child with deficits in social understanding, medication may not directly assist the individual with improved social understanding, but may be helpful with certain social or emotional behaviors, such as aggression, or hyperactivity.) Further, some evidence purports that medication is most effective when combined with other support services (Efron, 2006; O'Brien & McKinnon, 2009; Okorie & Connaughton, 2011). If the individual with NVLD is taking medication, coaches can be helpful with prompts or designing organizational systems to help individuals take medication consistently and in appropriate dosages. Further, a coach can assist the client with NVLD with understanding how taking medication or skipping dosages can affect mental health stability. A coach can provide objective feedback about the student's behaviors throughout the day when on and off medication to assist with monitoring and analyzing effectiveness. See the Developmental Pediatrician chapter 6 for more detail.

Summary

In summary, children with learning disabilities such as NVLD require unique supports such as assistance with psychosocial and executive functioning skills. These issues are not typically addressed during the K–12 years in the special education system. Further, these issues are typically not accommodated in college, unless the individual also has a documented disability in attention or a psychological disability. Therefore, it is critical to provide these supports early on for individuals with NVLD to facilitate independence and decrease dependence on familial support. The consistent attention to the unique educational and developmental needs of an individual with NVLD can be stressful for the entire family. Parents should consider employing a coach that can implement strategies across multiple home, school, social, and community domains to provide familial respite and encourage independence in the youth with NVLD. Furthermore, family member should also be sure to take care of their own needs by seeking social support from others who are familiar with the challenges of raising a child with NVLD.

References

Academic Coaching Services. (2010). Retrieved September 16, 2011, from http://academiccoaching.com.

Adreon, D., & Durocher, J. S. (2007). Evaluating the college transition needs of individuals with high-functioning Autism spectrum disorders. *Intervention in School and Clinic, 42*, 271–279.

Albert, U. B., Maia, G., Saracco, P., Brunatto, C., & Mataix-Cols, D. (2010). Family accommodation in obsessive–compulsive disorder: Relation to symptom dimensions, clinical and family characteristics. *Psychiatry Research, 179*(2), 204–211.

Alloway, T., & Warner, C. (2008). Task-specific training, learning, and memory for children with developmental coordination disorder: A pilot study. *Perceptual and Motor Skills, 107*(2), 473–480.

Ambery, F. Z., Russell, A. J., Perry, K., Morris, R., & Murphy, D. M. (2006). Neuropsychological functioning in adults with Asperger syndrome. *Autism, 10*(6), 551–564.

Antshel, K. M., & Joseph, G. (2006). Maternal stress in nonverbal learning disorder: A comparison with reading disorder. *Journal of Learning Disabilities, 39*(3), 194–205.

Autism Speaks. (2005). *Applied Behavior Analysis (ABA)*. Retrieved October 01, 2011, from Autism Speaks: http://www.autismspeaks.org/what-autism/treatment/applied-behavior-analysis-aba.

Baker, D. B., & McCal, K. (1995). Parenting stress in parents of children with attention-deficit hyperactivity disorder and parents of children with learning disabilities. *Journal of Child and Family Studies, 4*(4), 57–68.

Barrett, P. M., Farrell, L., Pina, A. A., Peris, T. S., & Piacentini, J. (2008). Evidence-based psychosocial treatments for child and adolescent obsessive-compulsive disorder. *Journal of Clinical Child and Adolescent Psychology, 37*(1), 131–155. doi:10.108.

Bear, G. G., Minke, K. M., Griffin, S. M., & Deemer, S. A. (1998). Achievement-related perceptions of children with learning disabilities and normal achievement: Group and developmental differences. *Journal of Learning Disabilities, 31*(1), 91–104.

Bedrossian, L., & Pennamon, R. E. (2007). *College students with Asperger syndrome: Practical strategies for academic and social success*. Horsham, PA: LRP Publications.

Bejerot, S., Edgar, J., & Humble, M. B. (2011). Poor performance in physical education – A risk factor for bully victimization. A case-control study. *Acta Paediatrica, 100*(3), 413–419.

Bender, W. N., Rosenkrans, C. B., & Crane, M. (1999). Stress, depression, and suicide among students with learning disabilities: Assessing the risk. *Learning Disability Quarterly, 22*(2), 143–156.

Bennis, C.L. (2011). A phenomenological study of homework from the perspectives of elementary special education teachers of students with learning disabilities. *Dissertation Abstracts International Section* A, 72.

BiswasDiener, R. (2009). Personal coaching as a positive intervention. *Journal of Clinical Psychology, 65*(5), 544–553.

Braaten, E. B. (2011). Learning disabilities. In E. B. Braaten (Ed.), *How to find mental health care for your child* (pp. 121–137). Washington, DC: American Psychological Association.

Bravo, L. (2001). Trastornos no-verbales y disfunción cerebral. *Psykhe: Revista De La Escuela De Psicología, 10*(2), 143–148.

Broota, A., & Sanghvi, C. (1994). Efficacy of two relaxation techniques in examination anxiety. *Journal of Personality and Clinical Studies, 10*(1–2), 29–35.

Brown, C.M. (2005). Parent home involvement and student achievement for Mexican-American and European American students with learning disabilities (Vol. 66). *Dissertation Abstracts International,* Section A.

Butler, D. L. (1998). The strategic content learning approach to promoting self-regulated learning: A report of three studies. *Journal of Educational Psychology, 90*(4), 682–697.

Caldwell, J. J., & Heller, T. T. (2003). Management of respite and personal assistance services in a consumer-directed family support programme. *Journal of Intellectual Disability Research, 47*(4–5), 352–367.

Case, S. (2001). Learning to partner, disabling conflict: Early indications of an improving relationship between parents and professionals with regard to service provision for children with learning disabilities. *Disability & Society, 16*(6), 837–854.

Casey, J. E., Rourke, B. P., & Picard, E. M. (1991). Syndrome of nonverbal learning disabilities: Age differences in neuropsychological, academic, and socioemotional functioning. *Development and Psychopathology, 3*(3), 329–345.

Cashin, A. (2008). Narrative therapy: A psychotherapeutic approach in the treatment of adolescents with Asperger's disorder. *Journal of Child and Adolescent Psychiatric Nursing, 21*(1), 48–56.

Chang, W. P., Davies, P. L., & Gavin, W. J. (2009). Error monitoring in college students with attention-deficit/hyperactivity disorder. *Journal of Psychophysiology, 23*(3), 113–125.

Cheek, J. R., Bradley, L. J., Reynolds, J., & Coy, D. (2002). An intervention for helping elementary students reduce test anxiety. *Professional School Counseling, 6*(2), 162–164.

Cheng, M., & Boggett-Carsjens, J. (2005). Consider sensory processing disorders in the explosive child: Case report and review. *Canadian Child and Adolescent Psychiatry Review, 14*(4), 44–48.

Christenson, S. L. (2005). Evidence-based parent and family interventions in school psychology: State of scientifically based practice. *School Psychology Quarterly, 20*(4), 525–528.

Coach Training Alliance. (2001). Retrieved October 08, 2011, from http://www.coachtrainingalliance.com

Cook, C. R., Crews, S., Wright, D., Mayer, G., Gale, B., Kraemer, B., et al. (2007). Establishing and evaluating the substantive adequacy of positive behavioral support plans. *Journal of Behavioral Education, 16*(3), 191–206.

Cosden, M., Brown, C., & Elliott, K. (2002). Development of self-understanding and self-esteem in children and adults with learning disabilities. In B. L. Wong & M. L. Donahue (Eds.), *The social dimensions of learning disabilities: Essays in honor of Tanis Bryan* (pp. 33–51). Mahwah, NJ: Lawrence Erlbaum Associates Publishers.

Cosden, M., Elliott, K., Noble, S., & Kelemen, E. (1999). Self-understanding and self-esteem in children with learning disabilities. *Learning Disability Quarterly, 22*(4), 279–290.

Crooke, P., Hendriz, R. E., & Rachman, J. Y. (2008). Brief report: Measuring the effectiveness of teaching social thinking to children with Asperger Syndrome (AS) and High Functioning Autism (HFA). *Journal of Autism Development, 38*(3), 581–91.

Cuijpers, P. P., van Straten, A. A., Hollon, S. D., & Andersson, G. G. (2010). The contribution of active medication to combined treatments of psychotherapy and pharmacotherapy for adult depression: A meta-analysis. *Acta Psychiatrica Scandinavica, 121*(6), 415–423. doi:10.1111/j.1600-0447.2009.01513.x

Dansinger, S. (2000). Academic Coaching for the Gifted Learner. *ERIC*, 1–5.

Davis, J. M., & Broitman, J. (2011). *Nonverbal learning disabilities in children: Bridging the gap between science and practice*. New York: Springer.

Dimitrovsky, L., Spector, H., Levy-Shiff, R., & Vakil, E. (1998). Interpretation of facial expressions of affect in children with learning disabilities with verbal or nonverbal deficits. *Journal of Learning Disabilities, 31*(3), 286–292, 312.

Dodge, K. A., Dishion, T. J., & Lansford, J. E. (2006). Deviant peer influences in intervention and public policy for youth. *Society for Research in Child Development, 20*(1).

Efron, D. (2006). Attention-deficit/hyperactivity disorder: Are we medicating for social disadvantage? (Against). *Journal of Paediatrics and Child Health, 42*(9), 548–551.

Elbaum, B., & Vaughn, S. (2003). For which students with learning disabilities are self-concept interventions effective? *Journal of Learning Disabilities, 36*(2), 101–108.

Epstein, T. T., Saltzman-Benaiah, J. J., O'Hare, A. A., Goll, J. C., & Tuck, S. S. (2008). Associated features of Asperger syndrome and their relationship to parenting stress. *Child Care, Health and Development, 34*(4), 503–511.

Espiner, D., & Guild, D. (2011). The Circle of Courage[TM] in transition planning. *Reclaiming Children and Youth, 20*(2), 44–49.

Etscheidt, S. (2006). Behavioral intervention plans: Pedagogical and legal analysis of issues. *Behavioral Disorders, 31*(2), 223–243.

Evans Getzel, E., McManus, S., & Briel, L. (2004). An effective model for college students with learning disabilities and attention deficit hyperactivity disorder. *Research to Practice Brief: Improving Secondary Education and Transition Services through Research, 3*(1), 1–6.

Evans, S. W., Schultz, B. K., & Sadler, J. M. (2008). Safety and efficacy of psychosocial interventions used to treat children with attention-deficit/hyperactivity disorder. *Psychiatric Annals, 38*(1), 58–65.

Evertson, C. M., & Weinstein, C. S. (2006). *Handbook of classroom management: research, practice, and contemporary issues*. Mahwah, NJ: Lawrence Erlbaum Associates.

Fairfax, H., & Barfield, J. (2010). A group-based treatment for clients with obsessive compulsive disorder (OCD) in a secondary care mental health setting: Integrating new developments within cognitive behavioural interventions – An exploratory study. *Counselling & Psychotherapy Research, 10*(3), 214–221.

Farmer, T. W., Hall, C. M., Weiss, P. M., Petrin, R. A., Meece, J. L., et al. (2011). The school adjustment of rural adolescents with and without disabilities: Variable and person-centered approaches. *Journal of Child and Family Studies, 20*(1), 78–88.

Fitzgerald, M. (1999). Differential diagnosis of adolescent and adult pervasive developmental disorders/autism spectrum disorders (PDD/ASD): A not uncommon diagnostic dilemma. *Irish Journal of Psychological Medicine, 16*(4), 145–148.

Fletcher, S. (2007). Educational research mentoring and coaching as co-creative synergy. *International Journal of Evidence Based Coaching and Mentoring, 5*(2), 1–11.

Forrest, K. (2003). Overcoming unintentional barriers with intentional strategies: Educating faculty about student disability. *Teaching of Psychology, 30*(3), 270–276.

Foster, C., & Banes, J. (2009). Use of a narrative therapy approach with a man with a learning disability: An alternative to cognitive behavioural therapy? *Advances in Mental Health and Intellectual Disabilities, 3*(1), 52–55.

Franz, C. (2000). *Diagnosis and management of nonverbal learning disorders*. New Orleans, LA: National Association of School Psychologists.

Gaddy, S. A., Bakken, J. P., & Fulk, B. M. (2008). The effects of teaching text-structure strategies to postsecondary students with learning disabilities to improve their reading comprehension on expository science text passages. *Journal of Postsecondary Education and Disability, 20*(2), 100–119.

Galway, T. M., & Metsala, J. L. (2011). Social cognition and its relation to psychosocial adjustment in children with nonverbal learning disabilities. *Journal of Learning Disabilities, 44*(1), 33–49.

Givon, S., & Court, D. (2010). Coping strategies of high school students with learning disabilities: A longitudinal qualitative study and grounded theory. *International Journal of Qualitative Studies in Education, 23*(3), 283–303.

Goldberg, R. J., Higgins, E. L., Raskind, M. H., & Herman, K. L. (2003). Predictors of success in individuals with learning disabilities: A qualitative analysis of a 20-year longitudinal study. *Learning Disabilities Research and Practice, 18*(4), 222–236.

Gray, C. (2000). *Writing social stories*. Arlington, TX: Future Horizons Inc.

Gray, C. n. (n.d.). *The Gray Center for social learning and understanding*. Retrieved December 31, 2011, from: http://thegraycenter.org/

Graziosi, E. (2010). Valuing support groups. *Exceptional Parent, 40*(4), 24–25.

Gunter, H. L., Ghaziuddin, M., & Ellis, H. D. (2002). Asperger syndrome: Tests of right hemisphere functioning and interhemispheric communication. *Journal of Autism and Developmental Disorders, 32*(4), 263–281.

Gutstein, S. E., & Sheely, R. K. (2002). *Relationship development intervention with young children: Social and emotional development activities for Asperger syndrome, autism, PPD and NLD*. London: Jessica Kingsley Publishers.

Hadley, W. (2006). L.D. students' access to higher education self-advocacy and support. *Journal of Developmental Education, 30*(2), 10–16.

Hardy, L. (2001). Mental help: Test-prep products promise to boost your students' scores, but do they really deliver? *American School Board Journal, 188*(1), 33–35.

Harrison, P. L., & Oakland, T. (2002). *Adaptive behavior assessment system* (2nd ed.). San Antonio, TX: Psychological Corporation.

Heiman, T., & Berger, O. (2008). Parents of children with Asperger syndrome or with learning disabilities: Family environment and social support. *Research in Developmental Disabilities, 29*(4), 289–300.

Herrera, C., Sipe, C. L., McClanahan, W. S., Arbreton, A. J. A., & Pepper, S. K. (2000). Mentoring school-age children: Relationship development in community and school-based programs. Philadelphia: Public/Private Ventures.

Holzer, M., Madaus, J. W., Bray, M. A., & Kehle, T. J. (2009). The test-taking strategy intervention for college students with learning disabilities. *Learning Disabilities Research and Practice, 24*(1), 44–56.

Individuals with Disabilities Education Act. (2004) 20 U.S.C § 1400, et. seq.

International Coaching Federation. (2011). Retrieved September 03, 2011, from Get Credentialed: http://coachfederation.org/getcredentialed/

Izzo, M. V., Yurick, A., & McArrell, B. (2009). Supported eText: Effects of text-to-speech on access and achievement for high school students with disabilities. *Journal of Special Education Technology, 24*(3), 9–20.

Kalyva, E., & Agaliotis, I. (2009). Can social stories enhance the interpersonal conflict resolution skills of children with LD? *Research in Developmental Disabilities, 30*(1), 192–202.
Kamps, P. (2001). Modifiability of the psychomotor domain. *Dissertation Abstracts International Section* A, 61.
Kelley, M. J., & Clausen-Grace, N. (2010). Guiding students through expository text with text feature walks. *Reading Teacher, 64*(3), 191–195.
Kenny, D. T., & Faunce, G. (2004). Effects of academic coaching on elementary and secondary school students. *The Journal of Educational Research, 98*(2), 115–126.
Kokina, A., & Kern, L. (2010). Social Story™ interventions for students with Autism spectrum disorders: A meta-analysis. *Journal of Autism & Developmental Disorders, 40*(7), 812–826.
Kouwenhoven, M. (2011). The strategic coaching matrix. *Transactional Analysis Journal, 41*(1), 77–91.
Krsti , N. (2001). Neverbalne smetnje u enja: Koncept i empirijska osnova. *Psihijatrija Danas, 33*(3–4), 133–147.
La Greca, A. M., & Mesibov, G. B. (1979). Social skills intervention with learning disabled children: Selecting skills and implementing training. *Journal of Clinical Child Psychology, 8*(3), 234–241.
Lackaye, T. D., & Margalit, M. (2006). Comparisons of achievement, effort, and self-perceptions among students with learning disabilities and their peers from different achievement groups. *Journal of Learning Disabilities, 39*(5), 432–446.
Landmark. (2011). *Inclusive communities self-determination and community integration*. Retrieved September 10, 2011, from Arizona State University: http://iic.asu.edu/services/areas
Lazarus, B. D. (1993). Guided notes: Effects with secondary and post secondary students with mild disabilities. *Education and Treatment of Children, 16*(3), 272–289.
Legoff, D. B., & Sherman, M. (2006). Long-term outcome of social skills intervention based on interactive LEGO© play. *Autism, 10*(4), 317–329.
Leplow, B., Murphy, R., & Nutzinger, D. O. (2002). Specificity of conditional associative-learning deficits in obsessive-compulsive disorder (OCD) and non-OCD anxiety disorders. *Journal of Clinical and Experimental Neuropsychology, 24*(6), 792–805.
Lewis, J. (2008). *NLD coaching*. Retrieved September 03, 2011, from NLD line: http://www.nld-line.com/
Lingam, R., Coad, J., Novak, C., & Emond, A. (2011). Identity and empowerment: A qualitative study of teenagers with developmental coordination disorder. *Archives of Disease in Childhood, 96*(1), A7–A9.
Little, L. (2003). Maternal perceptions of the importance of needs and resources for children with Asperger syndrome and Nonverbal learning disorders. *Focus on Autism and Other Developmental Disabilities, 18*(4), 257–266.
Little, L., & Clark, R. R. (2006). Wonders and worries of parenting a child with Asperger Syndrome and nonverbal learning disorder. *The American Journal of Maternal/Child Nursing, 31*(1), 39–44.
Lyle, M. (1998). *The LD teacher's IEP companion: Goals, strategies, and activities for LD students*. LinguiSystems, Inc: East Moline, IL.
Magiati, I., Moss, J., Charman, T., & Howlin, P. (2011). Patterns of change in children with autism spectrum disorders who received community based comprehensive interventions in their preschool years: A seven year follow-up study. *Research in Autism Spectrum Disorders, 5*(3), 1016–1027.
Mandell, S., Xie, M., Morales, K. H., Lawer, L., McCarthy, M., & Marcus, S. C. (2012). The interplay of outpatient services and psychiatric hospitalization among medicaid-enrolled children with Autism Spectrum disorders. *Archives of Pediatric Adolescent Medicine, 166*(1), 68–73.
Marek, W. K. (2004). Review of 'Asperger syndrome'. *American Journal Of Forensic Psychology, 22*(2), 75–78.
Margalit, M., & Heiman, T. (1986). Family climate and anxiety in families with learning disabled boys. *Journal of The American Academy of Child Psychiatry, 25*(6), 841–846.

Marti, L. (2004). Helping children with nonverbal learning disability: What i have learned from living with nonverbal learning disability. *Journal of Child Neurology, 19*(1), 830–836.

Martin, M. (2007). *Helping children with nonverbal learning disabilities to flourish: A guide for parents and professionals*. London: Jessica Kingsley Publishers.

McKinney, J. D., & Hocutt, A. M. (1982). Public school involvement of parents of learning-disabled children and average achievers. *Exceptional Education Quarterly, 3*(2), 64–73.

McNamara, J. K., & Willoughby, T. (2010). A longitudinal study of risk-taking behavior in adolescents with learning disabilities. *Learning Disabilities Research and Practice, 25*(1), 11–24.

Mikami, A., Lerner, M. D., Griggs, M., McGrath, A., & Calhoun, D. C. (2010). Parental influence on children with attention-deficit/hyperactivity disorder: II. Results of a pilot intervention training parents as friendship coaches for children. *Journal of Abnormal Child Psychology, 38*(6), 737–749.

Missiuna, C., & Pollock, N. (2000). Perceived efficacy and goal setting in young children. *Canadian Journal Of Occupational Therapy/ Revue Canadienne D'ergothérapie, 67*(2), 101–110.

Moon, M., et al. (1992). *The community leisure facilitator. Project REC.* Training and Research Institute for Children and Disabilities. Boston, MA: Children's Hospital.

More, C. (2008). Digital stories targeting social skills for children with disabilities: Multidimensional learning. *Intervention in School & Clinic, 43*(3), 168–177.

Murray, M., Baker, P., Murray-Slutsky, C., & Paris, B. (2009). Strategies for supporting the sensory-based learner. *Preventing School Failure, 53*(4), 245–251.

Nesselrodt, P., & Alger, C. (2005). Extending opportunity to learn for students placed at risk. *Journal of Education for Students Placed at Risk, 10*(2), 207–224.

Nydén, A. N., Ståhlberg, O., Anckarsäter, H., Dahlgren-Sandberg, A., Wentz, E., & Råstam, M. (2010). Adults with Asperger syndrome with and without a cognitive profile associated with "non-verbal learning disability." A brief report. *Research in Autism Spectrum Disorders, 4*(4), 612–618.

O'Brien, G., & McKinnon, I. (2009). Medication in people with learning disability and mental illness. *Psychiatry, 8*(10), 413–415.

O'Conner, E. (2009). The use of social story DVDs to reduce anxiety levels: a case study of a child with autism and learning disabilities. *Support for Learning, 24*(3), 133–136.

Okorie, E., & Connaughton, C. (2011). Antipsychotic prescribing in a residential facility for clients with learning disability. *British Journal of Developmental Disabilities, 57*(113 (Pt2)), 117–122.

Otterbourg, S. D. (1996). *Education today parent involvement handbook* (2nd ed.). Atlanta, GA: Atlanta Book Company.

Ozonoff, S., & Cathcart, K. (1998). Effectiveness of a home program intervention for young children with autism. *Journal of Autism and Developmental Disorders, 28*(1), 25–32. doi:10.1023/A:1026006818310.

Packer, L. E., & Pruitt, S. K. (2010). *Challenging kids, challenged teachers:Teaching students with Tourette's, bipolar disorder, executive dysfunction, OCD, ADHD, and more*. Bethesda, MD: Woodbine House.

Panerai, S., Ferrante, L. L., & Zingale, M. (2002). Benefits of the treatment and education of autistic and communication handicapped children (TEACCH) programme as compared with a non-specific approach. *Journal of Intellectual Disability Research, 46*(4), 318–327.

Paris, S. G., & Oka, E. R. (1989). Strategies for comprehending text and coping with reading difficulties. *Learning Disability Quarterly, 12*(1), 32–42.

Parker, D. R., & Boutelle, K. (2009). Executive function coaching for college students with learning disabilities and ADHD: A new approach for fostering self-determination. *Learning Disabilities Research and Practice, 24*(4), 204–215.

Petti, V. L., Voelker, S. L., Shore, D. L., & Hayman-Abello, S. E. (2003). Perception of nonverbal emotion cues by children with nonverbal learning disabilities. *Journal of Developmental and Physical Disabilities, 15*(1), 23–36.

Prevatt, F., Welles, T. L., Li, H., & Proctor, B. (2010). The contribution of memory and anxiety to the math performance of college students with learning disabilities. *Learning Disabilities Research and Practice, 25*(1), 39–47.

Price, J., & Fisher, J. (2010). *Take control of Asperger's syndrome: The official strategy guide for teens with Asperger's syndrome and nonverbal learning disorder*. Waco, TX: Prufrock Press.

Purcell, J. (1999). *Children, adolescents, and obsessive–compulsive disorder in the classroom.* ERIC, EBSCOhost (Accessed January 15, 2012).

Quinn, M. M., Gable, R. A., & Fox, J. (2001). Putting quality functional assessment into practice in schools: a research agenda on behalf of E/BD students. *Education & Treatment of Children, 24*(3), 261–275.

Raines, J. C. (2006). The new IDEA: Reflections on the reauthorization for social workers. *School Social Work Journal, 31*(1), 1–18.

Ratey, N. (2002). Life coaching for adult ADHD. In S. Goldstein (Ed.), *The Clinician's guide to adult ADHD* (pp. 261–277). New York: Elsevier Science.

Ratey, N., & Sleeper-Triplett, J. (2011). Strategic coaching for LD and ADHD. In J. A. S. Goldstein (Ed.), *Learning and attention disorders in adolescence and adulthood: Assessment and treatment* (2nd ed.). Hoboken, NJ: John Wiley & Sons Inc.

Riddell, S., Baron, S., & Wilson, A. (1999). Social capital and people with learning difficulties. *Studies in The Education of Adults, 31*(1), 49–65.

Ris, M., & Nortz, M. (2008). Nonverbal learning disorder. In J. H. J. E. Morgan (Ed.), *Textbook of clinical neuropsychology* (pp. 346–359). New York, NY: Psychology Press.

Risdall, D., & Singer, G. (2004). *Marital adjustment in parents of children with disabilities: A historical review and meta-analysis.* Retrieved December 12, 2011, from TASH: http://www.atypon-link.com/TASH/doi/abs/10.2511/rpsd.29.2.95

Robinson, C., & Gahagan, J. (2010). Coaching students to academic success and engagement on campus. *About Campus, 15*(4), 26–29.

Roman, M. A. (1998). The syndrome of nonverbal learning disabilities: Clinical depression and applied aspects. *Current Issues in Education, 1*(7), 1–26.

Rothman, H. R., & Cosden, M. (1995). The relationship between self-perception of a learning disability and achievement, self-concept and social support. *Learning Disability Quarterly*, 18(3), 203–212.

Rourke, B. P., Young, G. C., & Leenaars, A. A. (1989). A childhood learning disability that predisposes those afflicted to adolescent and adult depression and suicide risk. *Journal of Learning Disabilities, 22*(3), 169–175.

Ruta, L., D'Arrigo, V., Vitiello, B., & Mazzone, L. (2010). Obsessive–compulsive traits in children and adolescents with Asperger syndrome. *European Child & Adolescent Psychiatry, 19*(1), 17–27.

Ryburn, B. B., Anderson, V. V., & Wales, R. R. (2009). Asperger syndrome: How does it relate to non-verbal learning disability? *Journal of Neuropsychology, 3*(1), 107–123.

Sallows, G. O., & Graupner, T. D. (2005). Intensive behavioral treatment for children with autism: Four-year outcome and predictors. *American Journal on Mental Retardation, 110*(6), 417–438.

Sanders, K. (2006). Overprotection and lowered expectations of persons with disabilities: The unforeseen consequences. *Work: Journal of Prevention, Assessment, and Rehabilitation, 27*, 181–188.

Santelli, B. (2002). *Basics for parents: Parent to parent support*. Washington, DC: National Information Center for Children and Youth with Disabilities.

Schaaf, R. C. (2011). Interventions that address sensory dysfunction for individuals with autism spectrum disorders: Preliminary evidence for the superiority of sensory integration compared to other sensory approaches. In P. D. B. Reichow (Ed.), *Evidence-based practices and treatments for children with autism* (pp. 245–273). New York: Springer Science+Business Media.

Schechtman, Z., & Katz, E. (2007). Therapeutic bonding in group as an explanatory variable of progress in the social competence of student with learning disabilities. *Group Dynamics, 11*(2), 117–128.

Schiff, R., Bauminger, N., & Toledo, I. (2009). Analogical problem solving in children with verbal and nonverbal learning disabilities. *Journal of Learning Disabilities, 42*(1), 3–13.

Schwenn, J. O. (1991). Students with high incidence exceptionalities. In J. O. Schwenn, A. F. Rotatori, & R. A. Fox (Eds.), *Understanding students with high incidence exceptionalities: Categorical and noncategorical* (pp. 3–29). Springfield, IL: Charles C Thomas.

Semrud-Clikeman, M., Walkowiak, J., Wilkinson, A., & Christopher, G. (2010). Neuropsychological differences among children with Asperger syndrome, nonverbal learning disabilities, attention deficit disorder, and controls. *Developmental Neuropsychology, 35*(5), 582–600.

Shessel, I., & Reiff, H. B. (1999). Experiences of adults with learning disabilities: Positive and negative outcomes. *Learning Disability Quarterly, 22*, 305–316.

Shireman, T. I., Reichard, A., & Rigler, S. K. (2005). Psychotropic Medication Use among Kansas Medicaid Youths with Disabilities. Journal Of Child And Adolescent Psychopharmacology, 15(1), 107–115. doi:10.1089/cap.2005.15.107

Shumaker, L. (2008). *A regular guy: Growing up with autism: A family's story of love and acceptance*. Lafayette, CA: Landscape Press.

Smith, C. (2003). *Writing and developing social stories*. Bicester: Speechmark Publishing Ltd.

Smith, T. (2010). Early and intensive behavioral intervention in autism. In A. E. Kazdin & J. R. Weisz (Eds.), *Evidence-based psychotherapies for children and adolescents* (2nd ed., pp. 312–326). New York: Guilford Press.

Smith, S. G., English, R., & Vasek, D. (2002). Student and parent involvement in the transition process for college freshmen with learning disabilities. *College Student Journal, 34*(4), 491–503.

Sosna, T., & Mastergeorge, A. (2005). Retrieved November 25, 2011, from California Institute of Mental Health: http://www.cimh.org/downloads/The%20Infant,%20Preschool,%20Family,%20Mental%20Health%20Initiative%20Compendium%20of%20Screening%20Tools%20for%20Early%20Childhood%20Social-Emotional%20Deve.pdf

Speckman, N. J., Goldberg, R. J., & Herman, K. L. (1992). Learning disabled children grown up: A search for factors related to success in the young adult years. *Learning Disabilities Research and Practice, 7*, 161–170.

Stanton-Salazar, R. D. (2011). A social capital framework for the study of institutional agents and their role in the empowerment of low-status students and youth. *Youth & Society, 43*(3), 1066–1109.

Starr, E. M., Foy, J. B., Cramer, K. M., & Singh, H. (2006). How are schools doing? Parental perceptions of children with Autism spectrum disorders, Down syndrome and learning disabilities: A comparative analysis. *Education and Training in Developmental Disabilities, 41*(4), 315–332.

Stewart, K. (2007). *Helping a child with nonverbal learning disorder or Asperger's disorder: A parent's guide* (2nd ed.). Oakland, CA: New Harbinger Publications.

Stothers, M. E., & Cardy, J. (2012). Oral language impairments in developmental disorders characterized by language strengths: A Comparison of Asperger syndrome and nonverbal learning disabilities. *Research in Autism Spectrum Disorders, 6*(1), 519–534.

Tanguay, P. (2000). Pervasive developmental disorders: A 10-year review. *Journal of the American Academy of Child and Adolescent Psychiatry, 39*(9), 1079–1095.

Teeter, P. (2009). Neurocognitive interventions for childhood and adolescent disorders: A transactional model. In C. R. Reynolds, E. Fletcher-Janzen (Eds.), *Handbook of clinical child neuropsychology* (3rd ed.) (pp. 427–458). New York, NY US: Springer.

The behavior analyst certification board. (1998). *BACB Newsletter.* Retrieved October 08, 2011, from The Behavior Analyst Certification Board®, Inc: http://www.bacb.com/newsletter/BACB_Newsletter_05_2011.pdf

Troiano, P. F., Liefeld, J. A., & Trachtenberg, J. V. (2010). Academic support and college success for postsecondary students with learning disabilities. *Journal of College Reading and Learning, 40*(2), 35–44.

Truesdale-Kennedy, M., McConkey, R., Ferguson, P., & Roberts, P. (2006). An evaluation of a family-centred support service for children with a significant learning disability. *Child Care in Practice, 12*(4), 377–390.
Tuller, B. J., Olvera, D. S., & Scott Kelso, J. A. (2007). The influence of instruction modality on brain activation in teenagers with Nonverbal learning disabilities: Two case histories. *Journal of Learning Disabilities, 40*(4), 348–359.
Valås, H. (2001). Learned helplessness and psychological adjustment II: Effects of learning disabilities and low achievement. *Scandinavian Journal of Educational Research, 45*(2), 101–114.
Vallabha, T. (2003). Perception of facial affect: A functional magnetic resonance imaging study of adolescents and adults with and without nonverbal learning disabilities. *Dissertation Abstracts International, 64*.
van der Mars, H., & Butterfield, S. A. (1987). The Effects of a Performance Base Curriculum on the Gross Motor Development of Preschool Children during Teacher Training: A Pilot Study.
van Garderen, D. (2006). Spatial visualization, visual imagery, and mathematical problem solving of students with varying abilities. *Journal of Learning Disabilities, 39*(6), 496–506.
Vogel, S. A., Hruby, P. J., & Adelman, P. B. (1993). Educational and psychological factors in successful and unsuccessful college students with learning disabilities. *Learning Disabilities Research and Practice, 8*(1), 35–43.
Walbeck, D., Menlove, R., Garff, T., Menlove, S., & Harris, S. (2003). *What preservice and first year teachers need to know to survive and thrive.* In: Rural Survival. Proceedings of the Annual Conference of the American Council on Rural Special Education (ACRES) (23rd, Salt Lake City, Utah, March 20–22, 2003).
Wang, K., & Dovidio, J. F. (2011). Disability and autonomy: Priming alternative identities. *Rehabilitation Psychology, 56*(2), 123–127.
Westendorp, M., Hartman, E., Houwen, S., Smith, J., & Visscher, C. (2011). The relationship between gross motor skills and academic achievement in children with learning disabilities. *Research in Developmental Disabilities: A Multidisciplinary Journal, 32*(6), 2773–2779.
Whitehead, J. (2007). Telling it like it is: Developing social stories[TM] for children in mainstream primary schools. *Pastoral Care in Education: An International Journal for Pastoral Care & Personal-Social Education, 25*(4), 35–41.
Wiener, J. A. (1998). Parents' perceptions of the quality of friendships of their children with learning disabilities. *Journal of Learning Disabilities Research, 13*, 242–257.
Williams, S. (2010). Student with Asperger's overcomes obstacles: Devon's journey to independence. *Exceptional Parent, 40*(9), 23–24.
Williams, J. K., Richmond, L. C., & Yarbrough, D. B. (1992). Comparison of visual-spatial performance strategy training in children with turner syndrome and learning disabilities. *Journal of Learning Disabilities, 25*(10), 658–64.
Wilson, P. H., & McKenzie, B. E. (1998). Information processing deficits associated with developmental coordination disorder: A meta-analysis of research findings. *Journal of Child Psychology & Psychiatry & Allied Disciplines, 36*(9), 829–840.
Winner, M., & Crooke, P. J. (2011). Social communication strategies for adolescents with Autism. *ASHA Leader, 16*(1), 8–11.
Winterowd, C. L., Street, V. L., & Boswell, D. L. (1998). Perceived social support, disability status, and affect in college students. *Journal of College Student Psychotherapy, 13*(2), 53–70.
Wright, D. C. (2008). Nonverbal learning disability in the classroom: An assessment of teachers' knowledge. *Dissertation Abstracts International Section A, 69*.
Young, K. (2008). Narrative practice at a walk-in therapy clinic: Developing children's worry wisdom. *Journal of Systemic Therapies, 27*(3), 54–74.
Zwart, L. M., & Kallemeyn, L. (2001). Peer-based coaching for college students with ADHD and learning disabilities. *Journal of Postsecondary Education and Disability, 15*(1), 1–15.

Chapter 8
The Role of the Educational Therapist: Academic Interventions for Reading and Writing

Marion Marshall

What Is an Educational Therapist?

"Educational Therapy serves children and adults with learning disabilities and other learning challenges and provides a wide range of intensive, individualized interventions designed to remediate learning problems." (http://www.aetonline.org). Educational therapy demystifies learning problems and stimulates clients' awareness of their strengths so they can use those strengths to their best advantage. "Educational therapists create and implement a treatment plan that utilizes information from a variety of sources including the client's social, emotional, psychoeducational, and neuropsychological contexts" (http://www.aetonline.org).

Educational therapists are trained to address a variety of issues that affect learning. These include learning disabilities (dyslexia, nonverbal learning disorder, reading, written language, math), attention deficit disorder, language processing difficulties, and difficulties with executive functioning. Some educational therapists also provide formal assessments, but all educational therapists engage in diagnostic teaching within each session and seek to maximize the learning possible in each session. "They recognize that additional issues may emerge over time or as demands increase or change .... There is ongoing analysis of data in order to adjust, adapt or revise a treatment plan" (http://www.aetonline.org). Learning goals are matched to the most effective strategies and materials for each individual client. An educational therapist may also serve as the case manager. In this capacity the educational therapist seeks to promote partnerships and collaboration among all relevant parties of allied professionals. The educational therapist "will also signal when it is time to refer to outside professionals and will help to locate and make appropriate referrals to other practitioners" (http://www.aetonline.org).

M. Marshall, M.S., B.C.E.T., F.A.E.T. (✉)
Holy Names University, 3500 Mountain Boulevard, Oakland, CA 94619, USA
e-mail: marionmarshall@comcast.net

J. Broitman and J.M. Davis (eds.), *Treating NVLD in Children: Professional Collaborations for Positive Outcomes*, DOI 10.1007/978-1-4614-6179-1_8,

In addition to the one-to-one work conducted in individual sessions, educational therapists can serve as *learning specialists* in independent schools. Some of these positions are full-time, but the greatest number is part or half-time positions. Learning specialists can benefit the entire school community. As every school (public or private) has a unique culture and a student body, serving as part of the staff ensures that an educational therapist knows that school's expectations and the recommendations made can match the school's culture. They support the workings of the school as a whole, serve as part of the admissions team, assess individual students, provide staff development and training, and have regular parent contacts. Some school learning specialists work with small groups of children to facilitate their learning and some work directly with individual students, depending on the school's model. They can also answer teachers' questions and problem-solve about individual students. Some teach in the regular classroom to model additional strategies. When a teacher knows how to effectively support an individual student, those skills becomes a part of their professional knowledge.

Many students with learning issues are already overwhelmed by having to work much harder to keep up academically; then, they see a specialist after school. This greatly extends their school day. Not only is this taxing, but it also does not afford them the same opportunities for sports, recreation, music, individual creative pursuits, or much-needed *downtime* as their peers, not to mention starting their homework. Meeting with an educational therapist at a school site can allow the student to be served during the school day.

Referral to an Educational Therapist

When students are referred to an educational therapist for academic interventions, strategies are individualized with the goal of addressing the underlying learning processes while improving skills. Students are taught *how to learn* in remediation sessions. An effective educational therapist stresses *when* and *how* to apply strategies so that the student can use them independently and outside of the clinical setting (Ahern & Marshall, 2005).

According to clinical observations, students are referred for difficulties with written output, *messy* papers, or disorganized work often before a formal identification of NVLD is made. If the handwriting is very labored, the ET may make a referral to an OTR. Commonly, the student with NVLD is referred to an ET because of math difficulties. Many will be referred with issues in reading comprehension. When reading narrative literature, skills such as understanding character development, perspective taking, and summarization are lacking. Other students are referred when their courses require them to understand expository texts. Notetaking is challenging due to difficulties with saliency determination. Lastly, some will come to an ET because of the demands of organizing essays. When social issues are evident, the student is referred onto a SLP or psychologist. The ET may serve as the case manager or as an integral member of the student with NVLD's *support team*.

Research on Reading and Writing Interventions

A careful review of the literature found few articles specific to students with NVLD (Chow & Skuy, 1999; Clayton & Dodd, 2005; Cornoldi et al., 1999; Davis & Broitman, 2006, 2007, 2011; Liddell & Rasmussen, 2005; Palombo, 1996; Rourke & Tsatsanis, 1996; Stein et al., 2004; Tuller et al., 2007; Vacca, 2001; Volden, 2004; Warren, 2006). Even so, most of these were concerned with describing NVLD or defining possible subtypes. Nearly all of these comingled students with NVLD with Asperger's syndrome. There were only two articles that described very general strategies for students with NVLD (Poole, 1997; Thompson, 1985). However, in this era of "research-based" interventions, there is ample research for "what works" to improve reading comprehension skills (National Reading Panel Report, 2000) and these same practices may well benefit students with a learning disability (National Reading Panel Report, 2000). Similarly, effective interventions for increasing writing skills have been studied (Writing Next, Graham & Perin, 2007) and there is strong link between effective practices for non-LD student and the student with a learning disability (Effective Instruction for Adolescent Struggling Readers: A Practice Brief, Boardman et al., 2008). Additionally, there is a growing body of evidence that when readers are instructed in writing and use their reading texts (fiction and expository), reading comprehension improves (Writing to Read, Graham & Hebert, 2010). However, giving the paucity of intervention research with children with NVLD, we cannot be certain that all these "proven" strategies will work well for this population.

Reading Comprehension Research

As a part of the National Institute of Child Health and Human Development, the National Reading Panel, 2000 (http://www.nationalreadingpanel.org/publications) was charged with studying effective, "research-based" instructional practices. It described reading comprehension as a complex process but defined it as the "essence of reading." The authors further defined it as intentional thinking during which meaning is constructed through interactions between text and reader, borrowing from the definition offered by Durkin (1993). According to this Durkin meaning resides in the intentional, problem-solving, thinking processes of the reader that occur during an interchange with a text. The content of meaning is influenced by the text and by the reader's prior knowledge and experience that are brought to bear on it. Reading comprehension is the construction of the meaning of a written text through a reciprocal interchange of ideas between the reader and the message in a particular text. The Panel reviewed 203 studies of instruction of reading comprehension that met their stringent criteria for a being a well-designed study. That report, "Teaching Children to Read: Evidence-Based Assessment of the Scientific Research Literature on Reading and Its Implications for Reading Instruction," is available online (http://www.nichd.nih.gov/publications/nrp/upload/ch4.pdf) or through NIH Publication (No. 00-4769). The Panel identified 16 different types of practices designed to increase reading comprehension. Of those 16 types of instruction,

Table 8.1

National Reading Panel strategies	Technique
Comprehension monitoring in which the reader learns how to be aware or conscious of his or her understanding	Collaborative Strategic Reading: *Click and Clunk*
Cooperative learning in which readers work together to learn strategies in the context of reading	Educational therapist as partner
Graphic and semantic organizers that allow the reader to represent graphically the meanings and relationships of the ideas	Reduce the number of types; simply all graphics; use 3-dimensional models first
Story structure from which the reader learns to ask and answer who, what, where, when, and why questions about the plot and, in some cases, maps out the time line, characters, and events in stories	Two-column notetaking; use of "sticky notes"; teach text structure
Question answering in which the reader answers questions posed	Question–Answer Relationships (QAR)
Question generation in which the reader asks himself or herself what, when, where, why, what will happen, how, and who questions	Right-hand column in two-column notetaking
Summarization in which the reader attempts to identify and write the main or most important ideas	Collaborative Strategic Reading: *Get the Gist*
Multiple-strategy instruction that is flexible as to which strategies are used and when they are taught over the course of a reading session	Teach each strategy in isolation until mastery achieved; use texts at independent reading level

only eight offered a clear scientific basis for concluding that they actually improved comprehension. Those eight strategies are summarized briefly in Table 8.1. The techniques covered in this chapter discuss how to adapt or modify these techniques for instructing students with NVLD. The Center on Instruction (COI) prepared a practice brief which evaluated research specific to reading comprehension strategies for the student with a LD. The COI is *a cutting-edge collection* of research-based effective practices. The COI is funded by the US Department of Education with the mission of disseminating scientifically based resources on instruction in pursuit of high-quality instruction. The brief on effective reading comprehension strategies is available online (http://www.centeroninstruction.org/effective-instruction-for-adolescent-struggling-readers-a-practice-brief). Finally, the COI concluded that the review of reading comprehension studies with students with LD supports the use of the strategies recommended by the National Reading Panel which parallel those previously identified by Mastropieri and Scruggs (1997).

Writing Strategy Research

Graham and Hebert (2010) performed a meta-analysis of hundreds of studies of strategies designed to improve writing of *low achievers*, including those with identified learning disabilities, and identified 11 elements effective in helping adolescent students learn to write well.

Writing Next (2007) is available at http://www.all4ed.org/files. Of these 11, seven were selected for this chapter because they had been shown to be effective in clinical observations for 20 years by this practitioner.

The evidence-based strategies selected are:

1. Explicit teaching of writing strategies
2. Teaching summarization
3. Collaborative writing (with the educational therapist, as a "partner" rather than a peer)
4. Teaching the student to construct more complex sentences
5. Prewriting strategies which engage the student in activities designed to help generate or organize ideas
6. Inquiry activities which engage students in analyzing content materials
7. Writing for content learning, which uses writing as a tool for learning content material.

Teaching Writing to Support Reading Comprehension

In *Writing to Read: Evidence for How Writing Can Improve Reading*, Graham and Hebert (2010) performed a meta-analysis investigating whether writing about a text can improve reading comprehension. The studies included students in grades 1–12 who received writing instruction that was distinct from, rather than integrated with, reading instruction. Then, they contrasted those results with others where students had received instruction in writing which linked *meaningful connection with written texts*. Studies were included for analysis if they were published between 1930 and 2008, used an experimental or quasi-experimental design, and contained a reliable outcome measure of reading comprehension, word reading, or reading fluency. Graham and Hebert (2010) identified four practices as being effective. Listed, in order of effectiveness, they were:

1. Having students respond to text
2. Having students write summaries of a text
3. Having students write notes about a text
4. Having students answer questions about a text in writing or create and answer written questions about a text

A key finding was that if students received the kinds of instruction that enabled them to develop strong writing skills, "the evidence rather consistently indicated that writing can be used to bolster reading achievement" (Writing to Read p. 2). Of note, the common practice of having a student complete an outline or use a graphic organizer in preparation to summarize text was generally effective in improving reading comprehension for students in grades 3–12. "However, the effect on reading comprehension was stronger for elementary students than for middle and high school students" (Writing to Read p. 2). Writing to Read is available at http://carnegie.org/fileadmin/Media/Publications/WritingToRead_01.pdf.

Link from Research to Clinical Practice

Common wisdom holds that good teaching is multisensory. Nearly every IEP or list of recommendations for students with learning differences states that instruction would be systematic, structured, and multisensory (ldonline.org). Yet, as Thompson (1997) suggested this is not the *best practice* for students with NVLD. One of the ways to think about the student with NVLD's needs is to realize each has significant difficulties processing visual and spatial information. In fact, Davis and Broitman (2011) and Cornoldi, Rigoni, Tressoli, and Vio (1999) suggest that visual spatial issues are the core deficit of NVLD. A multisensory approach usually relies heavily on visual and verbal input. But it is considered *best practice* for children with NVLD to limit and/or simplify visual materials such as charts, graphs, tables, and graphic organizers.

For most educators, including special educators and educational therapists, the admonition not to use a visual combined with verbal instruction goes against the much of their previous teaching. The profile of the student with NVLD is difficult to understand. An example will illustrate this. Just prior to working with a NVLD student, this educational therapist had begun assisting a school to understand the unique needs of a child with low vision. Acting upon the recommendations of a vision specialist, we began experimenting with just how large a font must be for this student to be able to see clearly. Similarly, it was nearly intuitive and easily grasped that this child would not benefit from viewing cluttered charts, graphs, and illustrations. Verbal explanation would be best. It followed that certain aspects of the school day would prove more challenging. Physical education activities needed to be modified. Art activities were simplified. Time to learn to navigate through the campus was expected. Books were made available on audiocassette or CD and extra time was readily granted as listening or reading took longer. All of these *special* modifications seemed intuitive, reasonable, and justified. There was no grumbling about the extra effort needed to accommodate the student's needs.

Having just worked through the needs of the visually impaired child, this educational therapist was struck by how similar these accommodations would be to those needed for the newly identified child with NVLD. The child with NVLD needed more white space on many of her papers, assignments needed to the enlarged, verbal explanation was needed to explain charts and graphs; PE and art would need to be modified and she would need some special training to navigate the campus. She, too, would benefit from audio books. It would take a similar amount of time to experiment and customize the accommodations and modifications that would work best for her learning. Ironically and sadly, the staff had more difficulty accommodating to the needs of the child with NVLD. Her learning differences did not seem to equate to the needs of the child with low vision. The staff did not respond as warmly or readily to this student's needs. It was evident that her learning profile was much harder to grasp.

The issue of how to use visual materials such as charts, graphs, tables, and graphic organizers with children with NVLD will be addressed later in this chapter.

This educational therapist has had success teaching students with NVLD to use these tools if three-dimensional practice occurred first. It seemed that the *hands-on* approach was not the key. Rather, it was the "real life" three-dimensional exploration that was critical to create understanding and usefulness (Bruner, 1966).

Writing

Although students with NVLD are highly verbal, they are not always articulate when writing for many reasons. Mastering basic handwriting skills is difficult. Many are drawn to novel or original ideas and do not like having their work edited. Some write in a very formulaic manner, more akin to making a list. Paragraphs are generally not well sequenced and may contain ideas that are not germane. Difficulties with sequencing, flow, and topic maintenance are usually evident. Often, all ideas seem to be of equal importance to the student with NVLD. Items of personal interest are viewed as valid and weighty as those that are more on-topic. Additionally, most students with NVLD struggle with writing because of the motoric component and because it requires simultaneous integration of skills (clinical observation).

Handwriting

Most highly verbal students with NVLD truncate their writing in order to decrease the effort required to use the pencil (clinical observations). Commonly, language is simplified and ideas are expressed in almost telegraphic style. In the beginning stages of writing, difficulties with visual motor integration and pencil control can mar their efforts. But the issue is not theirs alone. According to Gladstone (2010. http://www.nea.org), many teachers received no instruction in how to teach handwriting in the teacher education courses leading to earning a teaching credential. In a study by Graham, professor of Special Education at the University of Maryland, about three-quarters of the elementary school teachers he surveyed, believed that they were inadequately prepared to teach handwriting (Graham, 2010).

Some schools do not instruct students in handwriting or in making the basic strokes, claiming that handwriting instruction is archaic and unnecessary. Others teach handwriting in isolation. Students will receive 20–30 min of instruction per week. Although basic letter formation and proper stroke techniques are demonstrated, they are not integrated into daily written work. So, students tend to go back to the ways that they intuited a letter must be formed. Usually, this results in inefficient and laborious handwriting. Even for students without fine motor difficulties, the ratio of minutes per week spent in handwriting practice and the minutes spent in writing is paltry. For the student, with NVLD, this amount of instruction is nowhere near adequate.

Written language disabilities are very common in students with learning identified learning disabilities (Berninger, 1998). The University of Washington research program on writing disabilities, funded by the National Institute of Child Health and Human Development, identified several reasons for writing difficulties. The second applies to those with NVLD, "processing problems related to handwriting, spelling and composition due to orthographic or phonological coding, fine motor planning, automatic letter retrieval and production, and working memory" (Berninger, 1998).

Many processes undergird handwriting. Postural control, the vestibular system, vision, fine motor development, and language are some of these (Olsen & Knapton, 2008). The students who struggle with fine motor control find that the pencil is not an efficient tool, nor is using it comfortable or natural. Many schools have embraced the handwriting program developed by Jan Olsen, occupational therapist, OTR, *Handwriting Without Tears* (HWT). According to Olsen and Knapton (2008), the following skills are needed to achieve speed and legibility: memory, the ability to visualize a letter or number quickly without seeing it; orientation, ability to print letters and numbers without reversals; placement, the ability to follow lines and place letters and numbers correctly on the baseline; size, make letters in a consistent size; start, begin all letters and numbers at the top; sequence, letter parts in the correct order and direction; control, print letter parts neatly with overlaps or extra motions; and spacing, keep letters in a word close enough and leave spaces between words in sentences.

According to clinical observation, group instruction in the classroom may not work for the student with NVLD. "Handwriting requires cognitive, motor, and visual recall skills. Therefore, the lesson should be multisensory" (Kindergarten Teacher's Guide (2008), Guide to Multisensory Lesson and Activities, p. 9).

All of the most commonly used handwriting programs, such as HWT, D'Nealian, Zaner–Bloser, and Loops and Groups, assume that the student knows basic directional positional skills and can, first, orient to their body and then to a chalkboard or writing surface. All employ the ability to visualize and translate the basic directional positional words onto paper and rely heavily on the student's ability to visualize the words governing spatial orientation in relation to self or to letter formation. These underlying skills emerge as significant impediments for the student with NVLD.

Another example from HWT illustrates this. It is the rhyme used to help students remember how to form the number 4. "Down and over, down once more, that's the way to make a four." Although the child with NVLD can readily recite the rhyme, it does not guide how to execute the numeral if the concepts "down" and "over" are not understood as they apply to a paper and pencil task.

Piaget & Inhelder (1971) theory might suggest that the lack of physical exploration and experiences in the toddler and preschool years contributes to struggles with handwriting. Most toddlers go through the sensorimotor stage where exploration of the physical world sets the stage for an inherent understanding of spatial positioning. This educational therapist recalls swinging in the backyard. If one pumped especially vigorously, the swing would be parallel to the rooftop of my single-story home. Basic directional and positional vocabulary such as "up," "above," "down," "below," and "beneath" became understood.

Research measuring handwriting fluency (Graham, Berninger, Abbott, Abbott, & Whitaker, 1998) of elementary students found that the lack of handwriting fluency accounted for 25–42% of the variance of writing quality. A lack of automaticity affected writing output and the overall quality of the students' written work.

Many students with NVLD will be referred for consultation or remediation with an occupational therapist (Davis & Broitman, 2011). Working with an occupational therapist to improve handwriting skills is often helpful. For others, it may lead to limited fluency. Then, the goal should be to stabilize handwriting skills so that work is legible to the student and others. Learning to word process is most beneficial for the long term. Without an understanding of the causes of the discrepancy between a very verbal child and limited written output, the student with NVLD may be viewed as messy, willful, lazy, or uncooperative.

The Link Between Reading and Writing

Most educators know the veracity of the phrase *learning to read* and then *reading to learn*. The phrase underscores that students originally learn basic reading skills but need to segue into comprehending written factual information independently to accumulate knowledge. Those students who have not established basic reading skills become overwhelmed when the expectation changes. Writing contains a parallel process. Initially, students learn the mechanics of writing and explore the processes of putting thoughts to paper. Students learning *to write* practice the mechanics of writing including handwriting, spelling, capitalization, and punctuation. Soon, students will be asked to write to demonstrate what they have learned. When writing is combined with reading, it enriches reading comprehension. If one must write about something just read, it increases the depth of thinking, allows for greater recall, and generally clarifies understanding of the material (Wallace, Pearman, Hail, & Hurst, 2007). Clinical observations had suggested that that there was a significant intersection between the strategies for increasing reading comprehension and in prewriting strategies. Recent research has confirmed this clinical practice (Wallace et al., 2007). Yet, most often reading comprehension instruction is not paired with writing instruction. Sadly, this is a missed opportunity. In general, linking *writing to learn* with reading can strengthen reading comprehension by developing pivotal skills such as summarizing, thinking from multiple perspectives, and organizing thoughts. Fortunately, the strategies to enhance reading comprehension also support writing. *Cross-training* is not only desirable; it is an efficient use of time.

Effective Practices

What follows is a discussion of various effective techniques and how to introduce or teach each. The use of graphic organizers as a tool to organize writing and support executive functioning is described. Graphic organizers that allow for isolating essential facts for comparing or contrasting are detailed. Graphic organizers that effectively teach rising action and cause and effect in a novel are illustrated. The graphic organizer for teaching the Four Square Writing Method is described; teaching elaboration of a student's written work is discussed. Effective techniques for improving reading comprehension of both narrative and expository texts are described. Techniques that teach essential skills such as summarization and notetaking are explained.

Graphic Organizers

For most developing writers, using graphic organizers is a well-regarded practice for organizing ideas (http://www.readwritethink.org, a joint publication of the International Reading Association and the National Council of Teachers of English). Despite their visual and holistic format, clinical observations suggest that students with NVLD can learn to use graphic organizers. However, each needs to be visually simplified and the purpose clearly identified to the student. Ample time should be allowed to practice with the graphic organizer. Each type should be very familiar before introducing a different organizer. Lastly, for this population, clinical observations suggest that, as with visual aids, it is necessary that the graphic organizer be experienced as a three-dimensional model first.

Compare and Contrast

Most educators find that compare and contrast is an important tool to organize student writing. In the book Organizing Thinking, it is the first type of graphic organizer presented because it "can be used to clarify content" (p. 6) and serve as a "metacognitive tool" (p. 2). Many educators use a simple T-shaped graphic organizer. Before teaching a student with NVLD to employ a two-dimensional paper and pencil graphic organizer of the T design, as suggested above, a three-dimensional model may be a better place to start. For instance, a wood and acrylic edged T square could be used to demonstrate this for the student. One clinical strategy is to use small "sticky notes" to label the contrasting sides. For a fifth-grader studying Colonial America, the left hand of the T bar might say "French colonies." The right-hand side would be labeled "English colonies." The student would revisit the text or class notes finding apt descriptions of each type of colony. Those pertaining to a French colony would be placed on the left side. Similarly, those describing an English colony would be placed on the right side. Using "sticky notes" affords the student with NVLD an opportunity to rearrange and re-sequence the notes on each side. Having spent time noting the essential aspects of each and specifying the differences enhances production. Once differences are demarked and understood, similarities can become more evident without blurring the distinctions. The descriptors of each colony that are similar are placed on the *neck* of the T. These items can be used to create the *similarities* paragraph. Once the student has had ample opportunity to practice and feels very comfortable with the physical model, a paper and pencil T graphic organizer can be utilized.

Kathy Allen (author of Star Shaped Pegs, Square Holes: Nonverbal Learning Disorders and the Growing Up Years, 1998) concurs with the use of three-dimensional models before moving to the typical visually based graphic organizers. She uses dominoes to represent cause and effect. She places four or five dominoes vertically so that when the first domino is pushed over it will start the tumbling action that eventuates in all the dominoes being knocked down. Then, they are righted. Note that is critical to select a reading passage that is at the student's independent reading level and that contains clearly demarcated events that lead to a conclusion. Later, Kathy rights the dominoes and asks the student to "place" a single event on each domino. As each event is stated, push it so that it topples into the next one. Typically, students very quickly understand the notion of cause and effect in a piece of literature, science, or history. Next, she creates a very simplified graphic organizer where there are erect dominoes and some beginning to tilt over. This becomes an effective graphic organizer for cause and effect.

For students with NVLD who struggle to follow the story line in a novel, this educational therapist employs a toy marble roll to demonstrate rising action. It is a vertical wooden structure with pathways that run zigzag down its face and ends with the marble rolling across a small xylophone. When the marble is placed on the first course, it quickly runs the zigzag and ends in a delightful tinny musical tumble across the keys of the xylophone. For students who have become accustomed to the domino graphic organizer, it is not a great leap to understand the rising action in a novel as viewed through a marble run. Once understood, a simple graphic organizer is employed which follows the zigzag pattern of the marble run. Although it may not look like a traditional graphic organizer to depict and record rising action, it is novel, memorable, and fun. As the toy has a limited number of courses for the marble to run, it becomes necessary for the student to judiciously select which are those events that create the rising action, and lead to the denouement and conclusion. This is an exercise in determining saliency.

The Four Square Writing Method

By far, the favorite technique of this educational therapist for teaching the writing process is the Four Square Writing Method, developed by Judith and Evan Jay Gould (1999). This educational therapist uses it because it is a highly effective way to teach organization of written language (McMackin & Witherell, 2005). Tomkins (2006) states that this methodology improves reading comprehension because it combines organizing writing while connecting thoughts. While all graphic organizers assist in organizing writing, few support the development of metacognitive

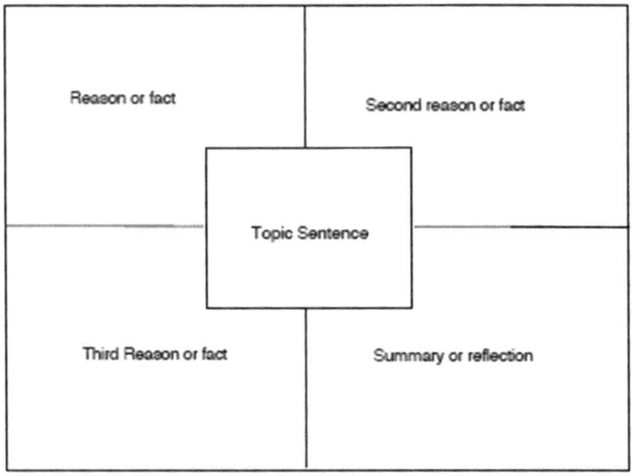

Fig. 8.1 Four Square Writing Method template

thinking as well as the Four Square method. "Writing facilitates learning by helping students explore, clarify, and think deeply about the ideas and concepts they encounter in reading" (Vacca & Vacca, 2004, p. 353).

The Four Square Writing Method is very versatile and useful for all types of writing: reading summaries, descriptive narratives, story writing, and expository tests. For students with NVLD their writing may be *list-like* and formulaic. This method may help students with NVLD to vary sentence structure, to improve vocabulary, and to elaborate simple ideas. It can be used to link four sentences together to create a simple paragraph. Later, it can be used to link paragraphs into cohesive essays. Clincial observation suggests that for many students with NVLD, their first well-constructed paragraph is a result of using this method. Later, a student can go back to each square adding additional detail thereby improving vocabulary or elaborating upon their initial ideas. A next phase of instruction would be to teach the explicit use of transitional or "signal" words to better link the writing in each square (see Fig. 8.1). For example, the topic sentence *Fall is my favorite season* is followed by a reason: *leaves change color* (upper left box); another reason: *the scent of wood burning fires* (upper right box); another reason: *apples ripen* (lower left); and a summary or personal reflection: *It is a cozy time of year* (lower right). This draft can be enhanced by the inclusion of transition words. The paragraph would now read, *Fall is my favorite season because the leaves change color. Next I enjoy the scent of wood burning fires. Also, apples ripen and are ready to be picked. Finally, it is a cozy time of year* (see Fig. 8.2).

Appendix B.6 (page 169) in the Wechsler Individual Achievement Test III manual gives a comprehensive list that can be customized to be appropriate for the grade level of your student. Students appear to enjoy having a long list or *menu* of transitional words and phrases from which to select. The list can be grouped into those that signal time (such as *finally, lastly, the next*) or words that are useful in mounting

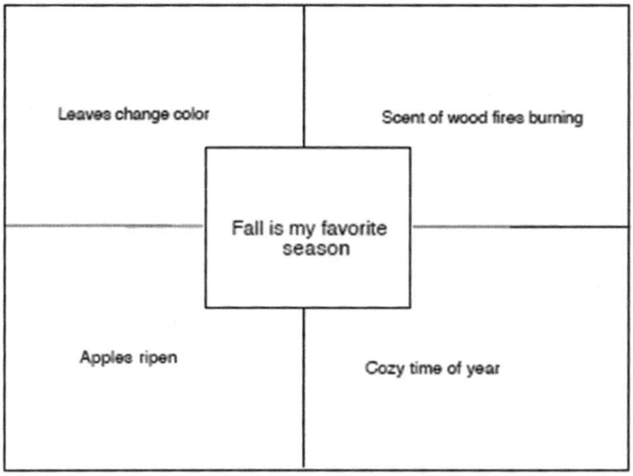

Fig. 8.2 Completed Four Square Writing Method template

an argument (such as *importantly, it follows that; consequently; not only; thus*) and those that are useful in compare and contrast papers (*similarly; conversely; on the other hand; in contrast*). In this way, the Four Square Writing process becomes more than a writing tool; it teaches organization of thought, which is essential for the student with NVLD who also often exhibit executive function issues (Davis & Broitman, 2011).

Some students are able to use the Four Square Writing Method immediately because the graphic organizer is so simple. Each of the four quadrants can be color coded for demarcation, as well. If not readily grasped, this practitioner employs a three-dimensional model. In the Bay Area, a bento box is commonly available. A bento box traditionally holds Japanese snack foods or a lunch. Each item is contained within a lacquered section. Its rigid walls and separation between foods is a good representation of the separation of ideas or "idea containment" within a paragraph (see Fig. 8.3).

If the student is writing about her dog, each space in the bento box will hold a strip of paper containing a phrase or sentence about her dog. Because the writing is on a slip of paper, they can be easily rearranged. This simple and physical introduction illustrates the development of a well-constructed paragraph. There is a topic sentence; sentences can be rearranged to create a better flow of ideas and each sentence can be augmented to improve vocabulary. Once the student has successfully used the bento box to create many well-crafted paragraphs, one can move to the visual graphic organizer typical in the Four Square Writing Method.

One of the problems utilizing this intervention is the issue of saliency determination, as many students with NVLD become enamored of some novel or idiosyncratically interesting idea (clinical observation). Most will argue vociferously for the inclusion of that idea, although it is off-topic or not germane. Attempts to discard or eliminate any such idea only yield more intensely emotional arguments. In order not

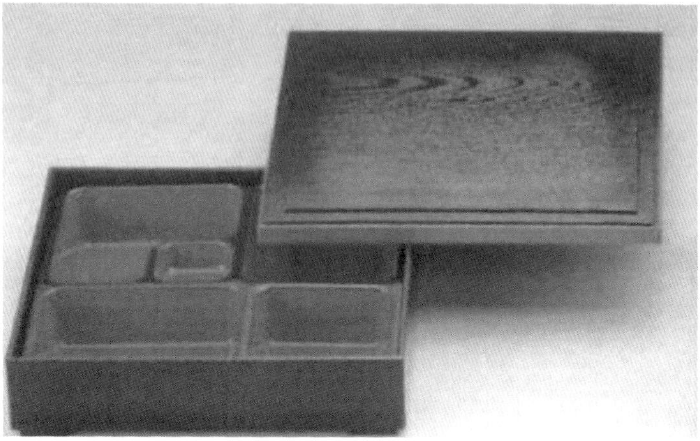

Fig. 8.3 Bento box from http://www.bookmice.net

to engage in wasteful time-consuming debates, one can create the space for these ideas to remain. Place them in the student's writing folder, or create a list of *really great ideas to explore later*. Or, write them down on *sticky notes* or slips of paper and safeguard these in a large envelope. This honors your student's interests and avoids wasting time, if those ideas are actually revisited at some point.

Teaching Elaboration

The Visualizing and Verbalizing (V and V) technique, authored by Nanci Bell (1991, 2007), is generally not successful in improving reading comprehension for the NVLD student, since it requires the ability to visualize (Thompson, 1997). But aspects can be a useful way to train students to augment their writing to become more descriptive. The list of *Structure Words* included in the V and V checklist is helpful. This educational therapist begins by using a physical object. The student describes it aloud. The student is encouraged to improve on the description by adding an element from the *Structure Words* list. For example, if the object was an apple and it had been described as *a red apple*, she could be asked to add in the shape or size.

Continue practicing with physical objects. Have the age-appropriate list of *Structure Words* available for reference. Use a laminated one but it can also be printed on a white board. Some students like to cross out or erase as they *punch up* their image. Next, one might select an object and describe it for the student. This educational therapist would purposely leave out some of the characteristics on the *Structure Words* list. To foster elaboration, this practitioner would ask the student to serve in the role of the teacher and prompt the practitioner to add to the description including more elements.

Later, this educational therapist would ask the student to choose some physical object from the room and place it behind a file folder that has been erected to service as a screen. Use some of the Lindamood–Bell terminology such as "Your description makes me see ...." Another variation is for the student to bring in a physical object from home, as some students reason that I'm familiar with all of the objects in my office and would have an unfair advantage in guessing. A detailed verbal description of her object is created, and one must guess what each object might be. This variation delights most students.

In the initial phases one should be prepared to prompt, praise, and record for the student. When the student becomes adept at using most of the age-appropriate descriptors, one can move on to asking the student to describe a picture, a character in a book, a specific place, or a memory. This type of practice answers the teacher's mandate to *describe, not tell* in creative writing.

Writing to Read

While educators may require students to answer comprehension questions related to a narrative passage or text, these tend to be short answer responses. Writing about texts in conjunction with the reading is one important way to significantly improve reading comprehension. Aukerman (2006) states that writing about texts helps readers solidify their interpretations and comprehension. Gammill (2006) finds that writing is "an excellent tool for building reading comprehension" (p. 754). "Writing to learn is writing for comprehension and provides students with an opportunity to recall, clarify and question what they have read" (Knipper & Duggan, 2006). Similarly, Fordham, Wellman, and Sandman (2002) note that "combining writing with reading enhances comprehension, because the two are reciprocal processes ... writing about it requires deeper processing than reading alone entails" (p. 151).

In the text, Writing for Comprehension, the authors, Wallace, Pearman, Hail, and Hurst (2007), state "many educators continue to treat reading and writing as separate subjects" (p. 41). These authors offer research-based writing strategies that teachers can use to improve student reading comprehension through writing. One key skill is summarization (Honig, Diamond, & Gutlohn, 2008). By definition, summarizing is where a reader can reduce a larger section of text into a much smaller one without any personal elaborations. The authors cite Winograd (1984) for this definition. Summarizing requires saliency determination which is the ability to separate important facts from less relevant information. According to clinical observations, summarization is particularly challenging for the students with NVLD. Specific facts may be recalled with great clarity but the main idea may be obscured facts of personal interest. Without understanding the whole, it is impossible to summarize. Like a skilled sophist, a student with NVLD will argue expressively to include some less than germane point.

Teaching Summarizing

Although students with NVLD are verbal, they can be overwhelmed by too much verbiage. That is why being able to summarize is so important. If one tries to hold onto and remember everything in a passage, the distinction between points becomes blurred. This can be likened to painting with watercolors; when one first dips the paintbrush into each separate color the colors are distinct. But if one continues to add more color or blend the colors, it can turn into a muddy gray. This is akin to what is happening when saliency is not easily determined.

When teaching a new skill such as summarizing, it is always important to use a text that is that at the student's independent reading level so that the student is concentrating on learning a new skill and not on decoding the passage (Honig et al., 2008). Select a passage that is likely to be of interest and is relatively short. After reading, ask the student to write down a single sentence that encapsulates the main idea of the passage. One may also scribe for the student. Sometimes it is helpful for you and the student to each write your own summary sentence independently. This allows for comparison. Some students learn to summarize by following your reasoning and examples. For others, learning this skill may take a great deal of time and patience. It is useful to ascertain whether the student can categorize. If this skill is missing or weak, it affects the ability to summarize (clinical observation). To address this, create a set. Have the student name the category and gradually include an item that does not belong. Ask him or her to identify what does not belong and state why not. Move to a list of facts. Include one that does not belong in the set. Make certain he or she can state why the fact is not relevant.

There is a playful way to try and mark the distinction between what is relevant and what is personally interesting. Ask the student to read the passage, instructing her to mark what is interesting. If done in tandem, practitioner and the student, it is likely that the exact same features were not highlighted. Then there can be a discussion about those differences. What one individual finds interesting may be unique to that person. One hundred different readers may mark different things in that same passage.

Next, select a topic. This is a first step prior to determining the main idea. Determine the topic and direct the student to find all related facts and mark those. At this point, one is practicing determining saliency and focal maintenance. Later, have the student mark what is interesting but require a second reading of the same passage. This time, give the instruction, "Mark what your teacher would put on a test." Compare the results. For many students this begins a glimmer of understanding between saliency and novelty.

In the Collaborative Strategic Reading model, a process called *Get the Gist* is employed. In this model, students are usually paired together to examine texts and to create an 11-word summary. For most students with NVLD learning this skill, collaborating with the therapist is more useful and productive than being paired with another student. The model asks the student to compare her summary to that of their partner. By limiting the number of words that can be used in the summary, the summarizer is forced to choose vocabulary carefully and identify only the key ideas (see page 30—how to teach *Get the Gist*).

Reading

Most students with NVLD appear to learn to *decode* readily especially when compared to their difficulties with handwriting and developing cohesive written language skills. However, as the text increases in length and the font size and becomes denser, many students with NVLD will struggle with reading fluency (clinical observation). Often this stems from an issue with visual efficiency. So, it may be useful to have a thorough vision exam that would include visual acuity, binocular vision, visual perception, visual efficiency, and tracking. Weaknesses can be addressed by exercises prescribed by a skilled developmental optometrist (Grisham, 1997).

Skilled readers employ several strategies to aid their reading comprehension. Prior to reading the passage, most students prepare by predicting what the title implies and accessing prior knowledge about that topic. While reading they engage in identifying main ideas and summarizing, evaluating their prior predictions, and measuring how well they are understanding the passage. After reading, he will reidentify main ideas, verify understanding, and attempt to synthesize new information with that already understood.

For many students with NVLD, there may be no reading difficulties until literature becomes more complicated and/or when students are asked to read expository text. Then, it may come as a surprise when the highly verbal student with NVLD struggles to comprehend what he or she has read. "The comprehension strategies, especially for struggling upper-grade students, needs to be explicit and scaffolded. The best intervention generally makes use of routines and repeated procedures, organizers, and visual aids. Instruction should include ample opportunities for monitored practice" (Honig, Diamond, Gutlohn, & Mahler, 2000, p. 16.16).

Reading comprehension is supported by visualization. Many readers seem to develop this skill naturally. Others can be taught to visualize as they read. Most educational therapists agree that attempting to teach visualization to the students with NVLD is not a useful practice (citation). So training in other techniques to improve reading comprehension becomes critical. The following strategies can be taught.

Notetaking as an Aid to Comprehension

To follow a detailed plot, the student should be encouraged to read "in chunks" and insert "sticky notes" at important passages or at the turning point in the plot. Together you can determine how long a "chunk" can be read and recalled. Different types of texts and those topics having disparate prior knowledge levels will determine the amount that can be read in one "chunk." This is an ongoing process to gauge and verify comprehension levels in different texts. Self-understanding may follow these type of metacognitive discussions led by the educational therapist. "This is your science text-right? What do you know/remember about ____________? How many paragraphs/pages do you predict you can read and remember the information?"

If the student is marking a chapter independently, the practitioner may be surprised to see how many places have been marked as "important." As noted above, many students with NVLD have difficulty determining saliency. All too often, nearly every word in a chapter will be highlighted. Reading comprehension suffers because saliency is not determined. Nothing stands out as important. All information is weighted equally. When this occurs, information is "blurred" in an indistinct mass. If this is the case, ask the student to use "sticky notes." This "sticky note" exercise can be very illuminating and diagnostic. The student must choose which parts to mark and be able to state why each selection was chosen. For some students you may choose to limit the number of notes for any one passage. In doing so, you are requiring the student to practice determining saliency. "Sticky notes" may need to be annotated. You may need to act a scribe. Most students benefit from creating a chapter summary using the succession of their "sticky notes." It is this clinician's experience that in the act of rereading the selected parts, the student will also have good recall for information or events not marked.

Annotated notetaking can be taught with the two-column method; this is a variation of the Landmark School's notetaking system, adapted for younger students, by this educational therapist. The left-handed column is where the student writes the page numbers and directly below records important ideas, plot development, and key information. In the second column (right side), the student records a question for the author, anticipates actions, or notes something that connects to prior knowledge or prior experience. Research has shown that reading comprehension is improved when the student makes a prediction about what will happen next (Honig et al., 2008). Interestingly, a prediction does not need to be accurate to increase comprehension and recall. By making a prediction, the reader is actively engaged with the text and that boosts comprehension.

By encouraging a student to formulate a question for the author, he or she can learn that authors often foreshadow important events or hint at character traits revealed in full, later. "Why did the author say the character had menacing eyes? Is the author hinting that person will do something mean?" "Oh! I was right! I was right! She so totally lied!" This type of active reading is the foundation of understanding inferences (see *Think like a Detective* in this chapter).

Teaching Question–Answer Relationships

Teaching Question–Answer Relationships (QAR) can be very helpful, as well. This technique was developed by Taffy Raphael in 1986 and was developed to enhance a student's ability to answer comprehension questions. This is based on the idea that there is a three-way relationship among the question, the text to which it refers, and the reader's prior knowledge (Honig et al., 2008). The effectiveness of the procedure lies in the way it clarifies how students can approach the task of reading texts and answering questions (Raphael, 1986). The QAR is a research-based technique that aims to clarify that the answers to questions come from different sources of information (Honig et al., 2008). Some answers can be found readily on one page of the text; others require the reader to piece together information located throughout the chapter. Another type of question assumes background knowledge. A different question is seeking an informed opinion. Both narrative and expository passages can be explored using the QAR strategy. Readers are taught to analyze the type of question being asked before searching for an answer (Raphael & Au, 2005). The simplest version of the QAR strategy teaches the student to sort questions into the following categories: Right There (the answer is located in a single sentence and reflects the wording of the question), Think and Search (the answer requires searching in different areas of the text or chapter), On My Own (the answer comes from the student's prior knowledge and may be an informed opinion), and the Author and Me (combines student's prior knowledge and text clues provided by the author).

Students enjoy separating analyzing the question from finding the answer. They find it curious and intriguing *not* to have to answer the question, merely to determine the question type. Clinicians can use file cards with each question type listed on a designated card. Practice identifying question types until each is recognized easily; then, the labeled cards are no longer needed. Using the QAR technique is one way to assist students in becoming strategic readers.

Additionally, students can be trained to *think like a detective*. Begin by displaying a picture of Sherlock Holmes, the famous deductive detective. Explain that many authors lay down clues for the reader to follow. This clinician lays a magnifying glass next to the text and asks the student to reread a passage where something of significance occurs. As the student improves in *detecting* clues and actively monitoring text in this way, engagement with the plot improves reading comprehension and recall. The second phase of this training requires only placing the magnifying glass on the table prior to beginning reading. This quietly reminds the student to *look for clues*. Later, student will use a blend of the *sticky notes* and will mark key places in the text with a quick sketch of a magnifying glass. So, as the student is reading, she is marking important information to recall the places where she believes the author has laid down an inferential clue. There are some commercial products that can be used to practice *thinking like a detective*. One example is the "Reading Detective" series with materials appropriate for grades 3–8 (Critical Thinking Company, publisher).

Text Types

To improve comprehension of expository texts, first instruct students to determine the type of text being read. This allows a student to read with greater understanding because he expects a text to reveal information in a predictable and predetermined manner. This sets up a schema for the reader to follow. A recent article published by the International Reading Association stated that "One of the most efficient strategies for which there is an influx of research and practice is training students on text structure knowledge to facilitate their understanding of expository texts" (*The Reading Teacher*, 64(5) p. 368).

There are specific types of texts and each has a unique organization. Knowing the organization allows for reading with increased understanding. For example, a descriptive passage is markedly different than a persuasive essay or a section describing a causal phenomenon. In determining what type of text will be read, the reader is better prepared to pay attention to the headings, key ideas, and features within the passage or chapter. The most common structures in textbooks are cause/effect, compare/contrast, description, problem/solution, and a time sequence. Teach students to recognize signal words that are typically linked with each type of text structure to help them learn the differences. For example, those associated with problem/solution are therefore, since, so, and as a result. Time order signal words include before, first, during, when, and finally.

Collaborative Strategic Reading

This educational therapist regularly employs two complementary strategies from *Collaborative Strategic Reading*: *Get the Gist* and *Click and Clunk* (Klingner, Vaughn, & Boardman, 2007) *Get the Gist* practices summarization. After reading a passage at the student's independent reading level, one writes a summary containing no more than 11 words. To accomplish this, one must select the most important ideas by determining saliency, refine one's thinking, use explicit vocabulary, and create complex sentences. It is more challenging than it sounds for all students and especially for the student with NVLD. The student creates a sentence and the educational therapist does the same. The two versions are compared and evaluated. Then, in collaboration, a new summarizing sentence is constructed. Individual vocabulary choices are weighed and essential ideas are debated.

Click and Clunk is an entry-level approach to teaching metacognitive skills. In a very playful way, it emphasizes self-monitoring while reading. Many students are in the habit of merely *reading until the end* of a chapter without realizing the *goal* of reading is to comprehend (clinical observations). Similarly many students with NVLD skip over words they can read but do not fully understand. In the *Click and Clunk* strategy, the student is instructed to say *Click* when something resonates with their prior knowledge or personal experience. One says *Click* when reading something that is recognized from another author, book, or source. The act of saying click and having to stop and explain the connection slows the reader down and emphasizes the connection. This educational therapist explains to the student that many reading comprehension strategies are like a *speed bump* on the street. What is a speed bump's purpose? To slow down the driver so she can navigate cautiously through a location. Similarly, metacognitive strategies slow a student down to encourage her to pay attention to *literary landmarks*, making the student a more careful and thoughtful reader. Stating the personal connections between prior knowledge or past learning reinforces the meaning in the text.

In contrast, one says *Clunk* if something is not clear or a word's meaning is not understood. Initially, the educational therapist may need to model the practice of saying *Click* and *Clunk* to demonstrate a *think aloud* approach to reading. This is a particularly useful technique for reading science and social studies texts where students are often reading *through the words* but not comprehending (clinical observation). It can be very illuminating for you and for the student to discover that *fluent sounding* reading actually contains many *clunks*. Recently, this practitioner read with a fifth grader who made no errors while reading his social studies text. But, when questioned he had understood very little. What happened? When asked to read back through the dense paragraph, it contained seven *clunks*. He explained he just “kinda skipped over words” he did not really understand. So that helped to explain the confusing discrepancy between his good reading comprehension for literature, where he had the background of the story, and his keen interest in each character to aid his understanding. But, when he skipped over seven key terms in the social studies text, he had little to no understanding and limited recall of what he had just read *fluently*.

Compare and Contrast While Reading

When teaching a new skill or strategy, it is always best practice to teach the new skill with material that is already familiar or at an independent reading level (Honig et al., 2008). This lowers the cognitive demand and creates more availability for thinking and attention to be directed towards the new skill (Ahern & de KIrby, 2012). In preparation for teaching the skill of comparing and contrasting information, especially in nonfiction texts, this educational therapist begins by using familiar folk stories such as Cinderella. The story of Cinderella is familiar to most English-speaking children. What many students may not know is that the Western European version derives its storyline from an ancient folktale that is known in nearly every culture. The educational therapist decides on the areas to compare (see Fig. 8.4). These are written in the center of the figure. The student reads through a text and finds the information. When the chart is completed, the content is well organized to make a comparison. It can be generated to compare similarities or differences. This type of graphic organizer spans many different curricular areas.

Perspective Taking

This is one of the most difficult aspects of reading comprehension to teach to the student with NVLD since viewing events from alternative perspectives can be very challenging (Davis & Broitman, 2011). Again, using a three-dimensional object, such as a stuffed lion, can be helpful. First, one faces the lion directly towards the student and asks him to describe it. The practitioner acts as scribe to record the student’s description. When the description is complete, the clinician turns the lion completely around so that only the back of the ears and tail are prominent. Repeat

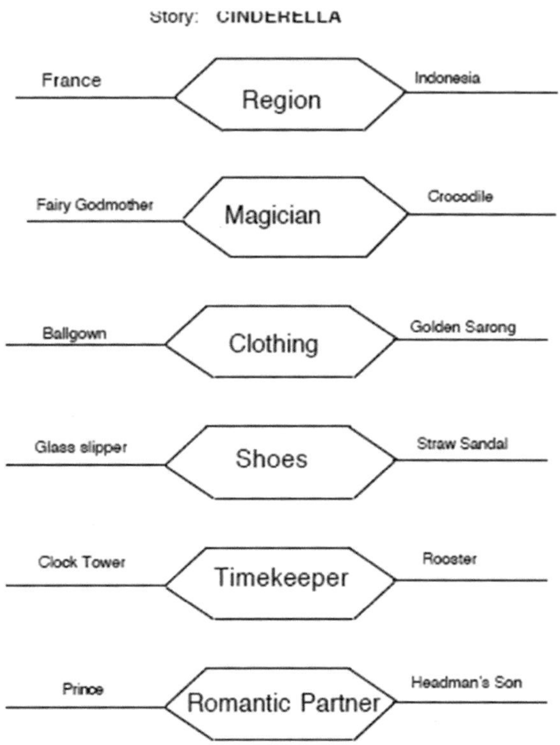

Fig. 8.4 Compare and contrast graphic organizer, adapted from organized thinking, book 2 (see Parks et al., 1990)

the request for the student to describe the lion. Record again. If successful, two completely different descriptions have emerged. Then the fun begins. Read aloud one of the descriptions and ask questions such as, "Is this is a correct description of the lion?" If the student agrees, read the second description aloud. Ask the same question, "Is this a correct description of the lion?" After receiving agreement, ask how that can be since the descriptions are so very different. One hopes to get the student to voice that each is description of the lion from a different perspective or viewpoint. If this is not clear, follow-up with other examples using concrete objects viewed from above or underneath.

A wonderful way to continue illustrating perspective is by using the book, *The True Story of the Three Little Pigs*!, as told by the wolf. Jon Scieszka (Viking, 1996) tells the familiar tale from the wolf's perspective. According to the wolf's recollection, what actually happened was that all that huffing and puffing was nothing but a bad cold that ended up in great big sneezes which unfortunately blew down the first two pigs' homes inadvertently crushing them. In the 10-year anniversary edition, dated 1999, there is a foreword by A. Wolf. In it the reader learns that *a confused little girl in a red riding hood* saw his picture in the paper and *made a tale* about the wolf dressing like her granny and scaring her with his big teeth. "Crazy. Would I do something like that?" This story illustrates the link between perspective taking and each character's perceptions in the same book.

For many students, these experiences are enough to begin to examine opposing viewpoints in history or in a piece of literature. Rosalyn Schanzer, author of the book *George vs. George—The American Revolution as Seen from Both Sides* (National Geographic Society, publisher, 2004), views the American Revolution as seen from the perspective of George Washington and the British King George III. In the introduction the following questions are posed: "Was King George a royal brute? American patriots said so but others hailed him as the father of the people. Was George Washington a traitor? The King supporters thought so. But many celebrated Washington as the father of his country. Who was right? There are two sides to every story" (p. 7).

For older students, using *Parallel Journeys* is recommended. This book is a factual account of two different youths during the same period of time—Nazi Germany during World War II. Each viewpoint is told in an alternating fashion, allowing for Helen's experience of being captured by the Gestapo to be contrasted with Alfons' obedience to Nazi ideals making him a high-ranking Hitler Youth (1995, Atheneum Books for Young Readers; Eleanor Ayer, author).

Conclusion

Although the learning profile for a student with NVLD is nuanced and complex, the remediation principles are not. Based on clinical observations conducted over the past 30 years, many of the recently identified evidence-based strategies and instructional methods can be successfully used or modified for the student with NVLD. During the past 10 years there has been a concerted effort to evaluate and document evidence-based instruction. The National Reading Panel published the *best practices* in reading (2000). Research-based strategies for improving student writing were published by Graham and Hebert in 2007. *Writing to Read* (2010) documented effective writing strategies that also improved reading comprehension. The National Reading Panel and *Writing to Read* reviewed the limited research for effective instructional practices for students with learning disabilities. Berninger and Graham have been documenting effective practices to improve handwriting. However, no research was located specific to *best practices* in language arts for students with NVLD. Until there is a repository of research specific to this group, practitioners will need to know the research about effective instructional practices, and adapt or modify them to provide effective interventions for the student with NVLD.

The educational therapist makes an ideal partner for practicing new techniques because she is more likely than a peer to follow the pace of the child with NVLD. Similarly, the educational therapist is likely more accepting and less judgmental of ideas and opinions than a fellow student. Further, the educational therapist's training in diagnostic and remedial instruction allows him to tailor the techniques to the individual student. So, while the student is learning these techniques, it is best to be done with the supportive adult.

To summarize, multisensory methodologies are not best practice. Reduce, eliminate, or *narrate* visual elements. Think about how you would modify a learning task for a student with low vision and be guided by that. Techniques that support reading comprehension also improve writing. Many students with NVLD need support in organizing and sequencing their writing before needing to improve reading comprehension. All the work you do in writing will support reading, too. *Cross training* is highly effective, in addition to being time efficient. Consider using three-dimensional models of graphic organizers before using simplified *paper and pencil* ones. Patient and playful interventions will yield results. Advances in assistive technologies (such as the *smart pen*) make capturing oral instruction and discussion possible while reducing the need for the student to *hold onto* everything. Teaching of essential skills, such as summarization and notetaking, has been detailed in this chapter. Clinical observations support that most of the evidence-based strategies to improve reading comprehension and written language are also useful for this population.

In conclusion, the educational therapist can be an effective educator for the student with NVLD. By using known *best practices*, and evaluating their usefulness with students with NVLD, a body of solid empirical knowledge about effective techniques will emerge that can be documented and shared.

References

Ahern, C., & de Kirby, K. (2012) Beyond individual differences organizing processes, information overload, and classroom learning. Springer.

Ahern, C., & Marshall, M. (2005). Understanding inconsistent academic performance in students: Integrating educational and neuropsychological perspectives. *The Educational Therapist, 26*, 1.

Allen, K. (1998). *Star Shaped Pegs, Square Holes: Nonverbal learning disorders and the growing up years*. Livermore, CA: Good Enough Books.

Association of Educational Therapists. (2011). *Educational therapy defined*. Retrieved February 11, 2011, from http://www.aetonline.org

Aukerman, M. (2006). Who's afraid of the big "bad answer"? *Educational Leadership, 64*, 34–41.

Ayer, E. H., Waterford, H., & Heck, A. (1995). *Parallel journeys*. New York: Antheneum.

Bell, N. (1991). *Visualizing and verbalizing: For language comprehension and for thinking*. Paso Robles, CA: Academy of Reading Publications.

Bell, N. (2007). *Visualizing and verbalizing: For language comprehension and for thinking*. Paso Robles, CA: Academy of Reading Publications.

Berninger, V. (1998). Assessment, prevention, and intervention for specific reading and writing disabilities. In B. Wong (Ed.), *Young children, learning about learning disabilities* (2nd ed., pp. 529–555). New York: Academic Press. Retrieved August 22, 2011, from http://www.wrightslaw.com.

Berninger, V., Graham, S., & Weintraub, N. (2001). The relationship between handwriting style and speed and legibility. *The Journal of Educational Research, 91*, 290–296. Retrieved August 22, 2011.

Boardman, A. G., Roberts, G., Vaughn, S., Wexler, J., Murray, C. S., & Kosanovich, M. (2008). *Effective instruction for adolescent struggling readers: A practice brief.* Portsmouth, NH: RMC Research Corporation, Center on Instruction.

Bruner, J. (1966). *Toward a theory of instruction*. Cambridge, MA: Harvard University Press.

Chow, D., & Skuy, M. (1999). Simultaneous and successive cognitive processing in children with nonverbal learning disabilities. *School Psychology International, 20*(2), 219.

Clayton, M. C., & Dodd, J. L. (2005). Nonverbal neurodevelopmental dysfunctions. *Pediatric Annals, 34*(4), 321–327.

Cornoldi, C., Rigoni, F., Tressoli, P., & Vio, C. (1999). Imagery deficits in nonverbal learning disabilities. *Journal of Learning Disabilities, 3*(1), 48–57.

Davis, J., & Broitman, J. (2006). A brief overview of nonverbal learning disorders. *The Educational Therapist, 27*(4), 5–10.

Davis, J., & Broitman, J. (2007). Nonverbal learning disabilities: Models of proposed subtypes, part II. *The Educational Therapist, 27*(4), 5–10.

Davis, J. M., & Broitman, J. (2011). *Nonverbal learning disability in children: Bridging the gap between science and practice*. New York: Springer.

Durkin, D. (1993). *Teaching them all to read* (6th ed.). Boston, MA: Allyn & Bacon.

Fordam, N. M., Wellman, D., & Sandmann, A. (2002). Taming the text; engaging and supporting students in social studies readings. *The Social Studies, 93*, 149–158.

Gammill, D. M. (2006). Learning the write way. *The Reading Teacher, 59*, 754–762.

Gladstone, K. (2010). *How to teach handwriting: Make handwriting instruction part of every school day*. Retrieved February 15, 2011, from http://www.nea.org/tools

Gould, J. S., & Gould, E. J. (1999). *The Four Square Writing method: A unique approach to teaching basic writing skills*. Carthage, IL: Teaching & Learning Company.

Graham, S. (2010). Want to improve children's writing? Don't neglect their handwriting. *American Educator, 33*(4), 23.

Graham, S., Berninger, V., Abbott, R., Abbott, S., & Whitaker, D. (1998). *The Journal of Educational Research, 91*, 5. Retrieved August 22, 2011, from http://www.sbac.edu.

Graham, S., & Hebert, M. A. (2010). *Writing to read: Evidence for how writing can improve reading. A Carnegie Corporation time to act report*. Portsmouth, NH: RMC Research Corporation, Center on Instruction.

Graham, S., & Perin, D. (2007). *Writing next: Effective strategies to improve writing of adolescents in middle and high school—A report to the Carnegie Corporation of New York*. Washington, DC: Alliance for Excellent Education.

Grisham, D. (1997). Which vision specialist should see your child? *International Dyslexia Association Newsletter*, 4–5.

Honig, B., Diamond, L., & Gutlohn, L. (2008). *Teaching reading sourcebook: For all educators working to improve reading achievement* (2nd ed.). Novato, CA: Arena Press.

Honig, B., Diamond, L., Gutlohn, L., & Mahler, J. (2000). *Teaching reading sourcebook: Sourcebook for kindergarten through eight grade*. Novato, CA: Arena Press.

Klingner, J. K., Vaughn, S., & Boardman, A. (2007). *Teaching reading comprehension to students with learning disabilities*. New York: Guilford Press.

Knipper, K. J., & Duggan, T. J. (2006). Writing to learn across the curriculum: Tools for comprehension in content area classes. *The Reading Teacher, 59*, 462–470.

Liddell, G. A., & Rasmussen, C. (2005). Memory profile of children with nonverbal learning disability. *Learning Disabilities Research and Practice, 3*, 137–141 (Blackwell Publishing Limited).

Mastropieri, M. A., & Scruggs, T. E. (1997). Best practices in promoting reading comprehension in student with learning disabilities: 1976 to 1996. *Remedial and Special Education, 18*(4), 197–214.

McMackin, M. C., & Witherell, N. L. (2005). Different routes to the same destination: Drawing conclusions with tiered graphic organizers. *The Reading Teacher, 59*, 242–252.

National Reading Panel. (2000). *Report of the National Reading Panel: Reports of subgroups*. Washington, DC: U.S. Department of Health and Human Services, National Institute of Health.

Olsen, J. Z., & Knapton, E. F. (2008). *Handwriting without tears: Kindergarten teacher's guide*. Cabin John, MD: HWT. http://www.hwtears.com.

Palombo, J. (1996). The diagnosis and treatment of children with nonverbal learning disabilities. *Child and Adolescent Social Work Journal, 13*(4), 311–332.

Parks, S., Parks, S., & Black, H. (1990). *Organizing thinking book II*. Pacific Grove, CA: Critical Thinking Press.

Piaget, J., & Inhelder, B. (1971). *Imagery and the child*. New York: Basic Books, Inc.

Poole, N. (1997). Remediation of nonverbal learning problems. *The Educational Therapist, 13*(3).

Raphael, T. E. (1986). Teaching question/answer relationships revisited. *The Reading Teacher, 39*, 515–522.

Raphael, T. E., & Au, K. H. (2005). Q.A.R. Enhancing comprehension and test taking across grades and content areas. *The Reading Teacher, 59*(3), 206–221.

Readwritethink.org. (2011). International Reading Association & National Council of Teachers of English. Retrieved on May 20, 2011, from http://www.readwritethink.org/classroom-resources

Rourke, B. P., & Tsatsanis, K. D. (1996). Syndrome of nonverbal learning disabilities: Psycholinguistic assets and deficits. *Topics in Language Disorders, 16*, 2.

Schanzer, R. (2004). *George vs. George: The American revolution as seen from both sides*. Washington, DC: National Geographic Society.

Scieszka, J. (1996). *The true story of the three little pigs*. New York: Viking Penguin.

Stein, M. T., Perrin, E. C., Wegner, L. M., Snyder, D. M., Glascoe, F. P., Wells, R. M., et al. (2004). Challenging cases: School problems with learning and behavior. *Pediatrics, 114*, 1448–1452.

Thompson, O. M. (1985). The nonverbal dilemma. *Journal of Learning Disabilities, 18*, 400–403.

Thompson, S. (1997). *The source for nonverbal learning disorders*. East Moline, IL: LinguiSystems, Inc.

Tomkins, G. E. (2006). *Literacy for the 21st century: A balanced approach*. Upper Saddle, NJ: Prentice Hall.

Tuller, B., Jantzen, K. J., Olvera, D., Steinberg, F., & Kelso, J. A. (2007). The influence of instruction modality on brain activation in teenagers with nonverbal learning disabilities: Two case histories. *Journal of Learning Disabilities, 40*(4), 348–359.

Vacca, D. (November 2001). Confronting the puzzle of nonverbal learning disabilities. *Educational Leadership, 59*, 26–31.

Vacca, R. T., & Vacca, J. L. (2004). *Content area reading: Literacy and learning across the curriculum* (8th ed.). Boston, MA: Pearson, Allen & Bacon.

Volden, J. (2004). Nonverbal learning disability: A tutorial for speech-language pathologists. *American Journal of Speech-Language Pathology, 13*(2), 128–141.

Wallace, R., Pearman, C., Hail, C., & Hurst, B. (2007). Writing for comprehension. *Reading Horizons, 48*(1), 41–56.

(2009) *Wechsler Individual Achievement Test* (3rd ed.). San Antonio, TX: Pearson.

Warren, R. (2006). Drawing on the wrong side of the brain: An art teacher's case for recognising NLD. *International Journal of Art & Design Education, 22*(3), 325–334.

Winograd, P. N. (1984). Strategic difficulties in summarizing text. *Reading Research Quarterly, 19*, 404–42. Resources.

Chapter 9
The Educational Therapist and Mathematics

Dianne Matthaei

Introduction

> I got a D- in algebra and it was a gift. A total gift. I have never been good at mathematics and I don't know why. I really do work at it, but things like fractions have never made sense. With a D- in algebra, how am I going to pass geometry? (Matthaei, 1)

How indeed? This quotation, from a tenth grader named Ryan, asks the questions many students with NVLD ask: "Why is mathematics so hard? How am I going to pass my math classes?" Students with NVLD often find, as Ryan did, that mathematics is a very difficult subject for them.

The core deficits of NVLD include visual–spatial and executive function difficulties; these difficulties significantly impact a student's progress in mathematics (Davis & Broitman, 2011; Forrest, 2004). The student with NVLD often presents with certain characteristics which affect his learning in mathematics.

D. Matthaei, M.Ed. (✉)
Annie Wright Schools, Tacoma, WA, USA
e-mail: dmatthaei@harbornet.com

J. Broitman and J.M. Davis (eds.), *Treating NVLD in Children: Professional Collaborations for Positive Outcomes*, DOI 10.1007/978-1-4614-6179-1_9,

Characteristics of an individual with NVLD

Characteristic	Description and examples
Difficulty with whole/part relationships	Often these students do not see the gestalt or overall picture. They seem to view all parts separately, not as a whole. They cannot accurately differentiate the parts from the whole. They see the *trees but not the forest* (Foss, 2006). They have an especially hard time learning math concepts, especially ones that rely on whole/part relationships such as fractions, decimals, and percentages.
Poor spacing and alignment	Individuals with visual–spatial difficulties often write calculation problems that drift over the page instead of staying proper vertical alignment.
Inaccurate skills for measurement	Individuals with NVLD experience difficulty lining up the ruler to accurately measure the length of a line. Concepts for units of measurement, such as an inch or a mile, frequently hold only a vague meaning for them. They struggle to accurately estimate length, distance, or weight (Neff, Neff-Lippman, & Stockdale, 2002).
Poor concept of time	Individuals with visual–spatial difficulties often cannot read an analog clock. They rely solely on digital clocks (Neff et al., 2002). They cannot estimate how long a given task might take. They report that they often are totally unaware of how much time has passed.
Difficulty with direction	Terms like north, south, east, and west have little meaning to these individuals. They can go from their home to point A and from their home to point B. They cannot go from point A to point B without returning home. They get lost often, even in their neighborhood or local grocery store. They report an inability to navigate even in familiar surroundings (Neff et al., 2002). Consequently, word or story problems involving direction, coordinate geometry, and trigonometry are very hard.
Inaccurate drawings even if motor skills are good	They often report frustration with their drawing. They will state that they know their drawing is not accurate, but they cannot figure out how to correct it. More severely affected individuals will report that their drawing is fine when it is fundamentally missing major elements.
Difficulty interpreting drawings and diagrams	Individuals with NVLD report that drawings are often just a bunch of lines. They need direct instruction in how a two-dimensional drawing relates to the three-dimensional object it represents. They often make errors in reading graphs and charts and tend to interpret them literally (Kozevnikov, Motes, & Hegary, 2006).

(continued)

Characteristic	Description and examples
Problems with visual overwhelm	Students with these difficulties cannot find the significant information on a workbook page with lots of distracting illustrations. A grade school youngster may not do all the problems on a workbook page because he did not even locate them. An older student may not be able to identify one angle in a group of angles. These individuals report fatigue and headaches when working with lots of visual information.
Deficits with imagery or the ability to form mental images	Students report difficulty with visual imagery, which is the mental representation of the visual appearance (shape, color, brightness) of objects. They experience some severe difficulty with spatial imagery, which refers to the spatial relationships of objects and the location of objects in space (Cornoldi, Rigoni, Tressoli, & Vio, 1999). The difficulty with imagery impacts a student's ability to form an accurate mental picture for the vocabulary of math and to visualize the relationships being described in a word problem.

The Research

Research into disabilities in mathematics did not emerge until the early 1990s (Berch & Mazzocco, 2007). Much of the research deals with mathematics at the elementary or middle school level. Little research has been conducted with high school students and the literature about mathematics-related disorders at the post-secondary level is scarce indeed (Sullivan, 2005). Even though there is "a paucity of research on MD (mathematical difficulties)" (Mazzocco, 2011), certain patterns are emerging about the relationship between mathematics and leaning disorders (Geary, 2004). These patterns guide practitioners to develop sound principles based on available research and best clinical practices.

Principles for Mathematics Instruction for Students with NVLD

> First, effective instruction to develop competency in mathematics needs to involve several important components including number sense, counting skills, math vocabulary, procedural skills, conceptual skills, fluency with math facts (number combinations), and skills for solving word problems (Steeves & Tomey, 1998).

These components can be represented in the following figure (Fig. 9.1).

These components must also be linked and connected with each other. For example, conceptual understanding must support procedural skills; otherwise, the

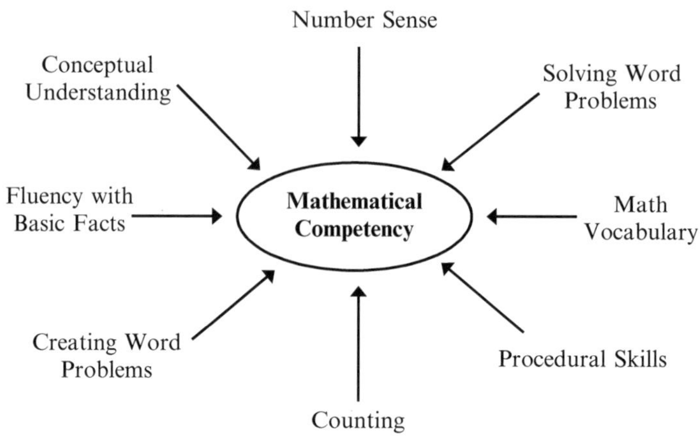

Fig. 9.1 Components of competency in mathematics

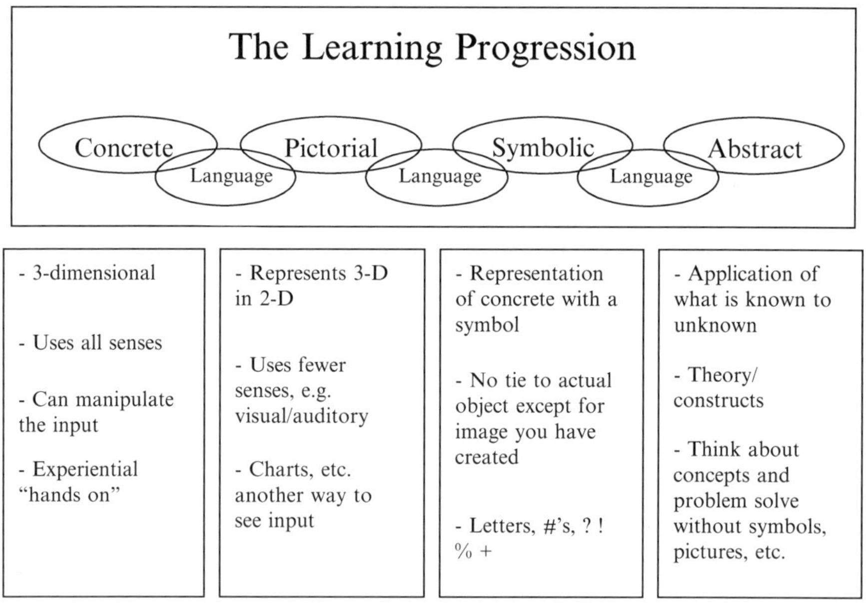

Fig. 9.2 The learning progression

procedural skills (calculation skills) will be learned rigidly and used narrowly (Steeves & Tomey, 1998).

Second, instruction needs to follow the progression of learning as shown in Fig. 9.2 (Matthaei, 2008). Specifically, instruction needs to start at the three dimensional, concrete level first before moving on the two dimensional level with pictures, diagrams, workbooks, and textbooks (Bruner, 1966; Steeves & Tomey, 1998).

The *learning progression* is also called the *abstractness continuum* (Miller, 2005). By either name, researchers agree that learning proceeds from the concrete level of actual three-dimensional objects, to the pictorial level using drawings, to the symbolic level using math symbols (=, +, −, %).

Physical objects and manipulatives need to be appropriately used with students with learning disorders for longer periods of time than is the common practice in most classrooms. Meaningful use of actual objects allows for better visualization when memory fails (Miller, 2005; Steeves & Tomey, 1998).

Since visualization or mental imagery is an especially difficult skill for individuals with NVLD (Cornoldi et al., 1999), starting with real objects becomes especially critical. After the student has had the opportunity to explore the objects, discuss their characteristics and how they look when drawn in two dimensions, they are ready to proceed with the mathematical concept or skill. They can make much more rapid progress than if instructors just start with the pictures in the workbook. For example, a middle school student with NVLD was struggling with the concept of total surface area of a box until he was given an actual box and encouraged to match the sides and vertices of the box with the drawing in his book. Then he said, "Oh, now I get it. There are six sides to this box even though you can't see all of them in the drawing. Top and bottom will be the same area. Opposite sides will be the same. You just have to find the area of all the sides and add them up." Instructors can move to the symbolic and abstract levels as long as they start at the concrete level for students with NVLD (Matthaei, 2008).

Third, the instruction must be specifically matched to the learning strengths as well as core deficits inherent to the profile of the individual with NVLD. Cornoldi et al. (1999) argue that there are strategies that are well matched to the student with NVLD, but they add an important caution; they state that, "Instructions which make tasks easier for other children were not only unable to help children with NVLD, the same instructions actually created confusion" (p. 55). Instructions and strategies must be fine-tuned to meet the needs of the learner with NVLD. For example, strategies need to be fine-tuned to help the student with NVLD acquire a comprehensive, applicable mathematical vocabulary.

Building Mathematical Vocabulary

In any discipline students need to learn the new terms that make up the vocabulary of that discipline. Marzano wrote about the dramatic difference that direct instruction in words specific to academic content can have on the students' abilities to learn that content (2003). To become competent in mathematics, students must learn the vocabulary of mathematics.

Students with NVLD are often adept at acquiring vocabulary. On quizzes and tests of math vocabulary such students often achieve high scores, especially if the test involves memorizing a definition or matching term and definition. Such high scores are desirable, of course, yet they often create the misleading impression that the student has an adequate, working knowledge of the vocabulary. Unfortunately for students with NVLD, this is not always the case.

Children and young adults with NVLD tend to memorize definitions well, but their understanding of the words is often rote, overly literal, and unable to see multiple dimensions (Foss, 2006). For example, a 9-year-old youngster may say, "The product is the answer to a multiplication problem." But if his homework assignment says, "Find the product of 3 and 6," he will often ask, "What am I supposed to do? Add?" The word "product" did not serve as a cue to multiply. Or a tenth grade student with NVLD may be able to write a perfect definition for "alternate exterior angles," but be unable to find them in a drawing.

Such high ability to recite accurate definitions coupled with low ability to apply those definitions is often baffling to regular education teachers. One geometry teacher describing his student said:

> Hailey could give definitions for the words, but she could not apply the vocabulary. She had a hard time understanding what a word or term looked like. She could repeat the definition, but not apply it … She couldn't correlate the vocabulary to a drawing. That was really hard for me as a teacher. Take for example, angle pair relationships. I would draw a pair of parallel lines cut by a transversal. She could give me a perfect definition of alternate exterior angles, but she couldn't find a pair of them on the drawing. That was just hard. (Matthaei, 2008)

This teacher identified a core characteristic of a student with NVLD. Students with this disorder have visual–spatial difficulties. The extent of the difficulty varies with each individual, but visual–spatial difficulties are a primary component of NVLD. So Hailey could define but not find the exterior angles. Her perception of visual–spatial tasks was not accurate or reliable for her; consequently, her memory for these tasks was not reliable either.

To help students like Hailey acquire a solid, useful vocabulary for mathematics, instruction often needs to start at the three-dimensional level as mentioned earlier. For example, to learn the terms "cube" and "cylinder," she needs to work with real cubes and cylinders. For some terms like exterior angles, she may only be able to start with a two-dimensional drawing, but it is vital that she links term, definition, and picture. The purpose of adding some kind of picture or drawing is to help ensure that the student forms a mental image for the term. Cornoldi et al. describe how difficult it is for NVLD children to form accurate, detailed images. They need instruction, tools, and practice to develop this skill carefully (1999).

Picture notes (Neff et al., 2002) are a valuable tool used to build imagery skills and link word to definition to image for math vocabulary. Picture notes are simple drawings or pictorial examples. They are one kind of nonlinguistic representation which Marzano (2003) listed as one of the nine categories of instructional strategies that yielded the greatest effect size in terms of student achievement. The picture is drawn on one side of a 3×5 in. index card, and the term is printed on the other side. Examples of picture notes are shown in Fig. 9.3.

The student looks at the picture and says the term. Sometimes the instructor would provide the definition orally and sometimes the student would give it. Saying the term (e.g., "cylinder") helped develop a more fluent recall. Often a student needed

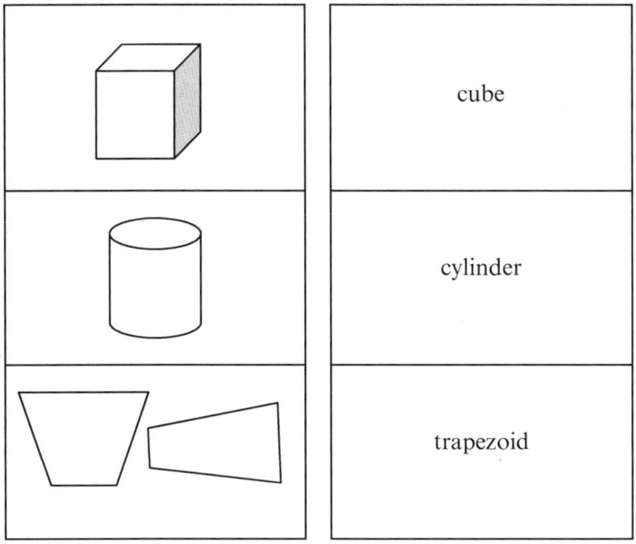

Fig. 9.3 Examples of picture notes

practice until he could quickly recall the correct term. For example, students would often say, "Radius? Is that the one that goes all the way across the circle or the one that goes half way across?" When a student spends time trying to recall the meaning of the word "radius," valuable time and space in working memory is being used. As one ninth grade student said, "I wasn't too sure about those picture notes at first, but they have really paid out. For the first time I can really follow what my teacher is talking about." His practice with picture notes helped him recall the meaning of the words fluently so that he could keep up with the pace of his teacher's instruction.

Since vocabulary development is an area of relative strength for NVLD students, picture notes provide a comfortable place to begin an instructional session. Educational therapists, teachers, and tutors sometimes vary the routine by saying the word and asking the student to draw the appropriate picture. Experienced practitioners ask students to deal with math vocabulary in different ways in order to develop flexibility and uncover overly literal misconceptions. For example, one educational therapist asked her student to underline all the pictures of diameters. The student only underlined a horizontal diameter. The student erroneously thought that there could only be one diameter per circle, the one just like his first picture. He needed prompting to expand his view of diameter to include a diameter that was vertical or diagonal; he needed to understand that there are an infinite number of diameters in any given circle.

Developing a solid, working vocabulary that links term, definition, and mental image is a critical first step toward mathematical proficiency, but it is only a first step. What about other components of mathematics, such as learning calculation or procedural skills?

Learning the Procedural Skills of Mathematics

Students with NVLD frequently describe feeling "lost" in mathematical calculations. When given tasks like dividing large numbers, multiplying fractions, or solving algebraic equations, they ask questions such as "Now, where do I start? What comes next? What is the answer supposed to look like?" Given the core deficits of executive functioning and visual–spatial skills, these feelings of "lostness" are readily understandable. Executive functioning includes the cognitive skills of planning, sequencing, holding information in working memory, and manipulating it; visual–spatial skills include ordering, sequencing, keeping track of direction (left/right or top/bottom) and position in space, and interpreting diagrams. Each of these executive functioning and visual–spatial components has a direct impact on learning the calculation skills of mathematics, but none more so than working memory.

Working memory has been described as "a limited capacity system responsible for temporarily storing, maintaining, and mentally manipulating information over brief time periods to serve other ongoing cognitive activities and operations" (Berch, 2011). A student uses her working memory to maintain the sequence of where to start and how to write down the numbers when multiplying 37 times 85; a student uses working memory to find the base of a triangle while maintaining that this information is only the necessary first step to solve the original problem which was to find the area of the triangle. There is "reasonably clear evidence of a generally strong association between working memory capacity and mathematics performance" (Berch, 2011). NVLD is a spectrum disorder so individuals will vary as to the extent of difficulties with working memory, but for many with NVLD the difficulties are significant. Strategies such as using scripts are vital to help these individuals deal with working memory difficulties and develop proficiency with mathematical procedures.

Scripts are instructions and examples of how to complete a mathematical procedure such as how to divide whole numbers or how to find the area of a triangle. The student starts by watching as the teacher or practitioner demonstrates and describes how to do the skill. Then the student with NVLD uses his verbal mediation skills to paraphrase how to complete the skill; he then writes his paraphrase on a 4×6 in. card which becomes his script. If handwriting is a problem for the student, the instructor can act as a scribe as long as she is recording, not supplying, the words for the student. The teacher needs to correct any errors the student makes, but must prompt the student to develop his own summary for the skill. Scripts can be made for simple or advanced mathematical skills.

A good script card would have:

- A title for the skill (e.g., How to Multiply Fractions)
- A series of steps necessary
- Examples and drawings

Figure 9.3 shows some examples of scripts created by students with NVLD.

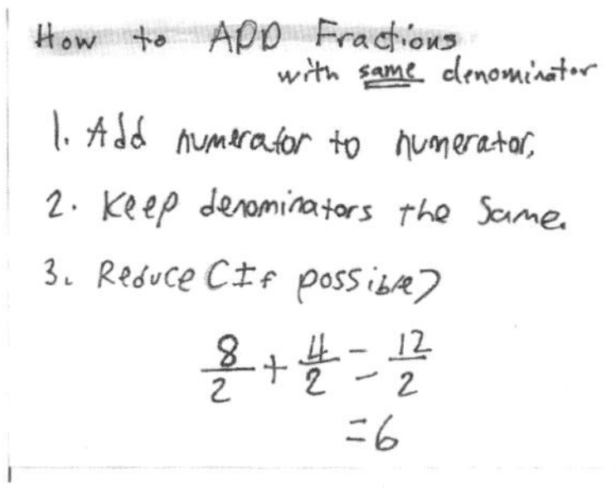

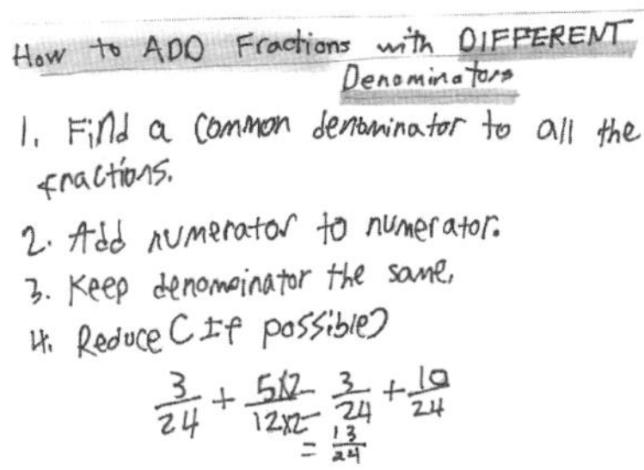

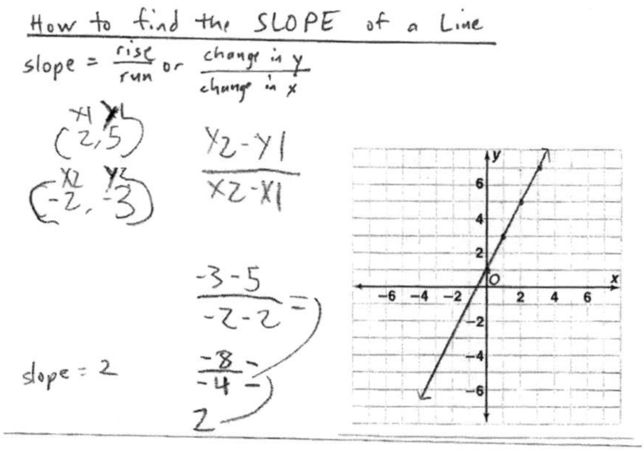

The script cards are kept together in a small photo album which becomes a personal reference book for the student. "It is essential for these students to compile strategies that they have used successfully in a notebook, allowing them to refer to their strategies whenever they need to use them and promoting the integration and generalization of those strategies" (Stein & Krishnan, 2007). Having a personal reference book allows the student to look back if he forgets a procedure and keeps the teacher from having to reteach the same skill over and over. Students often express that knowing they have such a reference book reduces their anxiety that they will forget important procedures. Reducing anxiety and the load on working memory by using scripts is an important strategy to learn procedural knowledge. To become proficient in mathematics, the student with NVLD must also learn the critical concepts of the discipline.

Learning the Conceptual Knowledge of Mathematics

Research has identified a number of advantages of strong conceptual understanding including having an easier time recalling new information, improved use of problem-solving skills, and improved reasoning when interpreting new information (Booth, 2011). Yet students with NVLD often struggle to grasp the major concepts of academic disciplines, especially mathematics. Of course, knowing the vocabulary and procedures of math will be very helpful, but not sufficient to understanding the major concepts. Fortunately, research has identified strategies which benefit the NVLD learner.

One important strategy is called the "whole-to-parts-to-whole" progression (Stein & Krishnan, 2007) where students are first given an overview or sense of the whole. Starting with the overview is also called "establishing the gestalt" or "building a frame of reference" (Neff et al., 2002). Students with NVLD frequently have difficulty distinguishing between main points and details; they tend to believe that all points are equally important and so they become overwhelmed with the total amount of information presented. They benefit from instruction that begins first with the overview, links the new information to prior knowledge, provides context and relevance for the learning, and emphasizes the main points. After establishing the overview and major concept, they can work with the parts or details, and end the instruction back with the major concept. "With respect to instruction within individual academic domains, students with nonverbal learning disabilities benefit greatly from a 'whole-to-parts-to-whole' progression in the curriculum, methods, and materials. This progression allows them to understand the connections among the parts and to conceptualize the whole as a sum of the parts" (Stein & Krishnan, 2007). Instruction in the classroom often goes "parts-to-whole," but students with NVLD will be able to learn the conceptual knowledge of mathematics much more effectively if the progression goes "whole-to-parts-to-whole."

Summary and Conclusion

To meet the requirements for graduation and become mathematically literate adults, students with NVLD need high-quality, evidence-based instruction.

Although the research for mathematics instruction for children and young adults with NVLD is still in the early stages, several principles have emerged:

- First, effective instruction to develop competency in mathematics needs to involve several important components including number sense, counting skills, math vocabulary, procedural skills, conceptual skills, fluency with number combinations (math facts), and skills for solving word problems.
- Second, instruction needs to follow the progression of learning by first starting at the three-dimensional, concrete level before moving on the two-dimensional level with pictures, diagrams, workbooks, and textbooks.

- Third, the instruction must be specifically matched to the learning strengths as well as core deficits inherent to the profile of the individual with NVLD.

To learn the *vocabulary* of mathematics, students with NVLD need to link term, definition, and image with special help on developing the image since that is often a difficult skill for them. One important tool is called "picture notes" (Neff et al., 2002). Picture notes are simple drawing or pictorial examples for terms.

To learn the *procedures* of mathematics, students with NVLD benefit from scripts, which are instructions and examples of how to complete a mathematical procedure such as how to divide whole numbers or how to find the area of a triangle. The script cards are kept together in a small photo album which becomes a personal reference book for the student.

To learn the *major concepts* of mathematics, students with NVLD need "whole-to-part-to-whole" progression where students are first given an overview or sense of the whole.

With support, students with NVLD can become competent at mathematics and achieve their learning goals. A student like Ryan who stated, "I got a D- last year in algebra and it was a gift," can be given hope that he can understand mathematics. As new research is undertaken in this emerging field, more students with NVLD can be given such hope. Hope can turn into academic success for more students.

Appendix A. Programs and Materials for Mathematics Interventions

Teachers, educational therapists, and parents need well-developed materials for mathematics interventions to use with students with NVLD. To date, no program or curriculum has been developed specifically or exclusively for those with NVLD. In the absence of such programs, instructors will want to evaluate each program to find the one most closely aligned with the principles for instruction delineated in Chap. 12 and age appropriate for the student. Every program will need some adaptations for the child or adolescent with NVLD. The following list is not an endorsement of any particular program, but rather a list of possibilities that educators and parents can investigate in their search for appropriate materials:

- *Grade-level mathematics textbooks*. All of the major educational publishers, such as Prentice Hall or Houghton Mifflin, have a series of mathematics textbooks for each grade or topic, such as geometry. These books and the teachers' editions which accompany them are available in bookstore or online at sites such as Amazon.com. New and used textbooks, workbooks, and teachers' manuals are available.
- *Making Math Real—David Berg*: *A Multisensory, Structured Program for Cognitive Development in Mathematics* (http://www.makingmathreal.org or 510 527-0720).

- *Math-U-See* (http://www.mathusee.com/) or 800 454-6284 (schools) or 888 854-6284 (parents).
- *Do the Math* by Marilyn Burns (http://teacher.scholastic.com/products/dothemath/) or 800 724-6527.
- *On Cloud Nine®* by Nanci Bell and Kimberly Tuley (http://www.ganderpublishing.com/On-Cloud-Nine/) or 800 554-1819.

References

Berch, D. (2011). Working memory limitation in mathematics learning: Their development, assessment, and remediation. *Perspectives, 37*(2), 21–26.

Berch, D., & Mazzocco, M. (Eds.). (2007). *Why is math so hard for some children?: The nature and origins of mathematical learning difficulties and disabilities*. Baltimore, MD: Paul H. Brooks Publishing Co.

Booth, J. L. (2011). Why can't students get the concept of math? *Perspectives, 37*(2), 31–34.

Bruner, J. S. (1966). *Toward a theory of instruction*. Cambridge, MA: The Belknap Press of Harvard University Press.

Cornoldi, C., Rigoni, F., Tressoli, P., & Vio, C. (1999). Imagery deficits in nonverbal learning disabilities. *Journal of Learning Disabilities, 3*(1), 48–57.

Davis, J., & Broitman, J. (2011). *Nonverbal learning disabilities in children: Bridging the gap between science and practice*. New York: Springer Science+Business Media, LLC.

Forrest, B. (2004). The utility of math difficulties, internalized psychopathology, and visual-spatial deficits to identify children with the nonverbal learning disability syndrome: Evidence for a visual-spatial disability. *Child Neuropsychology, 10*(2), 129–146.

Foss, J. (2006). *Students with nonverbal learning disabilities*. Nonverbal learning disabilities online. (Online). http://www.nldline.com/jean_fos.htm

Geary, D. (2004). Mathematics and learning disabilities. *Journal of Learning Disabilities, 37*(1), 4–15.

Kozevnikov, M., Motes, M., & Hegarty, M. (2006). Spatial visualization in physics problem solving. *Cognitive Science, 31*, 549–559.

Marzano, R. (2003). *What works in schools: Translating research into action*. Alexandria, VA: Association for Supervision and Curriculum Development.

Matthaei, D. (2008). *Strategies for success in geometry for students with a visual-spatial disorder: I got a D- in algebra—now what*? UMI Dissertation Services, UMI Number 145916. Proquest LLC.

Mazzocco, M. (2011). Theme editor's summary: Mathematical difficulties in school age children. *Perspectives, 37*(2), 7–8.

Miller, K. (2005). The principles of effective numeracy development: What the research reveals. *The Educational Therapist, 26*(1), 8–11.

Neff, B., Neff-Lippman, J., & Stockdale, C. (2002). *The source for visual-spatial disorders*. East Moline, IL: LinguiSystems.

Steeves, K. J., & Tomey, H. A. (1998). Mathematics and dyslexia. *Perspectives, Fall*, 14–15.

Stein, J. A., & Krishnan, K. (2007). Nonverbal learning disabilities and executive function: The challenge of effective assessment and teaching. In L. Melzer (Ed.), *Executive function in education* (pp. 106–132). New York, NY: Guilford Press.

Sullivan, M. (2005). Teaching mathematics to college students with mathematics-related learning disabilities: Report from the classroom. *Learning Disability Quarterly, 28*(3), 205–220.

Chapter 10
Promoting Social–Emotional Competency in Children with NVLD

Bernadette Evans-Smith

Nonverbal learning disability (NVLD) captures the profile of children who struggle with the perception, mental spatial manipulation, and reasoning of visual information. Additional symptoms have included deficits with tactile perception, sensory integration, and psychomotor skills. Such processing challenges have been associated with social–emotional difficulties, and problems with math calculation/reasoning, reading comprehension, and written expression, as examples.

This chapter will provide an overview of the social–emotional learning needs of children with NVLD from two complementary theoretical perspectives, neurodevelopmental behavioral (Lipton & Evans-Smith, 2006; Lipton & Nowicki, 2009; Siegel, 1999; Stern, 2000) and interpersonal neurobiology (Palombo, Bendicsen, & Koch, 2011; Schore, 2005; Siegel, 1999). Primary psychotherapeutic approaches that address these social–emotional needs are described along with a way to conceptualize their integration in therapy. These methods include cognitive-behavioral therapy (CBT), dialectical behavior therapy (DBT), mindfulness, relaxation, relational, and systemic interventions. Studies assessing peer group interventions, in particular, are then briefly reviewed with a special emphasis on the I-SELF (intervention-social–emotional learning framework).

Although there is agreement among some about the general symptoms of NVLD, controversy persists among professionals as to whether NVLD is a disability in and of itself. Is it a learning disorder that is unitary without subtypes as Rourke (1995) suggested, implicating differential development of the right and left hemispheres? Is NVLD common to specific genetic disorders or acquired medical conditions such as Fragile X, Turners Syndrome, congenital hypothyroidism, hydrocephalus, or in children who have received chemotherapy, in which

B. Evans-Smith, Ph.D. (✉)
Rush Neurobehavioral Center, 4711 West Golf Road, Suite 1100,
Skokie, IL 60076, USA
e-mail: bernadette_evans-smith@rush.edu

J. Broitman and J.M. Davis (eds.), *Treating NVLD in Children: Professional Collaborations for Positive Outcomes*, DOI 10.1007/978-1-4614-6179-1_10,

cerebral white matter disintegration is implicated (Rourke, 1995)? Is NVLD diagnostically distinctive from a pervasive development disorder (PDD) such as Asperger's syndrome (Davis & Broitman, 2011)? These questions are being explored in order to provide greater clarity as to the diagnostic symptomatology and differentiation of NVLD.

In order to properly conceptualize assessment and interventions designed to help children with NVLD, it is important to have some understanding as to the neurobiological underpinnings of the symptoms. "Nonverbal disorders of learning" was first identified by Johnson and Myklebust (1967). They recognized that there were children who had learning challenges that were not due to language processing deficits. Johnson and Myklebust identified various dissociative characteristic symptoms including problems with visual perception, spatial orientation, motor learning, and regulation of attention. Rourke (1995) continued to explore this type of learning disorder and determined that there was some coherency among symptoms implicating the involvement of the right hemisphere. He specifically identified "weaknesses" with visual-spatial organization, tactile perceptual abilities, and psychomotor skills. Current studies emanating from developmental neurobiological research reveal that the right hemisphere is associated with the processing of social, visual, and emotional information (Chiron et al., 1997; Decety & Jackson, 2004; Heberlein, Adolphs, Pennebaker, & Tranel, 2003; Semrud-Clickman & Hynd, 1990) and, more precisely, the visual cortex and amygdala (Adolphs, 2003). For example, with positive emission tomography studies the right hemisphere is activated in infants when attending to faces, gaze direction, auditory emotional signals, and tactile emotional stimuli (Le Grand, Mondloch, Maurer, & Brent, 2003; Schore, 2003; Yamada, Sadato, & Konishi, 2000). The right hemisphere undergoes the greatest amount of development through the first 2 years of life relative to the left hemisphere. During this developmental span, visual, tactile, and motor learning are most active.

What is the potential impact, therefore, of deficient neurological growth in the right hemisphere during infancy? With social–emotional learning, there is a distinct possibility that the understanding and implementation of social–emotional cues could be compromised (Chiron et al., 1997; Decety & Jackson, 2004; Heberlein et al., 2003; Schore, 2005). Its impact could be observed as an infant is beginning to perceive, interpret, and imitate facial expressions, gestures, and intonation, and use his body to communicate intent and regulate his response to internal/external discomforts and needs, the latter dependent on motor coordination. The scaffolding nature of development suggests that early deficits may have ongoing negative consequences on the acquisition of more complex skills (Decety & Jackson, 2004). Beyond the development of observed skills, a child's need for security is gradually being attained through his attachment with his primary caregiver. At this early stage, the reciprocating relationship of caregiver and infant begins. Problems linked to poor social–emotional understanding and reciprocation can lead to insecurities associated with attachment and trust. Theory suggests that these issues can contribute to increased emotional/behavioral dysregulation, anxiety/discomfort, depressed mood, distorted social self-image, poor self-esteem, and interpersonal mistrust (Palombo et al., 2011; Rourke, 1995; Schore, 2005; Semrud-Clickman & Fine,

2008; Siegel, 1999; Stern, 2000). There is no current evidence, however, indicating that children with NVLD have insecure attachments, rather may present with the latter issues.

Conceptualization of Social–Emotional Learning Needs

In this chapter, the author chose to conceptualize the social–emotional needs of a child with NVLD through a developmental behavioral (Annaz, Karmiloff-Smith, & Thomas, 2008; Greenspan & Wieder, 2005; Lipton & Evans-Smith, 2006; Lipton & Nowicki, 2009; Prizant, Wetherby, Rubin, Laurent, & Rydell, 2006a) and interpersonal neurobiological (Schore, 2005; Siegel, 1999; Stern, 2000) approaches. The assessment and treatment is therefore directed by these conceptualizations. A developmental behavioral approach allows for individualized assessment and treatment such that a child's strengths can be identified and enhanced and their challenges specifically addressed. An interpersonal neurobiological approach considers a child's relational development with special emphasis on attachment and emotional regulation.

Social–Emotional Learning Framework: Neurodevelopmental Behavioral Approach

The social–emotional learning framework (SELF) model is a theoretical framework for assessing and treating children with social–emotional learning (SEL) challenges such as those with NVLD (Lipton & Evans-Smith, 2006; Lipton & Nowicki, 2009). It follows a neurodevelopmental behavioral framework and allows a clinician to assess a child's social–emotional strengths and challenges relative to typical developmental expectations along the span of birth to 16 years old. The developmental expectations for the SELF were determined by conducting a thorough study of the neurodevelopmental literature for specific social–emotional functions. By referencing the SELF, a clinician can assess both a child's understanding ("comprehension") and implementation ("execution") of social–emotional behaviors. This differentiation between comprehension and execution parallels what Gresham and Elliot (2009) termed "acquisition deficits," a lack of understanding, and "performance" deficits, problems demonstrating a behavior even though the child understands the social expectations.

The SELF identified function areas that were considered most problematic for children notable for SEL deficits, such as those with NVLD and autism spectrum disorders (ASD). Behaviors associated with each of these areas are listed by age, in order of developmental onset and primary time of growth spurt. Not all children with NVLD will manifest deficits in each of these function areas, rather the SELF allows clinicians to assess which area(s) is less developed.

The comprehension portion of the SELF examines domains of function which include nonverbal awareness of basic and social emotions in self and others, perspective-taking, empathy, and higher order reasoning. Higher order reasoning considers a child's ability to understand social rules and causal relations between social events, integration of information about others over time such as their traits and values, and humor. Nonverbal awareness of emotions in others, for example, refers to a child's ability to fluidly read emotion from nonverbal social cues such as facial expressions, voice intonation/volume/prosody, gestures, interpersonal space, and touch (Duke, Nowicki, & Martin, 1996). Nonverbal awareness in self references the ability to experience and sense a range of emotion in oneself. Perspective-taking is a component of Theory of Mind (Baron-Cohen, Leslie, & Frith, 1985; Miller, Kessel, & Flavell, 1970; Selman, 1976; Wellman, 1992), the ability to assume someone else's perspective in a particular context without that person verbalizing his view or necessarily demonstrating it in his behavior. Higher order reasoning relies on earlier social–emotional development such that cognitively one can integrate increasingly complex experiences.

Domains of function for execution on the SELF include the ability to effectively use nonverbal social expressions to communicate feelings; apply executive function skills, such as regulate attention and emotional and behavioral responses, and process social–emotional information at a reasonable rate; apply pragmatic language skills; solve social problems; and engage in cooperative and reciprocal relations. An example of how this might be reflected on the SELF profile with emotion and behavior regulation is as follows: A 3-year-old child who is frustrated may be more apt to walk away or push something; at 4 or 5 years old, the child begins to seek help with an increasing reliance on language to express the feeling; and a child at 11 years old may begin to use metacognitive strategies to calm down.

Interpersonal Neurobiology

Dr. Alan Schore (2003, 2005) theorized that one of the functions of the right hemisphere is to process emotional interchanges between an infant and caregiver, that it is the social part of the brain where one forms internal working models of self, caregiver, and others. An infant's attachment is therefore influenced by his neurobiological condition and the caregiver and infant's social–emotional reciprocation. Schore (2005) hypothesizes that attachment serves an affective regulatory function. Infants/children with secure attachments are more likely to effectively regulate their emotional state. Children with insecure attachments have a greater propensity to become easily dysregulated.

Schore's (2005) theory has implications for children with NVLD. Assuming symptoms are present at birth or have an early onset, the theory suggests that an infant who experiences problems with right hemisphere development may be at risk for developing an insecure attachment, affective dysregulation, and poorly developed internal working models of self and others. With maturity, the experience of not feeling secure in the world and with less skill in managing one's emotions, one could increasingly manifest symptoms such as anxiety, mood instability, behavior "meltdowns," and/or prolonged tantrums. Also, the child's internal working models of self and others could be distorted such that his mental organization of social and affective information related to both would be deficient. This faulty cognitive integration and organization has the potential to negatively impact a child's self-image, identity, and relatedness to others (Palombo, 2001; Schore, 2003).

Psychotherapy

The social–emotional issues of children and adolescents with NVLD can include skill deficits, poor self-esteem, susceptibility to anxiety and depressed mood, possibly less well-developed internal working models of self and others, and the potential to be less emotionally/behaviorally regulated and trusting of others. It is not yet known if children with NVLD have difficulties establishing a secure attachment with caregivers but worthy of further exploration and consideration when working with them. Skill deficits commonly include problems with interpreting social nonverbal cues, effectively demonstrating those cues, inferential interpretation of information, using pragmatic language, perspective-taking, and sometimes behavioral/mood dysregulation potentially related to sensory sensitivities and anxiety (Davis & Broitman, 2011; Palombo, 2001; Stewart, 2002). Some primary treatment approaches to address the above issues include cognitive-behavioral therapy (CBT), dialectical behavior therapy (DBT), mindfulness and stress reduction (MBSR), relaxation, and relational therapies originating from psychoanalytical theory. These therapies can occur in the context of individual, family, or peer group therapy. There are also additional therapies that guide clinical methods used in family (as discussed earlier) or group, e.g., gestalt.

Context

The context of treatment is an important consideration as emphasized in Bronfenbrenner's work on ecological systems theory (Bronfenbrenner & Evans, 2000). Any child who has had social (relational) problems would benefit from systemic approaches at some point in therapy, i.e., family and/or peer. In addition, sometimes what is learned in individual therapy is not necessarily generalized to other settings such as school or home. Therefore, interventions that occur with the family, peers, and at school (classroom to district-wide) can be critical to promoting a child's social–emotional development. Family, school, and individual psychotherapy will be briefly discussed here. Peer group interventions will be addressed in more depth in the remainder of this chapter.

Family

What can family therapy offer? There are a range of therapeutic approaches that therapists adopt when working with families. In essence, though, engaging in family therapy enables the therapist to learn about the parent(s), siblings, and child's social–emotional strengths and challenges; their nonverbal and verbal communication patterns; alliances that may have formed; the structure of family subsystems (parental and sibling roles, boundaries); level of empathy and affection that is expressed in the family; each others' perspectives of situations; type of attachment; whether expectations of each other are realistic or not; and parental disciplinary responses to challenging behavior, as examples. By observing these family "traits," the therapist has the opportunity to intercede and improve each family member's understanding and response towards one another, strengthen healthy parental and child roles, validate experiences, change dysfunctional patterns of communication, build trust and stability, and overall strengthen their relations. In particular, when working with children with NVLD in a family context, there is an emphasis on emotional understanding of self and others and building trust and security in the relations.

There are numerous theoretical approaches to family therapy, each with their own philosophy for change and methods (Goldenberg & Goldenberg, 2012; Minuchin, Lee, & Simon, 1996). This author prefers to integrate psycho-education, cognitive-behavioral (skill), and relational psychoanalytical approaches to address different needs of a family who have a child with NVLD, as described later in this chapter. To enhance skills, for example, parents can learn techniques and strategies to use at home as modeled and practiced in sessions. To build emotional understanding and communication, therapists may ask parents to initially exaggerate their nonverbal responses, for example, in order to help a child with NVLD more effectively understand the parent's feelings. The child with NVLD may be asked to practice imitating facial expressions and gestures in role-plays with his parents or the family may complete a journal documenting emotional experiences. The journal may include photos of each member demonstrating a range of emotion, list of situations that trigger those feelings, and thought bubbles with accompanying thoughts. Families may generate a feeling chart to use at home to encourage greater attention to how each one feels and to increase the emotional language in the home. Children with NVLD tend to literally interpret information. With increased awareness, families learn to check for their child's understanding and provide more inferential/abstract interpretations, as appropriate. Social language skills can be enacted in family sessions either in vivo or reenacting a scenario common to school. Such skills as initiating and reciprocating conversation can be practiced. Families can be videotaped in session followed with a feedback session in which the tape is reviewed and discussed. The therapist facilitates understanding of each other, coaches members on how to verbally and nonverbally respond, and validates experiences, as examples. To foster improved trust, greater security in family relations, and empathy various therapeutic methods and activities within the family context are used that encourage understanding, nurturance, empathy, fun, and affection (Goldenberg

& Goldenberg, 2012; Minuchin et al., 1996). All of these experiences have the potential to lead to improved internal models of self and others (Palombo, 2001).

In addition to family therapy, a therapist may opt to work solely with the parents. In this instance, parents will benefit from meeting with a therapist who understands the impact NVLD can have, not only on their child but also on them personally and as a couple. Common parental experiences include feeling blamed, experiencing the loss of a dream of who your child could have become, rejection by family and friends, isolation, increased marital conflicts, disenchantment with professionals, financial stressors, guilt, and doubt. The therapist can offer parents emotional support and guidance about decisions they will need to make. In addition, a therapist can inform parents about reasonable developmental expectations, encourage parents to identify their child's strengths, explore ways to expand their child's experiences so that he is involved in rewarding activities, plan ways to manage transitions, and discuss ways to make play dates successful (Stewart, 2002).

Beyond the benefits of family therapy, there can be some limitations in choosing this as the primary treatment context. For example, some families may not be comfortable meeting together which may result in therapy being sabotaged. Marital conflict can be so dominant that those issues need to be addressed before family therapy resumes. Some parents may have significant personality disorders which disrupt the treatment focus on directly helping their child with NVLD. In some instances, one or both of the parents could have a social–emotional learning disorder such as NVLD or ASD. These parents may benefit from individual therapy first. In addition, some children may display/express a significant mistrust of their parents. In such instances, the child may need to first experience a trusting relationship or more secure attachment with the therapist before family therapy can be effective.

School

Appropriate peer group interventions conducted in a school environment offers a child the opportunity to apply his newly learned behaviors within this context hopefully aiding generalization and transfer of skills. These interventions can occur in the mainstream classroom, be part of the overall school milieu, and/or occur in a pullout friendship group facilitated by the school social worker, speech/language therapist, and/or school psychologist. Ideally, a child's social–emotional strengths and needs have been accurately identified and objectified for targeted treatment and outcome measurement. Importantly, too, relevant school staff will know the child's social goals [possibly through an individual education plan (IEP) or a Section 504 Plan] and have the necessary skill set to teach a child with NVLD.

School-based interventions, however, may not always be optimally effective. Currently, there a number of social curriculums used in the mainstream classroom (Durlak, Weissberg, Dymnicki, Taylor, & Schellinger, 2011) typically designed to address bullying and social problem solving. These curricula can be helpful to some degree for any child who has social challenges as well as foster better overall peer relations. These curricula are not intended, however, to help children with notable social challenges such as those with NVLD. As noted earlier and throughout this book, children with NVLD have some commonly shared deficits which require specialized instruction. Some schools offer smaller social groups for children to participate that contain elements of instruction valuable to children with NVLD, e.g., emotional awareness, communication, and problem solving. These groups, however, greatly vary in their focus, treatment methods, and effectiveness since there are few empirically supported manualized materials designed for short-duration groups as are common in schools, e.g., 20–30 min sessions, once per week (Evans-Smith, Allen, Johnson, & McKown, 2011). For school-based groups, time is typically spent working on skills. There is not enough time to address deeper relational/attachment issues.

Currently, there is a trend in educational policy towards developing an integrated model of social interventions in schools which would also benefit children with special needs (Durlak et al., 2011). Ideally, in the future, children with NVLD will benefit from the integration of a school-wide social–emotional curriculum with smaller, specialized groups either conducted in the classroom or as a pullout service. In this way, interventions will either indirectly or directly extend beyond skills per se and foster deeper relations and improved internal working models of self and others.

Individual

Given the potential benefits of receiving therapy in a social context, is individual therapy ever indicated? There are instances when individual therapy is warranted and very beneficial. Some children with long-standing histories of social rejection and isolation, for example, can present as clinically depressed, highly anxious, and/or severely dysregulated with mood, behavior, and attention. In these instances the child may not be ready to participate in family or peer group therapy. Individual therapy offers a child the unique experience of feeling understood and appreciated and discovering strategies to improve his/her social skills. The therapist can more effectively individualize skill instruction and use her relationship as a means of teaching the child about social–emotional issues, e.g., provide insight about her feelings and perspectives, her impression of the child's responses, practice role-plays, videotape interactions, and review for feedback. Attachment and regulation issues can be addressed as the therapist provides a comfortable, trusting, and predictable space along with opportunities to express oneself. Through the therapeutic relationship, a healthy internal image of oneself can develop (Palombo & Berenberg, 1997; Schore, 2003). The therapist can also coach parents and teachers in an effort to foster skill generalization across settings, improve adult and peer relations, and build friendships. She can provide strategies to improve parent and teacher skills and mold a positive alternative perspective of the child, if needed.

There are times when the effectiveness of individual therapy may be compromised. Sometimes a child's problems may not be evident. The interaction with parents and peers is minimally observed. Also, a child with NVLD may relate better to adults than peers. Therefore, the therapist may not observe the problem behaviors to the same degree that they interfere with the child's peer relations. In other instances, the child may not be able to report on the issues that are critical to address given his limited social understanding. This restricts the depth and focus of treatment. Some children struggle to generalize what they have learned in one-to-one therapy; so, in some cases, it extends the timeline needed for treatment and potentially, success. Children with NVLD can also present as highly anxious and mistrusting of others. When children chronically present this way, a child may strongly resist any change, and the therapist may hesitate to recommend family or group therapy, although it could be clinically indicated. Parents can also depend on the therapist for guidance and support such that they would not want to make any changes. The therapist is then left with a challenging decision as she contemplates next therapeutic steps.

Collaboration

Regardless of the therapeutic context, it is critical that psychotherapists collaborate with other professionals who work with the child. Through collaboration, professionals gain the perspective of others—how their client is seen through the eyes of someone else; it is an opportunity to share insight, goals, strategies, and progress. Through a more cohesive and complementary focus on clinical goals, a child has a greater chance of succeeding.

For the remaining portion of this chapter, therapeutic approaches and interventions that can be used in a peer group context will be emphasized. These include primary psychotherapy techniques that address skill development, anxiety, mood, self-image, and relational/attachment issues.

Primary Psychotherapy Approaches

Development of Skills

Cognitive-Behavioral and Dialectical Behavior Therapies

Cognitive-behavioral therapy (CBT) is one of the more common approaches to treating children with social–emotional learning problems. Most studies and practitioners integrate these techniques either in individual, family, or group psychotherapy (Beck & Beck, 2011).

Behavioral approaches focus on external situational cues or triggers, observable behavior, and outcomes such as forms of reinforcement, rewards, and punishment. Measurable behavior goals and objectives are commonly determined so that a particular social skill, for example, can be monitored. Outcomes shape the behavior such that important motivators to the child are identified as incentives for behavior change. Behavior change is "contingency shaped." For example, primary reinforcements of food may be a strong incentive for a child to practice a new skill. Other common methods associated with behavioral approaches to shape or fade behaviors include the use of time-out, role-plays, systematic desensitization, and modeling prosocial behavior (Miltenberger, 2011).

Cognitive therapy focuses on a child's thoughts and beliefs and its impact on behavior. The way someone perceives a situation affects the way he might respond to a situation. If someone believes another person likes him, for example, he is apt to respond more favorably towards that person than if he believes the individual does not like him. He will also attribute more positive qualities to that person. Techniques include exploration of one's beliefs and thoughts, cognitive reframing, and the use of "stop" strategies, as examples (Beck & Beck, 2011).

Dialectical behavior therapy (DBT) places greater emphasis on emotional experiences than does CBT. DBT initially evolved as a method to treat adults with borderline personality disorders (Marra, 2005). Over time, it has been increasingly used, mostly with adults, to treat various disorders including personality, anxiety, mood, impulse control, and eating disorders, as examples (Marra, 2005). Its effectiveness with children has not been studied or used to the degree it has with adults, but has the potential to address issues associated with NVLD. DBT is designed to improve emotion regulation and assist the client so that s/he accepts her/his emotional experience. Through this process, the client learns to cope in more effective ways rather than avoid intense and painful experiences. The therapist is direct and helps the child refocus on the issue (situation, thoughts, and emotion), to the degree that the child can tolerate the emotional experience. Unlike psychodynamic approaches that use transference as a means of promoting change, a DBT therapist uses self-disclosure and is clear about the strategies she is using. Schemas (mental belief systems that guide one's behavior) are explored and discussed (Elliot & Lassen, 1997; Marra, 2005).

The above treatment methods offer a structure to the therapeutic approach and directly impact skill development. To be an effective psychotherapist with children with NVLD, one needs to also integrate knowledge about the unique strengths and needs of these children and not be misled by the child's strong language abilities. For example, a child with NVLD tends to learn best when visual information is explained through spoken language. The therapist would want to remain mindful that it is important to describe her nonverbal reactions and provide verbal feedback to the child about his nonverbal responses. It is helpful to describe social situations in depth by noting situational cues and social forms of communication such as facial expressions, gestures, posture, interpersonal space and touch, and objectives. Some children with NVLD are also susceptible to becoming emotionally and behaviorally dysregulated. Sensory issues may contribute to these problems. Therapists who work with children with NVLD would be assessing the child's sensory world and his response. This information then informs intervention strategies, e.g., consult with occupational therapist, provide materials that address sensory needs, and/or remove items that overstimulate the child. Once the sensory issues are addressed, other matters that could contribute to anxiety, for example, can be addressed. In addition, children with NVLD may have fine motor delays, problems with written expression, reading comprehension, and math. A therapist would want to be aware of these potential deficits to address the impact of these problems at school and home, and on his self-image, mood, and motivation, for example. Optimally, the therapist will act as an advocate at his school regarding academic and social–emotional needs and provide parental guidance (Stewart, 2002; Winner, 2002).

Mindfulness

Mindfulness is a meditative practice that increases awareness of one's sensory experiences and thoughts, focuses attention on the present moment, and encourages nonjudgmental acceptance of one's experiences (Allen, Blashki, & Gullone, 2006; Kabat-Zinn, 1994). The practice of mindfulness is increasingly considered an effective intervention to treat a range of medical and psychological conditions (Baer, 2003). For example, mindfulness has been successfully employed to reduce chronic pain or stress associated with illness such as cancer or multiple sclerosis, and to treat anxiety, depression, or eating disorders (Allen et al., 2006; Kabat-Zinn, Lipworth, Burney, & Sellers, 1987; Kristeller & Hallett, 1999; Segal, Williams, & Teasdale, 2002). Common mindfulness techniques are attending to one's breath, body scanning, being mindful of your thoughts, and sensory experiences such as what you hear, see, touch, or eat (Kabat-Zinn, 1994; Semple, Lee, & Miller, 2006; Thompson & Gauntlett-Gilbert, 2008). Using these techniques can lead to improved attention and a greater awareness of self and the environment. It also encourages an acceptance of present moment experiences (Kabat-Zinn, 1994; Marra, 2005). Other popular and empirically supported therapies are now integrating mindfulness exercises into their practice, e.g., CBT, DBT, and Acceptance and Commitment Therapy (Baer, 2003; Germer, Siegel, & Fulton, 2005; Marra, 2005).

Although most mindfulness literature focuses on adults, there are several articles that discuss the implementation of mindfulness intervention for children and adolescents. Many of these studies are approach-based discussions with anecdotal evidence or case studies (Hooker & Fodor, 2008; Ott, 2002; Semple et al., 2006; Thompson & Gauntlett-Gilbert, 2008; Wall, 2005). Children participating in these studies were either neurotypical and without an identified problem, or they presented with anxiety, poor concentration, chronic pain, or depression (Linden, 1973; Semple et al., 2006; Semple, Lee, Rosa, & Miller, 2010; Thompson & Gauntlett-Gilbert, 2008). Practicing mindfulness helped improve these children's concentration, focus, mood regulation, self-control, and management of anxiety, pain, and stress.

Recently, this author and her colleagues completed a pilot study to study the effectiveness of a 9-week mindfulness-based and stress reduction (MBSR) group intervention on improving attention and mood/behavioral regulation in children with autism spectrum disorders (ASD) and attention deficit hyperactivity disorders

(ADHD). We hypothesized that children in the treatment groups would show improved attention, mood/behavior regulation, and self-awareness relative to a wait list control group.

Children (8–12 years) with average intellect and either ASD or ADHD were eligible. The study included two treatment groups split by age and diagnosis, and one wait list control group ($n=6$ each group). Outcome measures for attention, behavior/emotion regulation, and self-awareness were measured with standardized direct assessments.

The content of the group intervention adhered to a set structure across sessions. The first portion of group included discussions regarding class exercises that had occurred throughout the week. The second portion emphasized a particular MBSR exercise through practice, discussion, and the use of additional materials such as watching a video or listening to music. During the third portion children participated in enjoyable activities intended to emphasize the mindfulness exercise and build group cohesion and trust. Exercises emphasized awareness of breathing and moment to moment sensory experiences such as visual, auditory, touch, taste, and physical movement with a focus on accompanying thoughts, feelings, and physical sensations. The children also learned about each others' perspectives and emotional experiences through discussions and sharing experiences. The MBSR group protocol not only focused on elements valuable to children with ASD and ADHD but contained exercises that could be theoretically helpful for children with NVLD, e.g., increasing attention and awareness of emotional experiences in self and others. Efforts to address generalization were also included. A MBSR exercise was practiced every day in each child's class and parents received weekly summaries of the week's group content and related strategies.

The MBSR group intervention successfully improved attention in children with ASD and ADHD. The treatment group scored significantly higher on self-report of attention at posttest compared to the control group as indicated by the large effect size ($U=4.0, p=0.012, d=1.21$). When looking at within-group effects for the treatment group, auditory and visual attention improved as observed with effect sizes ranging from small to large ($d=0.3$–0.7, $p=0.032$–0.001). The MBSR group intervention successfully improved attention in children with ASD and ADHD. These data provide preliminary empirical support for MBSR as an effective intervention to improve attention in pediatric ASD and ADHD populations. Given the paucity of mindfulness studies that evaluate children with neurologically based challenges, these results are promising. Children with NVLD, in this age range, who have comorbid conditions of attention deficits, could potentially benefit from this type of intervention.

Relaxation

Relaxation techniques can also be introduced in therapy to help children with NVLD become more attuned to their physiological responses and, in turn, exercise improved awareness and self-regulation, if needed. Common relaxation strategies usually involve practicing deep, slow breathing as a method of calming the body and mind. This form of breathing is different than what is emphasized with mindfulness in which a child is encouraged to attend to his natural rhythm of breathing. Other relaxation strategies include body scans with systematic relaxation of each muscle group and visualization techniques. For the latter, the therapist directs a child to imagine the sensory details of a scene or image that triggers a calm state, e.g., laying on the grass and looking at the sky and sitting on the beach (Davis, Eshelman, & McKay, 2000).

Children with NVLD vary in their receptivity and ability to engage in relaxation exercises. In particular, many of them find visualization exercises difficult. There are alternatives to help children with NVLD think about calming imagery by tapping their preference for verbal descriptions or creating concrete visual images on paper. For example, the therapist could create an audiotape or podcast that can be downloaded onto a child's iPod which describes a scene in depth or make a collage with personal photos or pictures from the web (reducing the reliance on fine motor output).

Relational

Relational psychoanalysis and relational therapy are two variations of psychotherapy that consider the significance of social–emotional connectedness. Relational therapies address issues related to attachment and internal working models of self and others. The scope of a discussion regarding relational therapies requires more than a chapter of explanation. For a more thorough review, see Palombo et al. (2011). In general, though, the therapist-client relationship is a critical component to promote change. In the case of groups, the relations of the group members are also a critical contributor to change.

Relational therapies focus on the creation and maintenance of fulfilling relationships. Given the assumption that children with NVLD have experienced greater distress and misunderstandings in their relations from a very early age, a therapist with this orientation would hope to provide a new, rewarding social experience for the child. She would be attentive to his social experiences, offer insight about self and others through an empathic and genuine therapist style. When in the context of a social group, the therapist also fosters this new social experience for all members by facilitating communication and understanding of one another, maintaining respect of all members towards each other. The facilitator establishes a safe and predictable group environment which promotes increasing trust and willingness to take risks in trying new behaviors. Children begin to learn that they are likeable, desirable individuals and gain confidence in their social judgment. Through this process, a child's self concept/image can be positively reshaped, internal models of others reconstructed, and harmful, repetitive patterns of relating are no longer reenacted. Children begin to experience a greater sense of security in the social world which leads to healing, self-confidence, comfort in expressing oneself, and motivation to improve. A child may no longer present with the same severity of emotional and behavioral dysregulation.

Control mastery theory (CMT) is one type of relational therapy (Weiss, 1993). It is particularly well suited for children with NVLD. A therapist adopting a control mastery approach will assess how well a child is interacting with his environment. She would consider the beliefs the child is developing about himself especially in the context of his processing difficulties and relations.

The theory behind CMT assumes that a driving force in individuals is to consciously and unconsciously feel safe, find acceptance, and experience a sense of mastery over maladaptive thoughts and behavior. It emphasizes one's ability to exercise control over one's mental life and one's strong desire to get better. Adaptation and attachment are seen as the two central organizing principles in the development of the individual psyche. Childhood experiences are a particularly potent agent in creating unconscious beliefs, which lead to ongoing negative experiences. They can, in turn, interfere with the achievement of life goals.

A child with a learning disability such as NVLD is vulnerable to feeling inadequate, not accepted, and sometimes having minimal control over himself or his life. Starting at a young age, the child may begin to form an image, self-narrative, and belief about himself and others that is potentially incoherent and unhealthy. He may often feel confused and anxious about how to respond in social situations. Problems and misunderstandings may frequently occur when attempting to relate to others as a result of deficits in reading social cues, perspective-taking, and literal interpretations, for example. As a child with NVLD matures, he usually has limited choices in that he may have to meet with an occupational therapist, psychotherapist, and/or educational specialist in and out of school. The child's parents may make more decisions for him sometimes in an effort to protect him. His social opportunities are commonly limited or marked with experiences of rejection. A child with a learning disability, in general, typically experiences limited control and mastery in his life that contributes to an inadequate sense of self (Palombo, 2001).

These types of experiences can give rise to unconscious convictions that, as a child, you are at fault for the problems that arise. The child's irrational self-blame and unconscious guilt stem from the responsibility he assumes for anything bad that happens to himself or significant others. These beliefs are powerful. For example, a child with NVLD who is kept close to the family may incorrectly believe that his parents want him to remain dependent upon them. The families' actual motivation might be to protect him from potential problems. This misunderstanding might cause the child to inhibit his desires to be strong and independent because he might have incorrectly assumed that he would displease his parents if he followed this desire (Broitman, 2002).

A therapist adopting a CMT approach would address these issues by establishing a safe and accepting environment, foster the child's understanding of himself and others, and help him to experience mastery over pathogenic beliefs and gain control in his life. She would encourage a cooperative working relationship between herself and the child to disconfirm these pathogenic beliefs. The child is highly motivated to disconfirm these beliefs in order to recover the capacity to pursue life goals.

This theory is well suited for conceptualizing the dynamics between a child with NVLD and his or her family, peers, and/or school staff. Family members, for example, may feel discouraged because the interpersonal dynamics are chronically static or conflictual. Weiss (2000) would hypothesize that the conflict or limited progress is a result of the child testing others. Weiss and Sampson (1986) believed that everyone tests each other as a means of developing and refining our beliefs about ourselves and others. Parents who can conceptualize the dynamic of the interaction as a "test" can better endure, remain sensitive to their child's needs, and respond in a way that promotes feelings of emotional safety.

When in therapy, children will also test in order to determine if the conditions of safety exist before making their beliefs conscious. For example, with the therapist, a child may test his belief that he is the cause of his parents' constant worry. He may act worrisome with the therapist, hoping the therapist will not respond in the same manner as his parents. As the therapist responds differently than his parents, the child would begin to disconfirm his belief that he was the cause. Over time with continued testing and successful responses from the therapist, the child would begin to feel safe and more likely remember significant events. Subsequently, the child becomes increasingly aware of his beliefs, impulses, attitudes, goals, and/or feelings that he had repressed. For example, a child who was impaired by the belief he deserved to be blamed and ridiculed may not remember being blamed by his teacher until he assures himself that the therapist will not blame or criticize him in the same manner that his teacher did (Broitman, 2002).

When working within a peer group context, a therapist who adopts a control mastery approach needs to facilitate an environment of safety for all members. She must intervene in ways that encourage each child to display respect for one another and encourage responses that do not confirm each child's pathogenic belief.

Systemic

Beyond the therapies discussed above, it is important to understand systemic therapeutic approaches to peer group interventions. A gestalt approach can be easily adapted for social groups.

Gestalt Group Process

Theoretical orientations to adult group psychotherapy have been explored by a number of psychotherapists. Dr. Irvin Yalom (1995) wrote extensively about adult group psychotherapy emphasizing the essentials in his classic text, *The Theory and Practice of Group Psychotherapy*. He supported a gestalt approach in which the "here and now" was processed. Essentially, the group gives the therapist permission to comment on their interpersonal process and experience, adding a new layer of awareness for the members. The facilitator acts as a historian for the group and maintains a temporal perspective. The therapist reminds clients of their group history and personal growth as a means of promoting ongoing motivation and change. S/he keeps focused on the clients' goals and encourages reflection on their status. Group members are encouraged to "be who they are …" (Marra, 2005) such that a gestalt therapist would avoid making statements of approval. Internalized conflict is identified and validated. Gestalt therapists also adopt an empathic, reflective, and direct style of communicating.

To this author's knowledge, there is no research or literature that examines the impact of group process in social skills groups. Beyond a focus on skill development and interpersonal relatedness, it is important that a "here and now" process be integrated in children and adolescent social skills groups. Children with NVLD can benefit from the immediate identification of self and others' behavior, affect, and perspectives; potential internal conflict; and experiential accounts. It is also advantageous that a historical tracking of the groups' experience and progress be labeled and identified given the social–emotional limitations children with NVLD experience.

Integrated Conceptualization of Treatment

The psychotherapeutic interventions described above address varying layers of social–emotional function and can be applied across different systemic levels, e.g., school milieu, family, peer group, and intrapersonally. Some therapies primarily address skill development while other ones focus on enhancing attachment, interpersonal trust, and internalized models of self and others. Given each holds importance for the child, it is possible to integrate elements of these approaches to best serve him. For example, in a social skills group, gestalt and relational therapy principles can be applied to process the interactional dynamics, and build trust and understanding of one another. A child begins to learn about himself through the therapist and other children's perspectives and gradually becomes comfortable making change. At the same time, skills and understanding can be concretely taught by using CBT, DBT, mindfulness, and relaxation techniques. The therapist's style in all instances can be direct, empathic, genuine, reflective, and when indicated, include self-disclosures.

Social Group Interventions

Relative to the number of other studies that assess effectiveness of treatment, there are fewer studies that examine the efficacy of social group interventions. The following is a brief summary of such research literature. Children specifically identified with NVLD are not included in this summary given the paucity of those studies.

The group intervention that adheres to the SELF, and relies on an integrated therapeutic approach, is subsequently described.

Research Findings

The efficacy of interventions to address social impairments is continually being explored (Bauminger, 2007; de Boo & Prins, 2007; Frankel, Myatt et al., 1997; Koenig et al., 2010; Pfiffner, Calzada, & McBurnett, 2000; Prizant et al., 2006a, 2006b; Reichow & Volkmar, 2010; Solomon, Goodlin-Jones, & Anders, 2004). Many interventions focus on skill training and occur in the context of diagnostically homogenous peer groups of children with ASD or attention deficit hyperactivity disorders (ADHD). These studies range in their scope of focus, intervention methods used, general group structure and duration, whether and how generalization was considered, outcome assessment, and whether skills persisted over time. For example, some groups primarily focused on regulation, others affect recognition and perspective-taking, while others taught children conversational skills, how to join groups, good sportsmanship, and how to handle teasing, as examples. Specific skill instruction typically included role-plays, coaching, feedback, modeling prosocial behavior, and discussion. Therapeutic techniques were commonly cognitive-behavioral. In spite of the variability with skill focus, several studies reported some improvement in children's social skills following such training in groups (Bauminger, 2007; Cook et al., 2008; Laugeson, Frankel, Mogil, & Dillon, 2009; Lopata et al., 2010; Pfiffner et al., 2000; Solomon et al., 2004; Stichter et al., 2010).

Bauminger (2007) established an intervention model, referred to as the Cognitive-Behavioral Ecological Model, which included peers with and without ASD. Each peer group included two typical peers and one to three children with ASD. Children with ASD also received weekly individual support. The intervention occurred weekly for 1 h sessions for 7 months. Her model integrated a cognitive-behavioral approach to train cooperative social interactions, social problem-solving, emotion knowledge and recognition, and perspective-taking or theory of mind. Improvements in children's social perception, social problem solving, theory of mind, and executive functioning were reported. The children, however, did not generalize their skills to spontaneous dyadic and group interactions in naturalistic settings.

Solomon and colleagues (2004) developed and evaluated their Social Adjustment Enhancement Intervention to promote children's emotional awareness, theory of mind, conversation skills, and social problem solving. Their intervention consisted of weekly 1.5 h sessions for a total of 20 sessions with a high staff to student ratio (3:5). They used cognitive-behavioral strategies but, in contrast to many other studies, integrated a process-oriented approach to the group dynamics as an aspect of the learning experience. This therapeutic approach required clinicians to identify and influence patterns of communication and foster a greater understanding of each other in the "here and now." In addition, they provided weekly psycho-educational parent training. Facial affect recognition skills improved significantly, but not social problem solving or theory of mind.

The Program for the Education and Enrichment of Relational Skills (PEERS; Laugeson et al., 2009) has been used with adolescents diagnosed with ASD, ADHD, and Fetal Alcohol Spectrum Disorders. Their program adopted a skill-based approach which targeted conversational skills, peer entry, expanding friendship networks, managing teasing and arguments, and good sportsmanship, for example. The PEERS training was for twelve 90-min sessions. Parents participated in separate concurrent sessions. Knowledge of social etiquette related to making friends, hosted get-togethers, and the rated quality of friendships significantly improved. The frequency of invited get-togethers did not change, however. Unlike the other mentioned studies, Laugeson et al. did not measure or treat skills at a more basic level such as affect recognition and perspective-taking.

Glass, Guli, and Semrud-Clikeman (2000) developed Social Competence Intervention Program (SCIP), a group intervention that integrates drama, to teach social perception and competency to children with such compromised abilities. The SCIP emphasizes learning about nonverbal forms of communication through drama and processing immediate responses towards one another. The authors contrast their method to those groups that only integrate skill-based instruction common to cognitive-behavioral interventions. The SCIP is a manualized intervention that consists of 1.5 h sessions twice per week over a period of approximately 12 weeks. It has a high staff to child ratio (~4:6–8 students). For their pilot study, they assessed progress before and after group, and maintenance after approximately 8 weeks. Three outcome measures were used. They measured social skills through a parent rating scale, directly measured children's awareness of child facial expressions and voice intonation, and coded audiotape to assess positive, solitary, and cooperative behaviors. They did not find significant improvements in social perception according to parent report and direct measurement. In contrast, however, they found significant improvements in positive (increased) and solitary (decreased) behaviors, which behaviors were maintained over approximately 8 weeks. (See Table 10.1 for a brief summary of group interventions described above.)

Social development groups for children with ADHD have also been developed and evaluated. In a comprehensive review, de Boo and Prins (2007) reported that, although significant variability in scope, focus, duration, involvement of parent or teacher training, or foundation in a theoretical model, there were notable commonalities among groups. Most groups included cognitive-behavioral interventions to support improved anger management. All groups were clinic-based and typically lasted 1 h. Groups were facilitated by two to three clinical staff. In addition, intervention methods included behavioral contingencies, modeling, and role-plays (Antshel & Remer, 2003; Miranda & Presentación, 2000), which are considered effective tools when addressing behavioral dysregulation and attention problems (DuPaul & Eckert, 1997). These interventions did not target nonverbal social communication, perspective taking, or pragmatic language skills, as examples.

Table 10.1 Summary of studies

Focus of study	Bauminger (2007) Cognitive-Beh Ecological Model	Solomon et al. (2004) Social Adjustment Enhancement Intervention	Laugeson et al. (2009) PEERS	Social Competence Intervention Program (SCIP)	Evans-Smith et al. (2011) Intervention-Social Emotional Learning Framework (I-SELF)
Skill					
NV Awareness	x	x		x	x
NV Execution		x		x	x
Regulation					x
Pragmatic Language		x	x		x
Perspective-taking	x	x		x	x
Problem-solving	x	x			x
Cooperative Relations	x		x		x
Friendship Networks			x		
Anger Management					x
Therapeutic Orientation					
Cognitive-behavioral (CBT) (role plays, modeling, beh reinforcement, video feedback)	x	x	x	x	x
Process Dynamics "Here and Now"		x		x	x
Outcome Measures					
Parent Report		x	x	x	x
Teacher Report			x		x
Peer Review					
Child Report		x	x		x
Direct Assessment	x	x		x	x
Coding Video or Audiotape	x			x	x

Intervention-Social–Emotional Learning Framework

The following describes a manualized peer group intervention (I-SELF) that addresses many of the deficits children with NVLD may express. The I-SELF integrates elements of therapeutic strategies designed to address the needs of children with social–emotional learning challenges. It incorporates skill instruction, process of group dynamics, with an emphasis on shaping healthier attachments and internal model of self/others. Many of the strategies can be used with children ages 7–16 years old, with some subtle modifications. The groups are not diagnostically homogenous, rather have some commonality of interests and complementary skill sets, although have social–emotional learning challenges. Some elements are detailed below. Subsequently, the results from a pilot study examining the effectiveness of the I-SELF are briefly discussed. For additional information regarding the I-SELF protocol and study, readers are referred to the author.

The I-SELF was developed to reflect the SELF model. The I-SELF is a manualized series of lessons for 32 weeks of 1 h sessions per week. The SELF skills occur in a developmental sequence which is reflected in the group sessions across 5 units. Each unit (approximately 5–7 weeks) emphasizes a particular skill area. Skills and units are sequenced so that latter units build upon earlier ones. Units, in order, include (1) nonverbal communication, (2) emotional and behavioral regulation, (3) pragmatic language, (4a) perspective-taking, (4b) social problem solving, and (5) cooperative relations. To balance skill didactics and group process, sessions are divided into thirds. The beginning of each session requires the clinician to adopt more of a relational/gestalt approach. It includes a group "check-in" when children discuss their week and the clinician facilitates conversation, fosters greater understanding of others' feelings and perspectives, uses an appropriate level of self-disclosure, and models effective communication and empathy as part of the in vivo dynamic process. During this time, over the 32-week span, the clinician also identifies group patterns and progress. The second portion of each session consists of direct instruction and activities related to the skill being taught. This segment relies more on CBT, DBT, mindfulness, and relaxation approaches such that therapy is direct and addresses behavior, cognition, affect, and physiological reactions in concrete ways. Peer and facilitator feedback, modeling, coaching, contingency management, role-plays, video feedback, computerized programs, review of movie/TV clips, discussion, visual depictions, and lecture are all methods used. Cross modality instruction is also integrated into the skill lessons. In addition, the clinician continually encourages awareness of self and others, building trust and understanding of one another. Last, children engage in free play or activities while the clinician guides the process, emphasizing skills learned during previous unit lessons. During this time, the clinician's therapeutic approach may vary depending on the need of the group.

In recognition of prior mixed success of skill application outside of the therapy setting, the I-SELF considers multiple strategies for increasing skill generalization. These include workshops for parents or unit summary letters sent to parents/teachers, individual meetings with parents and teachers, progress monitoring of individualized goals and objectives, and inclusion of children with complementary strengths and deficits. In addition, the I-SELF is not only designed for use in a clinic setting, but can be used in school settings, with modifications.

The following are examples of techniques used to address particular skill deficits. In some cases, clinicians will have some initial conceptualization of the child's social–emotional strengths and challenges. This information may have been obtained from prior evaluations, behavior rating scales, and clinical interviews with caregivers, child, and teachers. During group, the clinician will also be gathering information about the child's functioning through observation and when engaging in social skill activities. When using the I-SELF, clinicians can use the SELF profile to structure their observations as they assess strengths and challenges, and then determine goals and objectives. Typically, goals and objectives are written around the sixth to eighth week of group, discussed with the children, and shared with parents and teachers. Three to four goals are commonly identified.

Introduction

During the first sessions of group, children learn about one another. They identify their interests and share information about themselves, encouraged through activities to remember information about one another. This information will be integrated into discussions and lessons throughout the year.

Nonverbal Awareness and Execution

In this unit, a child's feeling vocabulary, understanding and use of facial expressions, voice intonation and volume, touch and personal space, and gestures and postures are explored and practiced. With all nonverbal social cues, emphasis is on attention to relevant information, accuracy, processing speed, and imitation. Preference is given to the use of active imagery such as video versus static pictures. As an example for teaching understanding and application of facial expressions, there are three computer programs that are used depending on the age of the child. These programs teach children how to more effectively read basic emotions (Micro Expression Training Tool/Subtle Expression Training Tool; Ekman, 2004) (Humintell Microexpression Recognition Training; Matsumoto, 2010) (Faceland, 2010). The programs are sometimes modified so that parts of the face are covered to emphasize the eyes, for example. Children are asked to imitate what they see either in a mirror or with each other. The latter two programs are designed to measure speed of processing. With practice, the child aims to attain a higher percentage of correct responses at faster speeds. To work on intonation and volume, children listen to voices that express a particular feeling. The voices are from a computer program (Mind Reading: The Interactive Guide to Emotions; Baron-Cohen, 2002) or audiotape (DANVA; Nowicki & Duke, 1994). Children practice imitating the voices and discuss interpretation. They also practice repeating sentences using variations of tone and volume according to the feeling they intend to communicate. Some of these sessions are also videotaped and reviewed at a later point as a feedback mechanism. After all nonverbal social cues are reviewed and practiced children look at muted selections of movie or YouTube video clips and analyze the characters' feelings. This awareness and execution of nonverbal social cues are continually emphasized throughout future sessions.

In addition to using some of these methods to teach nonverbal social communication, children with NVLD benefit from others verbalizing their observations of others and related interpretation. By verbalizing observation of social cues (including situational cues), the therapist, caregivers, and teachers are accessing the strength of a child with NVLD.

The above are just a few examples of strategies that we use with the I-SELF. Besides what we have incorporated in our training, Duke et al. (1996) offer a range of ideas for teaching children about nonverbal social information in their book, *Teaching Your Child the Language of Social Success.*

Emotional and Behavioral Regulation

Lessons within this unit help children learn to identify their stressors. They recognize the impact situations can have on thoughts, feelings, and one's physical state and, in turn, their actions. Types of coping strategies are identified. In addition, a behavior plan is sometimes implemented and discussed.

After the above takes place, a cueing system is introduced that helps children become aware of their activity level and attention. Methods to effectively manage activity, attention, anxiety, and depressed mood are taught. Children learn about deep breathing, progressive relaxation, visualization, and mindfulness. Various teaching tools are used to introduce and practice these strategies. One example is encouraging children to become repetitively silly and then calm so that they learn to more easily shift between these emotional/physical states. Depending on the group's developmental level and ability, they also learn additional cognitive strategies including "self-talk." In some instances, a clinician may record these tips on a podcast, download it as an MP3, and send it to each group member to access on their iPod. Children are encouraged to use these strategies throughout the span of the group.

Pragmatic Language

There are many skills within this domain that can be addressed. For the I-SELF, we address active listening, what the listener and speaker's responsibility is, and how to start and organize a conversation. Children learn about these skills by pausing and analyzing video clips, observing self on video, and practicing through role-plays, for example.

As part of the lessons within this unit, there is an emphasis on mental organization of ideas. Some children with NVLD can present with problems when mentally organizing social information. A method to address this organizational challenge is by asking the group to generate and organize topics for conversational starters, e.g., movies, music, school (teachers, homework, classes). Children are encouraged to reflect on what they know about each other—interests, values, experiences—to determine topics they could initiate in conversation. Also, children learn to categorize conversational starters as either means of seeking or offering help, attempts to hang out, chitchat, or encourage/compliment, as examples. All of this information can be depicted in a conversational flow chart so that the initial statement/question and topic is listed at the top of the flow chart. Then, as with graphic organizers, varying responses can be tracked by connecting boxes that contain each potential subsequent comment or question. During this process, the clinician is also facilitating a more coherent mental working social model of others and self by emphasizing each other's interests, values, and personality.

Conversational rules of thumb are also introduced. For example, children may be encouraged to keep their responses to approximately five statements versus being too verbose (twenty sentences) or minimalists (one brief response) and to then pause for a few seconds to allow others to interject. Children are reinforced for using "wh" formed questions and a script for times when they are uncertain about what is being stated. There are a number of resources that provide additional ideas to address pragmatic language skills (My School Day computer program, Gajewski, Hirn, & Mayo, 1998; Gray, 2000; Jacobs & Jacobs, 2002; Mannix, 1993).

During these activities, children's feelings and thoughts are explored. Do they find themselves feeling nervous, insecure, worried about not succeeding when attempting to speak to others? Do they worry they won't be able to sustain a conversation? Methods to manage emotions are discussed and practiced as reviewed in the regulation unit.

Perspective-Taking

There are a number of tools that we use to teach perspective-taking, understanding that others may have different views and perspectives. Thought bubbles are introduced as a way to conceptualize that others have thoughts that may not be evident by what the person says or does. Cartoon strips such as Garfield, Webber Photo Cards (Super Duper publications), and Social Skills Picture Book (Baker, 2001); computer programs such as Mind Reading (Baron-Cohen, 2002); and the review of selected movie clips are used. All of these materials (except movie clips) contain static images with thought bubbles. After the concept is established with the static pictures, then movie clips are used. They offer a more realistic experience to assess others' perspectives. As with the nonverbal communication unit, sound is initially off to draw the children's attention to the nonverbal gestures and situational cues, which are clues to the potential perspectives of the characters. Afterwards, the movie is played back with sound so the children can assess their accuracy. After this series of instructions, the group engages in activities that address personal impressions (Winner, 2002). Perspective taking is also continually emphasized during our process at the beginning and latter portions of group throughout the year.

Social Problem Solving

There are a number of lessons that comprise social problem solving. Initially, the group brainstorms categories of social problems, e.g., being teased, being excluded, and dealing with someone who controls the play or conversation. This exercise is intended to help children form an organized mental schema for problems. Many children with NVLD struggle to describe a problem that they are having; this schema can act as a heuristic for them. Children are then introduced to two simple frameworks that guide their conceptualization of the problem and decision-making. One of the frameworks depicts issues that need to be considered with the problem: situation, thoughts, feelings, physiological reaction, and potential resulting behavior with self and others. The other framework extracts elements of what Lemerise and Arsenio (2000) and Crick and Dodge (1994) considered as important elements with social information processing. (1) A social problem is identified: what setting are you in, what are the implicit rules for behavior, and what are the feelings and thoughts of others and self; (2) brainstorm options for solutions by considering what self and others could think and feel with each option while taking into consideration the situation; (3) what could be the consequences of each option; and (4) choose the best option. Potential solutions and methods of resolution are taught such as conflict resolution/negotiation skills, how to compromise, and what it means to be assertive and empathic, for example. These skills are considered more complex interpersonal skills and integrate all the previous learning from prior sessions. Children engage in role-plays which can be videotaped and reviewed in future sessions. Also, problems that arise between people in video clips or computer programs such as My School Day (Jacobs & Jacobs, 2002) are reviewed and discussed.

Cooperative Play/Relations

The primary focus in this unit is on good sportsmanship and the use of humor. Issues related to cooperative relations have been informally addressed throughout the group's sessions, especially during the last portion of each session when the children play or engage in a mutually agreed upon fun activity. During this unit examples of good and bad sportsmanship are shared and role-played. Video clips depicting both are reviewed and discussed. The group also learns about different types of humor through discussion and review of video clips. Different perspectives are shared. In addition, children are given tips for telling jokes and opportunity to practice.

Closure

The last few sessions are focused on creating and writing cards for one another, sharing their progress, and having a party.

Pilot Study with the I-SELF

Method

The intent of the study was to assess the effectiveness of the I-SELF across therapy settings and ages by using multiple assessment methods (Evans-Smith et al., 2011). The I-SELF was implemented in both an urban school and clinic setting for the school year. A number of the children did not strictly meet the criteria for any childhood diagnosis. Children presented, however, with symptoms commonly associated with ASD, ADHD, and NVLD. The clinic group involved six boys ranging in age from 11.3 to 12.10 years old, most of whom were Caucasian. Their group was for 1 h each week across 30 weeks. The school group had four boys and two girls 8.1–9.5 years old of diverse ethnic backgrounds. The I-SELF was modified to accommodate the school schedule. It was for one-half hour each week across 16 sessions. Each group had two facilitators. Generalization was addressed by conducting parent workshops for the clinic group and integrating lessons in the classroom for the school group. Outcome measures included video coding, direct skill assessment, and rating scales. Nonverbal awareness accuracy and processing speed, perspective-taking, pragmatic language, and social problem solving were directly assessed. These skills along with emotional and behavioral regulation and cooperative relations were also assessed through behavior rating scales completed by parents, teachers, and the child. Nonverbal communication (including execution), regulation, pragmatic language, and social problem solving were coded from group videotape.

Brief Summary of Results

We found clinically significant improvement for most of the skills assessed. Problem solving and cooperative relations improved the most with significantly large effects observed across multiple assessments and settings, age, and symptoms. With respect to social problem solving, for example, the clinic group offered more ideas to solve problems ($d=1.47$) and sought clarification more often ($d=0.66$), according to video observation. Children from the school group demonstrated significantly improved scores on the direct measure ($d=0.89$). Moderate to large effect sizes were observed with cooperative play according to parent and teacher reports (clinic parent $d=0.80$, school parent $d=0.68$, school teacher $d=0.53$). Depending on which assessment measures were referenced, significant improvements were also noted with (1) regulation (video observation, large effect size, $d=-1.09$); (2) nonverbal communication—comprehension of others' emotions (video observation, large effect size, $d=0.93$) and improved execution of gestures and eye contact (large effect size, $d=1.42$) (other nonverbal communication assessment measures revealed small to medium effect sizes (direct assessment clinic $d=0.25$, school $d=0.33$, parent report clinic $d=0.36$, and teacher report school $d=0.51$)); and (3) pragmatic language (direct assessment, small to medium effect sizes, clinic $d=0.52$, school $d=0.31$) (video coding, large effect size, $d=0.72$), (parent report clinic, medium effect size, $d=0.48$, teacher report school, large effect size, $d=0.61$).

Conclusion

Despite differences between the clinic and school group participants, settings, and scope and depth of treatment, some similar positive outcomes were obtained. With respect to outcome measures, coded videotape was found to be one of the most sensitive and meaningful forms of measurement. Our findings also supported the involvement of both parents and teachers in training programs which was consistent with the literature (Reichow & Volkmar, 2010). Overall, these findings supported the continued exploration of this intervention as an effective tool for change for children with social–emotional learning challenges.

We also recognized the inherent limitations with this quasi-experimental design, especially in that it limited our ability to draw causal inferences about the intervention's effectiveness. We intend to conduct a larger scale study in which the design can be improved, e.g., control group and larger sample size, and assess for maintenance and generalization of skills.

Implications for the Future

Children with NVLD, in which the right hemisphere is implicated, present with problems in fluidly processing and reasoning with visual-spatial and social–emotional information, motor delays, sensory sensitivities, and, in some cases, struggle with emotional and behavioral regulation. With any delays or injuries to regions of the right hemisphere, especially in early development, the infant/child becomes susceptible to attachment problems and having gaps in his mental organization or schemas of others and self. As Schore (2003) theorizes, these children are likely to be vulnerable to dysregulation, whether manifest in anxiety, mood, or behavior. A developmental behavioral, interpersonal, and neurobiological orientation, therefore, provides a comprehensive perspective to a child's social–emotional needs. Utilizing a theoretically integrated therapeutic approach has the potential to greatly benefit the child. Clinical techniques that originate from cognitive-behavioral, dialectical behavior, mindfulness, relaxation, relational, and gestalt therapies can address these more global needs. Such techniques can be used in individual, family, and group psychotherapy. Children with NVLD present with notable skill deficits which remediate best with concrete, direct clinical interventions. They also have internalized struggles whether they are related to insecure attachments with caregivers and/or poorly developed internal working social models of self and others. These children are more vulnerable to feeling inadequate, unwanted, mistrusting, and anxious, as examples. These latter clinical issues are better addressed with relational forms of therapy.

As discussed, the SELF is one such model that can be used to conceptualize a child with NVLD's social–emotional strengths and challenges. Through this assessment, interventions directed towards skill development can be individualized. The I-SELF extends the conceptualization of the child with NVLD's social needs to consider his relational attachments and internal schemas of others and self through an integration of therapeutic methods as described earlier in this chapter.

The ongoing question of whether NVLD is a disability or differentiated from a pervasive developmental disorder, for example, will require continued clinical review, research, and advocacy. Regardless of the outcome, however, children can be best treated when clinicians adopt a more individualized approach to the child's social and emotional learning needs, knowing areas of skill function that a child with nonverbal and motor processing problems is most likely to struggle. The ongoing and subsequent impact on self-image and relationships also needs to be assessed and treated. The effectiveness of these treatments requires continued exploration and empirical support.

References

Adolphs, R. (2003). Cognitive neuroscience of human social behavior. *Nature Reviews Neuroscience, 4*, 165–173.

Allen, N., Blashki, G., & Gullone, E. (2006). Mindfulness-based psychotherapies: A review of conceptual foundations, empirical evidence and practical considerations. *Australian and New Zealand Journal of Psychiatry, 40*, 285–294.

Annaz, D., Karmiloff-Smith, A., & Thomas, M. (2008). The importance of tracing developmental trajectories for clinical child neuropsychology. In J. Reed & J. Rogers (Eds.), *Child neuropsychology: Concepts, theory, and practice*. London: Blackwell.

Antshel, K. M., & Remer, R. (2003). Social skills training in children with attention deficit hyperactivity disorder: A randomized-controlled clinical trial. *Journal of Clinical Child and Adolescent Psychology, 32*(1), 153–165.

Baer, R. A. (2003). Mindfulness training as a clinical intervention: A conceptual and empirical review. *Clinical Psychology: Science and Practice, 10*(2), 125–143.

Baker, J. (2001). *The Social Skills Picture Book: Teaching play, emotion, and communication to children with autism*. Texas: Future Horizons.

Baron-Cohen, S. (2002). *Mind reading: The interactive guide to emotions*. London: Jessica Kingsley Publishers.

Baron-Cohen, S., Leslie, A., & Frith, U. (1985). Does the autistic child have a "theory of mind?". *Cognition, 21*, 37–46.

Bauminger, N. (2007). Brief report: Group social-multimodal intervention for HFASD. *Journal of Autism and Developmental Disorders, 37*(8), 1605–1615.

Beck, J., & Beck, A. (2011). *Cognitive behavior therapy, second edition: Basics and beyond*. NY: Guilford.

Broitman, J. (2002). *Using control mastery theory to treat the child with NVLD. Symposium on nonverbal learning disorders*. Berkeley, CA: NLDA.

Bronfenbrenner, U., & Evans, G. (2000). Developmental science in the 21st century: Emerging theoretical models, research designs, and empirical findings. *Social Development, 9*, 115–125.

Chiron, C., Jambaque, J., Nabbout, R., Lounes, R., Syrota, A., & Dulac, O. (1997). The right brain hemisphere is dominant in human infants. *Brain, 120*, 1057–1065.

Cook, C. R., Gresham, F. M., Kern, L., Barreras, R. B., Thornton, S., & Crews, S. D. (2008). Social skills training for secondary students with emotional and/or behavioral disorders: A review and analysis of the meta-analytic literature. *Journal of Emotional and Behavioral Disorders, 16*(3), 131–144.

Crick, N. R., & Dodge, K. A. (1994). A review and reformulation of social information-processing mechanisms in children's social adjustment. *Psychological Bulletin, 115*(1), 74–101.

Davis, J., & Broitman, J. (2011). *Nonverbal learning disabilities in children: Bridging the gap between science and practice*. USA: Springer.

Davis, M., Eshelman, E., & McKay, M. (2000). *The relaxation and stress reduction workbook* (5th ed.). Oakland, CA: New Harbinger Publications, Inc.

de Boo, G. M., & Prins, P. J. M. (2007). Social incompetence in children with ADHD: Possible moderators and mediators in social-skills training. *Clinical Psychology Review, 27*(1), 78–97.

Decety, J., & Jackson, P. (2004). The functional architecture of human empathy. *Behavioral and Cognitive Neuroscience Reviews, 3*(2), 71–100.

Duke, M., Nowicki, S., & Martin, E. (1996). *Teaching your child the language of social success*. Georgia: Peachtree Publishers, Ltd.

DuPaul, G. J., & Eckert, T. L. (1997). The effects of school-based interventions for attention deficit hyperactivity disorder: A meta-analysis. *School Psychology Review, 26*(1), 5–27.

Durlak, J. A., Weissberg, R. P., Dymnicki, A. B., Taylor, R. D., & Schellinger, K. B. (2011). The impact of enhancing students' social and emotional learning: A meta-analysis of school-based universal interventions. *Child Development, 82*, 405–432.

Ekman, P. (2004). *Micro expression training tool/subtle expression training tool*. San Francisco: Mozgomedia. http://www.emotionsrevealed.com/

Elliot, C., & Lassen, M. (1997). A schema polarity model for case conceptualization, intervention, and research. *Clinical Psychology: Science and Practice, 4*(1), 12–28.

Evans-Smith, B., Allen, A., Johnson, J., & McKown, C. (2011). *Promoting social competence in children with social emotional learning challenges: A developmental group model*. Manuscript submitted for publication.

Faceland. (2010). USA: Do2Learn.

Frankel, F., Myatt, R., Cantwell, D. P., & Feinberg, D. T. (1997). Parent-assisted transfer of children's social skills training: Effects on children with and without attention-deficit hyperactivity disorder. *Journal of the American Academy of Child and Adolescent Psychiatry, 36*(8), 1056–1064.

Gajewski, N., Hirn, P., & Mayo, P. (1998). *Social skill strategies: A social emotional curriculum for adolescents*. WI: Thinking Publications.

Germer, C., Siegel, R., & Fulton, P. (2005). *Mindfulness and psychotherapy*. NY: Guilford.

Glass, K., Guli, L., & Semrud-Clikeman, M. (2000). Social competence intervention program: A pilot program for the development of social competence. *Journal of Psychotherapy in Independent Practice, 1*(4), 21–33.

Goldenberg, H., & Goldenberg, I. (2012). *Family therapy: An overview*. Belmont, CA: Brooks/Cole Cengage Learning.

Gray, C. (2000). *The new social story book*. TX: Future Horizons, Inc.

Greenspan, S., & Wieder, S. (2005). *Infant and early childhood mental health: A comprehensive, developmental approach to assessment and intervention*. Washington, D.C.: American Psychiatric Publishing, Inc.

Gresham, F. M., & Elliot, S. N. (2009). *Social skills improvement system: Teacher rating scales*. Bloomington, MN: Pearson Assessments.

Heberlein, A., Adolphs, R., Pennebaker, J., & Tranel, D. (2003). Effects of damage to right-hemisphere brain structures on spontaneous emotional and social judgments. *Political Psychology, 24*(4), 705–726.

Hooker, K., & Fodor, I. (2008). Teaching mindfulness to children. *Gestalt Review, 12*(1), 75–91.

Jacobs, J., & Jacobs, L. (2002). *My School Day*. Leesburg, VA: Social Skill Builder.

Johnson, D., & Myklebust, H. (1967). *Learning disabilities: Educational principles and practices*. NY: Grune & Stratton.

Kabat-Zinn, J. (1994). *Wherever you go, there you are: Mindfulness meditation in everyday life*. New York: Hyperion.

Kabat-Zinn, J., Lipworth, L., Burney, R., & Sellers, W. (1987). Four-year follow-up of a meditation-based program for self-regulation of chronic pain: Treatment outcomes and compliance. *The Clinical Journal of Pain, 2*, 159–173.

Koenig, K., White, S. W., Pachler, M., Lau, M., Lewis, M., Klin, A., et al. (2010). Promoting social skill development in children with pervasive developmental disorders: A feasibility and efficacy study. *Journal of Autism and Developmental Disorders, 40*(10), 1209–1218.

Kristeller, J., & Hallett, B. (1999). An exploratory study of a mediation-based intervention for binge eating disorder. *Journal of Health Psychology, 4*(3), 357–363.

Laugeson, E. A., Frankel, F., Mogil, C., & Dillon, A. R. (2009). Parent-assisted social skills training to improve friendships in teens with autism spectrum disorders. *Journal of Autism and Developmental Disorders, 39*(4), 596–606.

Le Grand, R., Mondloch, C., Maurer, D., & Brent, H. (2003). Expert face processing requires visual input to the right hemisphere during infancy. *Nature Neuroscience, 6*, 1108–1112.

Lemerise, E. A., & Arsenio, W. F. (2000). An integrated model of emotion processes and cognition in social information processing. *Child Development, 71*(1), 107–118.

Linden,W. (1973). Practicing of meditation by school children and their levels of field independence–independence, test anxiety, and reading achievement. *Journal of Consulting and Clinical Psychology, 41*, 139–143.

Lipton, M., & Evans-Smith, B. (2006). *Social emotional learning framework (SELF): Conceptual, clinical, and research aspects*. University of California, Davis, CA: The Summer Institute on Neurodevelopmental Disorders, MIND Institute.

Lipton, M., & Nowicki, S. (2009). The social emotional learning framework (SELF): A guide for understanding brain-based social emotional learning impairments. *Journal of Developmental Processes, 4*(2), 99–115.

Lopata, C., Thomeer, M. L., Volker, M. A., Toomey, J. A., Nida, R. E., Lee, G. K., et al. (2010). RCT of a manualized social treatment for high-functioning autism spectrum disorders. *Journal of Autism and Developmental Disorders, 40*(11), 1297–1310.

Mannix, D. (1993). *Social skills activities for special children*. NY: The Center for Applied Research in Education.

Marra, T. (2005). *Dialectical behavior therapy in private practice*. Oakland, CA: New Harbinger Publications, Inc.

Matsumoto, D. (2010). *Microexpression recognition training tool*. CA: Humintell, Inc.

Miller, P., Kessel, F., & Flavell, J. (1970). Thinking about people thinking about people thinking about …: A study of social cognitive development. *Child Development, 41*, 613–623.

Miltenberger, R. (2011). *Behavior modification: Principles and procedures* (5th ed.). Belmont, CA: Wadsworth Cengage Learning.

Minuchin, S., Lee, W., & Simon, G. (1996). *Mastering family therapy*. NY: Wiley.

Miranda, A., & Presentación, M. J. (2000). Efficacy of cognitive-behavioral therapy in the treatment of children with ADHD, with and without aggressiveness. *Psychology in the Schools, 37*(2), 169–182.

Nowicki, S., & Duke, M. P. (1994). Individual differences in the nonverbal communication of affect: The diagnostic analysis of nonverbal accuracy scale. *Journal of Nonverbal Behavior, 18*(1), 9–35.

Ott, M. (2002). Mindfulness meditation in pediatric clinical practice. *Pediatric Nursing, 28*(5), 487–490.

Palombo, J. (2001). *Learning disorders and disorders of self in children and adolescents.* NY: Norton & Co.

Palombo, J., Bendicsen, H., & Koch, B. (2011). *Guide to psychoanalytic developmental theories.* USA: Springer.

Palombo, J., & Berenberg, A. (1997). Psychotherapy for children with nonverbal learning disabilities. In B. Mark & J. Incorvaia (Eds.), *The handbook of infant, child, and adolescent psychotherapy: New directions in integrative treatment* (Vol. 2, pp. 25–67). London: Reiss-Davis Child Study Center.

Pfiffner, L. J., Calzada, E., & McBurnett, K. (2000). Interventions to enhance social competence. *Child and Adolescent Psychiatric Clinics of North America, 9*(3), 689–709.

Prizant, B. M., Wetherby, A. M., Rubin, E., Laurent, A. C., & Rydell, P. J. (2006a). *The SCERTS model: A comprehensive educational approach for children with autism spectrum disorders* (Vol. 1). Baltimore, MD: Paul H Brookes Publishing.

Prizant, B. M., Wetherby, A. M., Rubin, E., Laurent, A. C., & Rydell, P. J. (2006b). *The SCERTS model: A comprehensive educational approach for children with autism spectrum disorders* (Vol. 2). Baltimore, MD: Paul H Brookes Publishing.

Reichow, B., & Volkmar, F. R. (2010). Social skills interventions for individuals with autism: Evaluation for evidence-based practices within a best evidence synthesis framework. *Journal of Autism and Developmental Disorders, 40*(2), 149–166.

Rourke, B. (1995). The NLD syndrome and the white matter model. In B. Rourke (Ed.), *Syndrome of nonverbal learning disabilities: Neurodevelopmental manifestations.* NY: Guilford.

Schore, A. (2003). *Affect dysregulation and disorders of the self.* NY: Norton.

Schore, A. (2005). Attachment, affect regulation, and the developing right brain: Linking developmental neuroscience to pediatrics. *Pediatrics in Review, 26*(6), 204–217.

Segal, Z., Williams, J., & Teasdale, J. (2002). *Mindfulness-based cognitive therapy for depression: A new approach to preventing relapse.* NY: Guilford.

Selman, R. (1976). Social-cognitive understanding: A guide to educational and clinical practice. In T. Lickona (Ed.), *Moral development and behavior: Theory, research, and social issues* (pp. 299–316). NY: Holt, Rinehart & Winston.

Semple, R., Lee, J., & Miller, L. (2006). Mindfulness-based cognitive therapy for children. In R. A. Baer (Ed.), *Mindfulness-based treatment approaches: Clinician's guide to evidence base and applications* (pp. 143–166). San Diego, CA: Elsevier Academic.

Semple, R., Lee, J., Rosa, D., & Miller, L. (2010). A randomized trial of mindfulness-based cognitive therapy for children: Promoting mindful attention to enhance social-emotional resiliency in children. *Journal of Child and Family Studies, 19*, 218–229.

Semrud-Clickman, M., & Fine, J. (2008). A meta-analysis of the neuropsychology of NVLD. Paper presented at the International Neuropsychological Society.

Semrud-Clickman, M., & Hynd, G. (1990). Right hemisphere dysfunction in nonverbal learning disabilities: Social, academic, and adaptive functioning in adults and children. *Psychological Bulletin, 107*(2), 196–209.

Siegel, D. (1999). *The developing mind: How relationships and the brain interact to shape who we are.* NY: Guilford.

Solomon, M., Goodlin-Jones, B., & Anders, T. F. (2004). A social adjustment enhancement intervention for high functioning autism, asperger's syndrome, and pervasive developmental disorder NOS. *Journal of Autism and Developmental Disorders, 34*(6), 649–668.

Stern, D. (2000). *The interpersonal world of the infant: A view from psychoanalysis and developmental psychology.* NY: Basic Books.

Stewart, K. (2002). *Helping a child with nonverbal learning disorder or asperger's syndrome.* Oakland, CA: New Harbinger Publications.

Stichter, J. P., Herzog, M. J., Visovsky, K., Schmidt, C., Randolph, J., Schultz, T., et al. (2010). Social competence intervention for youth with asperger syndrome and high-functioning autism: An initial investigation. *Journal of Autism and Developmental Disorders, 40*(9), 1067–1079.

Thompson, M., & Gauntlett-Gilbert, J. (2008). Mindfulness with children and adolescents: Effective clinical application. *Clinical Child Psychology and Psychiatry, 13*(3), 395–407.
Wall, R. (2005). Tai Chi and mindfulness-based stress reduction in a Boston public middle school. *Journal of Pediatric Health Care, 19*(4), 230–237.
Webber photo cards. South Carolina: Super Duper Publications.
Weiss, J. (1993). *How psychotherapy works: Process and technique*. New York: Guilford.
Weiss, J., Sampson, H., & The Mount Zion Psychotherapy Research Group. (1986). *The psychoanalytic process: Theory, clinical observations, and empirical research*. New York: Guilford.
Wellman, H. (1992). *The child's theory of mind*. MA: MIT.
Winner, M. (2002). *Thinking about you, thinking about me*. San Jose, CA: Michelle Garcia Winner Publications.
Yalom, I. (1995). *The theory and practice of group psychotherapy* (4th ed.). NY: Basic Books.
Yamada, H., Sadato, N., & Konishi, Y. (2000). A milestone for normal development of the infantile brain detected by functional MRI. *Neuroscience, 55*, 218–223.

Chapter 11
College Counseling with the NVLD Student

Jane McClure

This chapter will provide practical suggestions for advising college-bound students with nonverbal learning disabilities (NVLD) and their families in the college selection and application process. A literature review found no research on this topic for students with NVLD, and little for specific learning disabilities. What was found will be included in this chapter, but the strategies and suggestions discussed herein are largely based upon the experiences of seasoned practitioners in the field. As they relate to selecting and applying to college, the impact of NVLD on academic, organizational, and social difficulties will be discussed.

Furthermore, this chapter will explore a variety of challenges facing the college-bound student with NVLD and his or her family. This will include the *typical* academic and social issues of students with NVLD, academic and social interventions and accommodations for working with college-bound and college-transitioning students with NVLD, a brief overview of relevant laws, and description of a model for how to think about differing levels of support provided by colleges for students with NVLD. Lastly, a case study illustrating this kind of work with a student with NVLD and her family will be presented.

Academic Issues

In order to understand the significant issues related to college-counseling students with NVLD, it is helpful to know what selective colleges (those that don't admit all students who apply) are looking for when reviewing applications in general. To begin with, college admission personnel are looking for students who have chosen *a challenging curriculum* within the context of what has been available to them at

J. McClure, M.A (✉)
McClure, Mallory, Baron & Ross, 200 Lombard Street,
San Francisco, CA 94111, USA
e-mail: janemcclr@aol.com

J. Broitman and J.M. Davis (eds.), *Treating NVLD in Children: Professional Collaborations for Positive Outcomes*, DOI 10.1007/978-1-4614-6179-1_11,

their high schools. It is to a student's advantage to take some honors or Advanced Placement courses. It is also viewed positively if students take more than what is minimally required, e.g., 4 or 5 years of math when 3 years are required or 3 or 4 years of foreign language when only 2 years are required. Grades earned in all courses are important, of course, but getting straight A's in a "weak" curriculum will not be impressive to a college admission counselor.

College admission counselors may have to help students with specific learning disabilities to make choices regarding a *challenging curriculum* because SLD students may not be able to do as well in all subjects. Students with NVLD, specifically, often have difficulty with math and/or science (Whitney, 2002). Writing essays and papers, especially with the level of complexity and concept formation/abstract thinking that is required during the last 2 years of high school, is also very challenging for many students with NVLD (Davis & Broitman, 2011). Finally, since many students with NVLD have executive function challenges, they may be struggling in several classes just because they are having difficulty with organization and time management. These students may, for example, be taking four academic courses instead of five because taking five courses is too stressful and would cause them to do poorly in some or all of their classes (Davis & Broitman, 2011).

When counseling these students, it is important to appreciate the challenges they typically face and to advise them cautiously. It is also important *not* to make generalizations about students with NVLD because NVLD is a spectrum disorder and students are affected to varying degrees and in different areas and disciplines (Davis & Broitman, 2011). A counselor cannot make assumptions when looking at a transcript. It is crucial to interview the student about the choices made; it can be extremely helpful to talk to parents and tutors and special education teachers as well. As mentioned above, college admission counselors evaluate students within the context of what is available to them at their high schools. They also evaluate students within the context of challenges they have faced, which would certainly include NVLD. (Issues about disclosure in the application process will be discussed in a later section of this chapter.)

Typical Areas of Weakness that Emerge During the High School Years: *Reading*. Despite precocity in the acquisition of language and decoding skills in the early years, reading comprehension may decline in the higher grades for students with NVLD. Single-word reading and vocabulary usually remain strong, but deficits in reading, especially for novel material, become increasingly problematic (Rourke, 1989). This can be extremely frustrating for a student who was excellent in reading and language skills in earlier years.

Math. Rourke (1989) also describes the acceleration of math difficulties as students with NVLD advance through school. Typically, math has *always* been significantly harder than language-based classes, but procedural math (computation, calculation, etc.) is usually very difficult for students, a problem that is exacerbated by the inevitable difficulty students then have with higher level math skills involving math reasoning and application of basic math skills to complex, multistep problems. By the time students are seen for college counseling, they are likely to have developed a strong dislike for math and are sometimes even math phobic.

Science. Problem solving and complex concept formation, such as those required for subjects like physics and chemistry, tend to be very challenging for students with NVLD. Students may do much better in certain aspects of science, like biology, where they may be required to memorize the names of the bones and muscles of the body or perform some other more rote academic tasks rather than more complicated and spatially challenging sciences such as chemistry.

Typically college counselors don't encourage students to take advanced level courses in areas that are impacted by their NVLD. Instead, the students are helped to evaluate how many courses and what kind of courses they can take which will provide them with an appropriate level of challenge, but also allow them to earn reasonable grades and to make their lives less stressful as well.

College Admission Tests: As might be expected, many students with NVLD have significantly lower math scores than those on critical reading or writing, but this isn't always the case. The critical reading section can be difficult for some of these students because of the inferential nature of many of the multiple-choice questions. The writing section calls for quick organizational skills and that's often difficult for students with NVLD, too. In sum, some students with NVLD do quite well on these tests while others really struggle. There is enormous variation in their performances, just as there is with neurotypical students. The best strategy is for students to take both SAT and ACT practice tests early in the junior year to determine which test is more comfortable and is the best fit for the student. A test preparation course or a tutor may also be helpful in providing the student with the best opportunity to do as well as possible. Since there are so many students with learning disabilities who are planning to attend college, many well-known test preparation companies (such as Princeton Review and Ivy West) have specific tutors whom they match with LD students. It is advisable for college counselors to be knowledgeable about test preparation programs and tutors in their area who have experience and (perhaps) special training and can work effectively with learning-disabled students. For example, if students have been granted extended time or other accommodations on the SAT or the ACT, it makes sense for them to take practice tests using those accommodations. If they take the usual six to ten practice tests under standard conditions, they will not be well prepared for the test as it will actually be administered to them. Studying for the SAT or ACT with one-on-one tutors is usually more effective for students with NVLD than taking regular classes because these students often learn differently and have a more difficult time grasping certain concepts. With regard to math, for example, learning step-by-step sequential methods which require less visual–spatial problem solving is beneficial for many students (Rubenstien, 2009).

For those students who don't perform well on standardized tests, either the SAT or the ACT, there is some good news. Each year, a few more colleges join the list of schools that are "test optional." Usually, this means that students can simply choose whether or not they wish to submit test scores as part of their application documentation. At some schools, however, certain criteria must be satisfied if a student does not submit test scores. For example, at Franklin and Marshall College, students who do not believe that their standardized test scores reflect their academic ability are able to submit two graded writing samples (from junior or senior year) in lieu of

SAT or ACT scores. Sarah Lawrence College has gone beyond "test optional" in that they no longer consider SAT or ACT scores, or subject test scores, in their admission process. If students send them, they won't be reviewed.

So how can counselors and students figure out what to do about testing if they would prefer not to send their scores? The website http://www.fairtest.org is a good place to start. It provides a frequently updated list of colleges and universities "that do not use SAT or ACT scores for admitting substantial numbers of students into Bachelor Degree programs." Once individuals have identified colleges on this list that are of interest to them, it is essential that they next go to the specific college websites to find out if there are other requirements to satisfy in lieu of SAT or ACT scores. If not, students can feel comfortable submitting their application materials without submitting test scores. An additional *caveat* to keep in mind: Students who most benefit from test-optional admissions are those whose test scores are significantly lower than their grades (http://www.petersons.com/college-search/college-admission-test-optional.aspx).

High School Interventions for Students with NVLD: In order to advise a student about which colleges will be a good fit, it is essential to determine the level of accommodations and/or services the student will need. This will be discussed in detail in a later section in this chapter. The first step in making this determination, however, is to assess the student's high school experience, evaluating the kind of help they have had, especially during senior year. *This must be a collaborative process*. Typically students are first spoken with to find out what academic areas or tasks are most difficult for them both at school and with homework assignments. But these students are often not very self-aware about their academic needs (Dalke & Schmitt, 1987), so it is important to find out what enables them to be successful from other sources. Parents can be instrumental, especially as relates to work students do at home. For example, do parents have to oversee and nag students to get their homework done on a regular basis? Do they feel they need to read all their papers before they are turned in at school? Do they help them with their math homework, or is there a tutor the student sees after school? Appended at the end of the chapter will be the Executive Function Survey which was created by Dr. Peggy Hock and this author to help get at these questions.

Resource teachers, classroom teachers, and tutors are also crucial resources for this kind of input. The resource teacher is in a position of knowing which subjects are most difficult for a student and what kind of assistance a student needs to get work done. Can students start a paper on their own, or must the resource teacher break it down into chunks for them and assign target completion dates? The classroom teacher can report about a student's engagement in the classroom, including focus of attention, participation in discussion, ability to grasp concepts relative to other classmates, and need for extended time on exams. Outside tutors can provide insight about how a student learns. Does the student simply need to have the concepts presented again because he wasn't able to grasp them when first presented in the classroom? Or does the student need to discuss a biology or chemistry concept with the tutor in order to grasp it. This is often the case because students with NVLD can compensate for their learning deficits by employing their strength in language.

While gathering the information, it is useful to find out which specific interventions work best for this student. The student's perspective, of course, is particularly relevant to this question. It is also important to be aware that interventions can become more or less appropriate as the student advances through school. For example, having long-term assignments broken down into sections may be essential during freshman and sophomore years, but by senior year a student may have internalized this process and can do it for himself. Gaining a thorough understanding about "what works for this student" will be an important aspect of a successful college-counseling process. What (if any) level of remediation is still required, and how well has the student been able to compensate for his or her NVLD? Most students will need the same level of support they are receiving at the end of high school during their first year of college (Dalke & Schmitt, 1987).

Once the picture becomes more clear, the college counselor can assess what level of services will be necessary in order for the student to make a successful transition to college, and, subsequently, successful progress toward graduation.

Self-Advocacy: There is no more important skill for a student who is headed toward college to develop than becoming a good self-advocate (Krebs, 2002; Lock & Layton, 2001; Skinner, 2004). The responsibility for acquiring accommodations or services shifts from the school to the student once a student moves from secondary to postsecondary education. This can be a shock to students who have been supported throughout their school careers by parents, teachers, tutors, and coaches. Now they not only have to be able to *recognize* when they are in academic trouble, but they also need to figure out what kind of help they need and how to get it. And they need to realize the importance of getting that help sooner rather than later, before it is too late. In almost all cases, this will require practice in high school (Durlak, Rose, & Bursuck, 1994).

Students don't usually figure this out completely on their own; in fact, this can be particularly challenging for students with NVLD because of impaired social competency, or at least social awkwardness (Davis & Broitman, 2011). Role-playing during junior and senior year can be very helpful for students. Working with them to write a script and providing real, authentic opportunities for them to seek help are excellent training for what they will need to be able to do in college. For example, one of this author's seniors was struggling in two of his classes. His resource teacher and his mother were communicating with his teachers because of his reluctance and, frankly, ineffectiveness at self-advocacy with his teachers. When the necessity of developing this student's self-advocacy was discussed at his IEP meeting, the mother and resource teacher realized that they needed to help this young man speak for himself. A new objective was initiated in which the resource teacher worked with him, first to put the words down on paper and second, to role-play the scenario so that the student could eventually feel comfortable communicating with classroom teachers on his own behalf.

Providing realistic and appropriate feedback will also help students understand how to express their needs effectively when communicating with someone who is expected to provide a service for them. Scheduling an appointment with a service provider to ask for help will work much better than interrupting a conversation that is taking place. Having some failures while still safely in their home environment can actually be a *good* thing. Working through these experiences and figuring out how to approach the situation differently next time are often how they learn best.

But it is so important to keep in mind that students with NVLD learn best from words. Since they often don't accurately grasp social cues from body language or tone of voice, they might not pick up what seems clearly obvious to others. Explanations should use very specific language because that's how they will best understand exactly what is meant. For example, it may be insufficient to merely tell a student to ask a professor after class if he can have a meeting to go over a test on which he did poorly. The student may need to role-play this conversation, after being instructed to wait until the professor has finished speaking to other students and to ask the professor if he has a moment to talk before his next class.

Counseling the College-Bound Student with NVLD

Organization: Deficiency in organizational ability is one of the hallmarks of NVLD. That makes applying to four to eight colleges, standard for high school seniors, extremely problematic. Most students find it daunting to stay organized while applying to college, especially in light of the fact that they are also trying to do well in their high school courses and manage a couple of extracurricular activities, or perhaps a job, on the side. For students with NVLD, this can be terrifying if they are aware of their organizational problems, or confusing and overwhelming if they are not. Parents are usually even more worried, even panicked, fearing that the applications will never be completed. The college application process can become a time of terrible stress, anxiety, and family discord. What can a college counselor do to help families get through this process with less angst?

First of all, it helps to start early. It is essential for students to begin thinking about college options during the junior year and to visit colleges, if at all possible, over spring break. This will enable students to have determined where they will apply by the summer between junior and senior year. Students should begin working on their applications during that summer. Many high schools offer "application boot camp" programs during the summer for this purpose, and independent college counselors are also available to assist students with essay development and application completion strategies.

If students have a good working relationship with their parents, parents can assist the students with organization. Setting up a filing system, constructing a timeline, and creating a calendar with specific dates assigned to the various tasks are just some of the ways that parents can help students with organization. This, however, will only be successful if, and this is a big "if," the parents are skilled at organizing and, more importantly, the students are willing to take direction from their parents. Most students at this age are not so inclined! It is essential for the student to willingly engage with the person who will provide them with an organizational structure for completing applications. If the student resists intervention by the parents, then the resulting conflict makes this an impossible situation and it becomes essential to find someone else to take on this project. It is a delicate balance because the student must write the application him- or herself. The organizational assistance can facilitate getting it done, but the responsibility for and engagement in the process must not be taken away from the student. Students should be involved in choosing the person who will work with them so that cooperation with the organizational tutor is more likely to occur.

As part of the organization process, it's important to identify how many different applications a student will need to complete. A large number of colleges—456 in 2011—accept the Common Application. Most students, especially those applying to at least some independent colleges and universities, will use the Common Application. It lightens the workload to some extent because the basic application and the main essay can be completed just once and submitted to the desired number of colleges who accept this application. Many colleges also require supplements, but these are often brief and easily completed. (Go to http://www.commonapp.org to learn more about this application.) The Common Application becomes available to students online on August 1, so students can have it completed, with the main essay and activity essay already uploaded, before school starts. Students may also be applying to state colleges and universities, most of which are not included on the Common Application, so students will need to find out when they are due, whether or not an essay is required, and what other credentials they will need to submit. Once again, much of this can be completed before school starts in the fall.

Social Issues: Many students look forward to moving away from home and living on campus in a dormitory environment. Students with NVLD are often fearful about this because they have experienced social difficulties in the past (Whitney, 2002). Perhaps their awkwardness has led to teasing and social isolation, so moving into a dorm is a scary prospect for them. On the other hand, some students with NVLD view their social problems in high school differently. They perceive that the problem lies in the behavior and attitudes of their classmates, and they may have an unrealistic belief that they will easily make new friends in college. Parents may worry, with good reason, that these fantasies will be dashed and that their child may be crushed.

Not all students with NVLD have social problems, but for those who do the housing aspect of college selection is very important (Rubenstien, 2009). Here are some important questions to consider:

- Is the student mature enough to move into a college dorm? Is he or she ready for the give-and-take that is required to live with a roommate or is a single room available?
- Will the student be able to handle exposure to sex, drugs, and alcohol? Many students who have had social difficulties in the past are so eager to make friends that they are particularly vulnerable to peer pressure around drugs and alcohol. Similarly, girls may be so eager to have a boyfriend that they place themselves in a situation where they can be taken advantage of.

- Can the student take on the organizational responsibilities that are necessary when living away from home? Managing money? Doing laundry? Eating healthy food? Getting enough sleep? Getting to class on time?
- Many students with NVLD have difficulty reading nonverbal social cues. Is the student aware of this difficulty and has he or she learned how to cope with the resulting confusion?

Many parents are so hopeful that their students can take the "normal" postsecondary route and go away to college that they are in denial about the challenges their kids will face socially. If you as the college counselor perceive that a student has deficiencies in social competence that are not being acknowledged by the student or the parents, it will be important to be direct and open about your concerns. Ask the hard questions so that they become more aware of the potential problems.

Sometimes parents, out of love and concern for their children, have tried to manipulate the environment as much as possible to prevent hurtful experiences (Rose & Bursuck, 1990). As a result, the student may not have learned how to cope with his or her inadequacies. For example, Sue is a freshman who has just moved into the dorm at Blue Lake College. She and her roommate are getting acquainted and Sue is eager to have a close relationship with Ann, her roommate. Sue likes to get up early in the morning and she likes to talk while getting dressed and ready for school. Ann likes to sleep in later and is not eager to talk before breakfast. She stays in bed with her eyes closed and responds very briefly to Sue's questions, but Sue doesn't get it. Ann gets irritated and starts avoiding Sue as much as possible. Sue is baffled; what did she do wrong? Sue needs to realize that this might happen because of her inability to read social cues. When things aren't going well, she needs to fall back on her verbal strength and ask to have a talk with Ann. She could explain to Ann that she has a type of learning disability that impacts her ability to read social cues. She could tell Ann that she is sorry if she has done something to annoy or offend, and ask Ann to tell her what it is so they can work it out. This requires maturity, self-awareness, and willingness to compromise. Role-playing or having actual experience with this kind of conversation before going away to college can be extremely helpful. But this requires openness within a family rather than denial. It requires facing the consequences of this learning disability straight on rather than pretending that they don't exist and that everything will somehow turn out OK.

If students are not ready to leave home and move into a college dorm, for any of the reasons described above, it might be better to live at home for the first year or two, to gain increased maturity and learn how to cope first with the academic requirements of college. However, there is a danger that the student will become socially isolated and even more dependent on parents. If students remain at home, they should be strongly encouraged to join clubs, sports teams, or volunteer organizations in order to meet other students who share their interests. This is important for students who live on campus, too, but even more important for students who are living at home.

Transition Challenges: Transitions can be very difficult for students with NVLD for several reasons (Rubenstien, 2009). To begin with they have a difficult time deciphering subtle, "invisible" rules. They've probably learned to rely on parents, tutors, siblings, resource teachers, or close friends to explain these rules to them when they are confused. Sue, in the previous section, didn't understand that you don't start talking to your roommate when she is trying to sleep because Sue had never had a roommate before. Students with NVLD have undoubtedly had experiences going into new situations where they make blunders and suffer the consequences, without understanding what they did wrong. This probably started in the early grades at school, making them feel that new situations are fraught with danger. These students can benefit from transition counseling before going to college, so they don't make blunders that leave them feeling confused, isolated, and anxious (Dalke & Schmitt, 1987). A small-group setting is ideal because it allows students to role-play various situations and give each other feedback. A skilled facilitator who understands how explicitly circumstances and behaviors must be described to students with NVLD is essential.

In the author's clinical experience, it is very important that this pre-transition counseling be conducted outside the home, away from parents, regular tutors, and resource teachers in order to maximize the opportunity for students to develop more independence (Dalke & Schmitt, 1987). For example, the mother of a student with NVLD may instruct a student to engage in conversation with someone "new" in a particular way, using specific words. Students are so accustomed to their mother (or teacher or tutor) telling them what to do and how to act that they don't think about why. Or perhaps pragmatics are so difficult for them that they don't know how to think about it! They just follow the instructions without internalizing the behavior sequence and learning to generalize this behavior to similar situations. This is very hard for students with NVLD to do anyway, so it is important to maximize their potential for this social learning. In a group situation, one that ideally includes other students with NVLD and some neurotypicals as well, an incident can be role-played, analyzed, broken down, and discussed (Rubenstien, 2009). Verbal explanations will facilitate understanding and appropriate behaviors can be reinforced. Students' confidence and independence are therefore likely to be enhanced.

Students who have been getting regular counseling and/or taking medication during high school need to be sure that they will have this kind of support available to them in college. It can be very helpful for parents to encourage students to make contact with the college's counseling center *before* school starts so the student feels comfortable scheduling regular appointments or occasional appointments as the need arises (Rubenstien, 2009). Students will need to take responsibility for taking medication on their own and should get into the habit of doing this while still living at home.

Interaction Between NVLD and Personality Traits and Features: While there are aspects of a nonverbal learning disability that are characteristic of most or all students who carry this diagnosis, that does not mean that all of these students will present in the same way or face the same challenges. A student who has an outgoing personality and likes being around people will suffer more from social isolation (due to making unwitting blunders) than will a student who is introverted and quite comfortable spending time alone. Some students are physically awkward because their NVLD has an impact on the way that they move their bodies through space, but this is not true for all students with NVLD. Many students have tremendous difficulty with math and/or some difficulty with organization when writing papers or essays, but other students do quite well in these academic areas. Therefore, each student is an individual and service providers must be careful not to make too many generalizations. It is important to get to know the student as a person, not just a diagnosis, before formulating a treatment plan or strategy for assisting them in reaching their goals.

Working with the Family System: As was mentioned earlier, the parents of high school students with NVLD are often providing a level of support that is no longer appropriate because the students have faced so many challenges—academically, socially, and organizationally—in the past. It is often the case that the parents either needed to be or felt that they needed to be overprotective, to a degree that might have interfered with the students' developing the independence and coping skills they will need upon leaving the home environment. On the other hand, these seemingly overprotective behaviors evolve because the parents noticed students' deficits. Since they love their children, they wished to avoid their getting hurt or experiencing failure. They are deserving of respect and empathy, even as you work with them to encourage them, when appropriate, to "back off" and allow the students to fail. You may need to be a good salesman as you convince a family that there is a delicate balance between helping and overprotection. What may be helpful to a student in the short term could be problematic and constraining in the long term. You may have more difficulty convincing parents to let the student take on more responsibility than you do with the student. At the same time, students are sometimes unrealistic about what they are ready to handle on their own. It is essential that their attempts to take on new responsibilities be closely monitored, and it is also important that both students and parents feel that they are being heard and understood by you and other support providers (specific examples are provided in a subsequent section).

Some parents are overly protective to the point of not disclosing the NVLD diagnosis to the student, and this can be especially problematic. As the college counselor, you learn of this choice early on because the parent usually tells you not to reveal the diagnosis because it will be "upsetting" to the student. This presents you with an impossible situation and will likely be very damaging, in the long run, to the student. How can the student be a good self-advocate and request appropriate interventions and accommodations if he or she does not understand the disabling condition (Rubenstien, 2009)? If the student makes social blunders in this new environment (college) but doesn't understand that it is due to a nonverbal learning disability, what will he or she assume? For most people, it's easier to accept difficulties if you can understand a reason for them rather than thinking you are "a fool" or "stupid" or that something is wrong with you. As the college counselor, you need to discuss openly and frankly with the student aspects of the college that will be important during the college selection process: campus layout, support services available, student body characteristics, distance from home, etc. This "elephant in the room" can't be ignored!

Visual/Spatial Deficits and Their Impact on College Selection: First of all, this is a feature which presents in various ways for students with NVLD. Eliciting feedback from students after college visits is a good way to learn how much of an impact it has on your student (Davis & Broitman, 2011). Some students are "directionally challenged" and will easily get lost. They may be unable to use a map and require lengthy, specific verbal directions in order to find their way around. Some students are therefore overwhelmed by large campuses, or even small- to medium-sized campuses located in large cities. If students with NVLD say, "I didn't feel comfortable on that campus," it is essential to ask why in order to obtain this kind of information. It may take patience on your part because a student can feel embarrassed to say, "I felt totally lost and couldn't find my way around." Another interesting aspect of a visual/spatial deficit is that a student with NVLD may not care about aesthetic aspects of the campus at all. While a parent might find the deferred landscaping maintenance distressing, the student might not even notice. If other aspects of the college environment make it a good fit for a student, the lack of ivy growing on the walls might be unimportant in this instance—and the parent might need some gentle persuasion to understand this perspective.

Other Housing Issues: This is often the most difficult aspect of transition from high school to college for students with NVLD. At times, parents and counselors may wish that they could handpick a student's roommate in order to select the most patient, tolerant, kind, and supportive freshman on the campus! While that might be ideal, it's probably not realistic. However, once a student has made the final choice, it may be appropriate to contact the housing office—and the learning disability support program director as well—to inform them that the student has a learning disability which impacts his or her social skills and makes living with a roommate more challenging than it is for other students. A request for a roommate with special characteristics can be made. It might be better for this student to live with a sophomore or upperclassman who is more mature and is willing to take on this challenge. The director of the housing office may know of students that could be approached for this purpose.

Students with Asperger's syndrome often request a single room because it is so stressful for them to interact with students constantly—during the day in classes and the rest of the time in a dorm room with a roommate (Adreon, 2009). They are overwhelmed by the constant stimuli in their environment and need a quiet and private place for some downtime. This can be an appropriate solution for some students with NVLD, but it can also lead to social isolation. Students with NVLD may want to form friendships but may have great difficulty doing so. Having a single-room freshman year may prevent them from meeting other students with which they could form friendships. This is an important topic for discussion during the college search and application process. Since students with NVLD can have difficulty "picturing" what it might be like to have a roommate, it will be helpful for them to have firsthand experience so that they can determine how well they can cope with it. If students have never shared a room with a sibling, attending a summer camp or summer school program during high school where they live with other students can be very helpful. Keeping a diary in which they write about interpersonal issues can facilitate discussion later.

It is very important for parents and college counselors to be straightforward with students with NVLD about potential difficulties in a community living situation. Pretending that these difficulties will not happen means sacrificing the opportunity to prepare students for what is likely to be the most difficult part of college for them. It is tempting for some parents to use the popular defense mechanism of denial because they are so hopeful that students will adapt to their new environments and because they find it hard to discuss this issue openly with their adolescent children. They don't want to upset them, they don't want to frighten them, and they may not even want to think about it. But thinking about specific situations and practicing coping skills for typical situations might mean the difference between a successful college residential experience and one that is a traumatic failure.

Strategies for Working with the College-Bound NVLD Student

An important aspect of advising the college-bound student with NVLD is to assess college readiness in general as well as how much and what kind of support a specific student will need. Babbitt and White (2002) take a broad approach in their recommendation that social skills, self-awareness, academic preparedness, social supports, and personal responsibility should all be targets of assessment when considering whether students are ready for college. Similarly, Conley (2007) describes "college readiness" as a multifaceted construct. Many students with NVLD have difficulty with executive function issues, a multifaceted construct in and of itself, as one of the most important aspects of college readiness. Executive function is a cognitive process that involves a person's ability to self-regulate. Typically, problems occur related to organization, planning, time management, prioritizing, adjusting to a new environment, developing a routine, and decision making (Davis & Broitman, 2011). When students make the transition from high school to college, particularly if they leave home and live in student housing, all of these skills are required. Most students have some difficulty in this transition, but a student with NVLD is more likely to struggle to a greater extent. An executive function disorder has been described as a symphony without a conductor. You could have a world-class symphony, but without a conductor, it is just noise rather than beautiful music. The potential is there but cannot be realized unless the cognitive process of executive function is in the driver's seat.

A colleague, Dr. Peggy Hock, and this author created a survey of executive function to use with college-counseling clients (see Appendix). Its purpose is to gain a better understanding of the behaviors and skills in which students have deficiencies so that the level and amount of support they will need in college becomes clearer. Having learned from experience that students and parents are often unaware of how much support a student is currently receiving in order to have success in high school, the author gives copies of the survey to at least three people, sometimes four: the student, a parent, a tutor, and a resource teacher. An obvious goal for seeking multiple reviewers is to determine if there is consistency in the way a student is viewed. It is especially important to establish how self-aware a student is about the level of support he needs as well as what he can or cannot do for himself. A wide variety of areas is covered in the survey, including sleep, personal hygiene, nutrition, time and money management, organization, academic skills, and test-taking skills. Delineation of the specific accommodations the student is currently using is also assessed.

The student, who is informed that there will be others assessing him as well, is asked to complete the survey thoughtfully and honestly. The survey requires the responder to "indicate the level of independence the student has demonstrated over the past 2 months." There is also room at the end for the responder to "indicate any additional support the student receives for activities of school or daily living." Once the surveys are returned—some prompting is often required, especially with the student—the responses are compared and analyzed. There are no norms for this survey, but it is very useful for the purpose described above. It also provides fruitful information for discussion, especially if there are significant differences between responders. For example, within the time management section, one item states the following: appropriately limits use of electronic media (computer, TV, games, cell phone). Students often have very different ideas about what is appropriate when compared to parents and tutors! These differences often extend to academic skills, such as "Can retain information from reading." A frank discussion of these differences can benefit the student's development of more accurate self-awareness.

An additional positive consequence of using this survey is that it often helps students—and parents —understand that there are significant areas in which a student is getting help that they had not previously recognized. As an example, students in college need to be able to get themselves out of bed and to classes in the morning. Students with time management challenges often find it difficult to get to bed at night and to get up in the morning. Parents may be in the habit of going back to prod them out of bed three or four times each morning. Becoming aware of these dependencies can aid the student and those working with him to establish important and realistic goals that will need to be achieved before the student can live on his own in a dorm. While several authors have described possible interventions at the postsecondary level (e.g., Brinckerhoff, 1994), little has been written about tools that can be used by counselors with high school students in preparation for their transition (Milsom & Dietz, 2009). The following suggestions are presented with this in mind.

Once the surveys have been analyzed and discussed, a list can be made of the behaviors a student will need to be able to perform independently with which he is currently getting help. This can be done collaboratively—with the student and one parent—and it is helpful to have an additional party present, too. The college counselor, the resource teacher, or a tutor who has a good relationship with the student can all be good choices for this task. The third party can provide a mediating influence in what could become an emotionally charged discussion. At this point, the student can be asked (by the "mediator") which task he is willing to take responsibility for in the future. Typically, when the student chooses something, the parent will say something like, "Oh, I don't think that's a good idea. I think you should choose this other task." That comment needs to be challenged immediately. The parent needs to be reminded that the whole purpose of this exercise is to facilitate the student in becoming more independent and more responsible. Telling him that his choice isn't a good one and that someone else knows a better choice is counterproductive. If the student fails, that will provide useful information to everyone. Was the task choice too big at this time? Did the student need to choose an easier task first? Was there insufficient structure to make it work? What went wrong and how might it go better next time? It is better that the student fail in this situation, in which he is provided with guidance and support, than when he is away at college. When the student makes his choice and a plan of action is devised, it's important that teachers be informed of the goals and strategies so they can play a facilitative role and provide feedback to the student along the way.

An example may better illustrate this strategy. Charlie, his mother, and his resource teacher all agree that he is not independent when it comes to learning material from class notes. Charlie has great difficulty determining what is essential and inessential during class lectures, so he has a classmate take notes for him in each of his classes. Charlie reads through these notes before tests but doesn't seem to benefit from this unless his resource teacher goes through the notes with him. He's become very passive in this environment, relying on his resource teacher to tell him what's important and what he needs to commit to memory, etc. He hasn't made an effort to do this for himself until now, but he chose this as the first task he wants to tackle. His mother is worried because she fears this will be very difficult for him and that his grades will drop because he will perform poorly on tests. This is a complicated task and it's understandable that his mother would be concerned. She informs Charlie's teachers about his goal and his determination to become more independent at learning material from class notes, so they will realize that a drop in test grades, if it occurs, is not due to "slacking off." The teachers are also informed of the gradual strategies being employed by Charlie, his resource teacher, and his tutor, aimed at helping him to develop this skill. For the next test, Charlie's teacher doesn't just tell him what he should study; she asks him pointed questions in order to elicit from him the most essential material. In doing so, she is teaching him how to figure this out for himself. His tutor also spends time going over the material but in a new way by teaching him how to review his notes and how to think about the information in a more analytic way. In effect, Charlie is learning how to learn within the narrow context of learning how to study from class lecture notes. It's an essential skill to have in college, and it's better to have some knowledge of how to go about it *before* going to college.

Charlie works hard and makes big gains, but his grades still drop from a B+ to a C+ in history class, with similar results in other classes. This practice was begun at the beginning of the second quarter, so these grades were averaged in with his better grades from first quarter. Therefore, the drop in grades was slight, and all agreed that the benefits gained were worth this consequence. And Charlie can describe the circumstances leading to these grades in his college applications.

But what if the results had not been this positive? What if he'd earned D's or even F's on all tests, and there was a dramatic drop in his grades? If this was still happening halfway through the quarter, it would have been important to stop the experiment and let Charlie choose an easier task with which to begin. Charlie and his supporters would have learned that he needs more help in this area and that it isn't realistic at this point in time for him to become completely independent at studying for tests from class notes. Charlie may need help with this even while in college, or he may need to spread out the learning strategy over a full year rather than just a quarter or a semester. But Charlie is learning for himself, from his own experience, rather than just following what others are telling him to do. He is taking responsibility for his learning and gaining an understanding of his learning process, including his strengths and weaknesses. Once one goal is achieved, a subsequent goal can be chosen. The survey of executive function can be a valuable first step in this process.

How the Laws Differ from K–12 to Postsecondary Education

The essential difference between the laws that govern K–12 education and the laws that govern postsecondary education is this: The Individuals with Disabilities in Education Act (which pertains to K–12 education only) is an education entitlement law while the Americans with Disabilities Act and Section 504 of the Rehabilitation Act are civil rights laws (see Chap. 5 for more detail). In a nutshell, while Section 504 and the ADA require postsecondary institutions to provide accommodative services to students with disabilities, *once the student has been admitted to a college*, it is the student's responsibility to self-identify and provide documentation of the disability. In grades K through 12, the school district is responsible for identifying, conducting assessments, providing interventions, and paying for services required so that students can graduate. There is no guarantee of postsecondary education, but students must have equal access to an education. This means that students are entitled to accommodations *on the basis of a disability* if that disability would prevent them from having equal access to an education. Equal opportunity, however, is not meant to "benefit" students with disabilities, or to provide them with opportunities that go beyond leveling the playing field.

Since students must be able to advocate for themselves once they get to college, it is essential that they understand their learning disability and be able to explain it, as well as what accommodations they will need in order to be successful in college. They cannot rely on teachers to come to them and urge them to go to the learning center. They cannot rely on the learning center director to contact them and invite them in for a meeting. Students have to be ready to take the initiative to garner the support they need. The laws are there to protect them and provide them with equal opportunity for a college education. They need the self-awareness, initiative, resourcefulness, and self-advocacy skills to make it happen (Luker & May, 2009).

Levels of Support Available on College Campuses

A review of guidebooks which describe the support services available at colleges and universities reveals that there are usually three levels of support, although the names given to these levels vary. Obviously, within each level there is a continuum of services; however, there are some specific distinctions that separate these levels, and it is helpful to understand them when counseling students with NVLD.

1. *Structured/Comprehensive*. This is the greatest level of support provided on college campuses, and there are not many institutions that offer it. Some of the hallmarks of this level are:

    (a) Staff trained to work with students with NVLD
    (b) Special orientation programs, usually a week or two before school starts
    (c) Some curriculum modifications offered, if this is supported by a student's documentation
    (d) Assistance with advocacy
    (e) Academic monitoring and counseling
    (f) Professional subject area tutors rather than student tutors as they may be better equipped to help students with NVLD, given their special needs

    The latter can be especially important for students who don't recognize that they are in academic difficulty. Students with NVLD can be unaware that they are doing poorly in classes. For example, Charlie in the above example had a difficult time distinguishing between essential and unimportant details. He might have written an essay that was lengthy and contained a great deal of specific, factual information. However, his essay may not have addressed the issues the professor wanted him to focus on, and it may have been poorly organized. If Charlie was in a structured/comprehensive program, he would have a special advisor assigned to him who would check regularly with all of his professors to see how he was doing. This could be monthly, every 2 weeks, or every week. The professor could alert the advisor about Charlie's difficulties and the advisor could make sure that Charlie meets with someone in the writing center before starting his next essay.

    Students in the structured/comprehensive programs may be required to sign a contract, agreeing to have a weekly meeting with a special advisor/mentor, and to spend a certain number of hours in tutoring each week. There is usually a substantial program participation fee. While this can be problematic for most families, the upside to it is that these programs don't go away when there is a budget crunch. The programs pay for themselves and are therefore less likely to be cut. Many of these programs also have a separate admission process. For example, a student may be asked to apply simultaneously to the college's admission office and to the program. The student may be asked to write an additional essay, usually something related to an understanding of his or her learning disability. If the student is admitted to the college, the program director will then review the program application and the student's documentation to determine if the student is eligible for the services and accommodations they provide and if the student would be a good fit for the program.

2. *Coordinated Services*. This middle level of services is available at a large number of colleges and universities, including most public institutions. These programs usually have a learning disabilities specialist, at least part time, who assists students in coordinating their academic accommodations and needed services. These services often include:

   (a) Instruction on learning strategies
   (b) Counseling/advising
   (c) Tutoring
   (d) Assistance with advocacy

   As is also true with the structured/comprehensive support programs, coordinated services programs always have a designated center on campus for students with disabilities in addition to the academic support center which is available to all students. Students are not part of a structured program; they will need to be in charge of requesting services and accommodations on an as-needed basis. (It is sometimes possible to request a regular meeting with a staff member, which can be accommodated if they have sufficient personnel.) When students self-identify and provide documentation (at a meeting) to a staff member of the LD support program, there is usually a collaborative approach to determining what accommodations the student is eligible to receive. The staff member writes a letter on the center's letterhead, outlining these accommodations. The student can make copies of this letter and give it to each professor. The professor can then, for example, send the student's exam to the support center so the student can have extra time in a distraction-free setting. The professor can make sure the student has a seat in the front row, or can facilitate finding a notetaker.

3. *Basic Services*. These programs provide the minimum support necessary in order to comply with the law. Usually, they provide accommodations but not services. There is not a separate support center for students with disabilities; learning-disabled students' accommodations are arranged within the regular academic support structure. Students must still provide documentation of their disability in order to receive accommodations and a staff member may provide a letter to be given to each professor. It is important that students find out how the program works and what accommodations will be provided before making the decision to attend a college that does not have a separate LD support program. The tutors usually have no special training for working with students with learning disabilities and there is rarely a learning specialist on staff. However, if a student is bright, has been mainstreamed in high school, has a good understanding of his or her learning disability which he or she can articulate to others, and is a good self-advocate, a college with a basic services program can work.

The Right Match?

- Structured programs work best for students who need close monitoring and high levels of support.
- Coordinated programs work best for students who want to be "mainstreamed" but know they will need support.
- Basic service programs work best for the highly motivated, independent self-advocators.

College Cultures

When you visit college and university support programs, which is strongly advised, it is evident that there are varying philosophies. At some colleges, counselors who work with students with learning disabilities welcome the students with open arms. The counselors are willing to spend considerable time with students, making sure the student understands what is being offered to them. In some instances, counselors are provided with an office to meet with students while the director steps out so that students can share their experiences freely. There is openness in this kind of program which puts the visitor and the student participants at ease. These colleges clearly see it as part of their mission to help students with learning disabilities become successful in their quest to become college graduates. In addition to the work they do with students, they make the effort to educate the faculty about different kinds of learning disabilities, so that professors can be more supportive in the classroom and lecture hall. The former director of disability services at a major university stated in a meeting with a group of counselors that she had initially encountered resistance when trying to educate the faculty about learning disabilities. With the support of the university president, she offered the faculty the opportunity to have a gourmet lunch in a special setting as part of the education program. The turnout increased dramatically as did the understanding of the faculty.

On other campuses, the director (or some other staff member) spends more time describing all the hoops that students must go through to obtain accommodations rather than providing information about what the college has to offer. Counselors, students, and parents may walk away from this kind of an encounter feeling that they had just met with a "gatekeeper" rather than a compassionate, supportive service provider. Sometimes the LD support center is located in cramped quarters which are poorly maintained and—in a word—unwelcoming.

Another sign of the college culture is related to how busy the centers are. In these times of severe budget cuts, the staff of LD support programs has often been cut drastically. When visiting, if you see long lines and lots of frustrated students, this is not a good sign. It's worthwhile to have a conversation with two or three students who are receiving services or accommodations to find out how easy (or difficult) it is to get the help they need.

How Much (or Little) to Disclose on the Application

This topic often causes students and parents considerable angst. Anxiety is usually caused by the fear that if the admission counselor knows of a learning disability, the student is less likely to be admitted. While this was occasionally true many years ago, it rarely, if ever, is true these days (Mamlet & Vandevelde, 2011). Admission officers are more interested in whether or not a student can be successful in college than in whether they have a learning or some other kind of disability. One of the qualities they like to see in students is resiliency, which can be demonstrated by overcoming a hardship (Milsom & Dietz, 2009). If a student describes in an application essay difficulties experienced during high school—academic, social, organizational, or otherwise—while also indicating the development of insight, self-awareness, and compensatory strategies, the story can be both compelling and impressive. In other words, disclosure of the nonverbal learning disability can actually help a student be admitted, as long as it is done in an appropriate way.

What is the right way to write about this? It's easier to describe the wrong way. Whining, complaining, and describing oneself as a victim don't work. It makes the student appear damaged and lacking in resilience. Overemphasizing difficulties is also problematic. A straightforward presentation of the ways in which the NVLD has impacted the student's academic performance along with a discussion of what the student has done to cope with these difficulties is the best approach. It is essential that students be specific. For example, if a student earned low grades during the first 2 years of high school in science and history courses because he required organizational skills that were very difficult for him, this can be disclosed. Perhaps the student worked with a tutor in the junior-year American history course and learned an organizational system that enabled him to study more efficiently. Perhaps having a note taker further enhanced his ability to assemble and learn the material presented in lecture format. Those are the kinds of specifics that will be convincing to an admission officer, especially if junior-year grades in American history support the student's story.

And How Does It All Work When Students Get on Campus?

The most important thing for students and parents to remember is that it is *students' responsibility* to disclose their disability once they arrive on campus. A parent can't make all the arrangements for a student. It is essential that counselors advising families understand how this process works, so they can explain it accurately to students and parents. While there are many variations depending on the college campus, there are some general principles that are followed most of the time.

Once students have decided which campus to attend, they should contact the office through which accommodations and services will be provided. This can be as early as the spring before they matriculate in the fall or during the summer months.

Documentation can be sent to the appropriate office, to make sure that there is no further testing or other kinds of information that must be provided for students to access the help they will need once school starts. A meeting should be arranged as soon as possible, ideally no later than freshman orientation, in order to have accommodations or services available immediately when classes begin.

Typically, at a meeting with a service provider, students will discuss what accommodations they need, and an agreement will be arrived at which works for the student and fits in with the institution's policies. A letter is then written, on appropriate letterhead, which identifies the services or accommodations for which the student is eligible: extended time on tests in a distraction-free setting, a note taker, editorial services on papers and essay exams, preferential seating, etc. Students can then make copies of this letter to give to each professor. This paves the way for students to avail themselves of what they need without having to get in a lengthy discussion with each professor. It signals to the professor that a professional has gone over a student's documentation and made a determination of what the student should receive, according to institutional policy. With this system, there is no need for students to feel that they must explain the nature of their disability in order to receive appropriate accommodations. The documentation is kept confidential in the disabled-student services office and professors need only comply with what is delineated in the letter.

In order for this system to work for students, they must be able to explain the following to the service provider:

What they need and why they need it.
How it has enabled them to be successful in the past.
What they have tried that doesn't work as well as what does work.

Their documentation needs to support the requests they make (Helmus, 2009). If the documentation is insufficient, it may be necessary to have further testing done. For example, if a student requests a substitution for a foreign language graduation requirement but there is nothing in the documentation that explains why the student would have difficulty learning a foreign language and there is no recommendation that the student be granted a substitution, additional testing may be necessary. Obviously, this is why the presentation of a student's documentation and a meeting with the service provider should be held as soon as possible.

While on the one hand the list of accommodations is too extensive to enumerate, students may not be able to obtain a requested accommodation in college, even if it was granted to them in high school. Institutions receiving funds from the federal government are required by the Americans with Disabilities Act to provide "reasonable accommodations" for disabled students, in order that they may have "equal access" to a postsecondary education. However, a college might decide that a student's requested accommodation goes beyond what they determine is "reasonable." Colleges also have the right to refuse to grant an accommodation if they believe that it will "fundamentally alter" the mission of the school or the way that it operates. Policies are established at each institution to govern their decisions and these can vary considerably from school to school.

If a faculty member is unwilling to implement a student's accommodation plan, here are some steps a student can take (Kravets & Wax, 2010):

- Try to work it out with the faculty member directly.
- Seek advocacy help from someone in the disabled-student services office.
- Go to the dean's office of the faculty person's department and seek support.
- Most colleges have some kind of grievance procedure. Find out what it is and initiate the process.
- If all else fails and the situation cannot be resolved amicably and cooperatively, the student has the right to file a complaint with the US Department of Justice.

A Final Note

The Buckley Amendment of the Family Rights and Privacy Act of 1974 (FERPA) was designed to prevent the release of educational records (and other information) to third parties without the permission of the student. As described earlier, many parents have been very involved in making sure that their son or daughter is receiving supportive services and accommodations and in monitoring their son or daughter's compliance and participation. During students' freshman year, service providers often find themselves in the position of explaining to parents why they cannot discuss how the students are doing and how often, for example, they participate in tutoring. This can be a very tough adjustment for parents and it is advisable for counselors to help families understand this reality before students matriculate. While students can sign a consent form, granting permission for a service provider to speak to his or her parents, not all service providers conform to this possibility. Many service providers believe that this interferes with students' development of independence and self-regulation (Hamblet, 2009).

Case Study

As might be expected, identifying details about this student have been changed for privacy reasons. Nonetheless, this student was chosen for presentation because she illustrates many of the challenges and specifics that have been previously described in this chapter.

The author first met Marjorie and her parents in the middle of her junior year, as she and her family were beginning to think about college placement after she graduated from high school. Marjorie attended an independent school in which she was receiving some college counseling. Her previous testing was very outdated, so the author was asked to complete a new comprehensive evaluation and to provide some supplementary advice about her college choices.

Background Information: Marjorie was born with some physical deformities to her torso which caused her embarrassment around her peers, particularly in middle school. She had successful reconstructive surgery midway through high school, but the years of teasing had a lasting impact on her perception of herself and her self-confidence. Language development was normal, although she did have some articulation problems for which she received speech therapy in early childhood. As a young child, she demonstrated a strong knowledge base and could easily comprehend narrative, but had difficulty producing language "with expressive requirements." Marjorie was described as "information thirsty," but had difficulty with reciprocity in conversation. Motor development was delayed, and at age 6, she began to receive occupational therapy. Marjorie had taken, over time, a number of medications to manage attention problems and to alleviate anxiety.

Marjorie was evaluated in third grade, even though she was doing well academically, because of anxiety-related behaviors. She was reevaluated in sixth grade due to concerns about academic performance and a suspected weakness in visual memory.

In high school, she earned A's and B's in most classes, except for C's in math, a subject that was more difficult for her. In addition, Marjorie explained that understanding science concepts and applying words and numbers were usually very hard for her. She also had problems with organization and was being assisted by a learning specialist who helped her to break down her homework assignments into manageable chunks. Prior to this assistance, she often did too much homework or the wrong homework, and had significant problems with prioritizing.

Within her family system, Marjorie was very attached to both parents and got along reasonably well with her older brother. She had always, however, had difficulty making friends and did not get invited to other children's houses. She was perceived as "odd" by other students and was often made fun of in elementary and middle school. The high school she attended placed great emphasis on tolerance and kindness, so she was accepted there, despite being "different." There were other students she could eat lunch with, although she didn't interact with these students outside of school. Marjorie did not appear to recognize that she lacked friends because she did not complain about it, so her level of self-awareness in this area is unknown. She was more comfortable in the company of other adults, probably because they were more tolerant of her "differentness." She had a strong desire to please and a very "sweet" nature.

Testing conducted in the third grade revealed verbal abilities that were significantly stronger than her nonverbal skills (93rd percentile on WISC-III: VCI vs. 58th percentile on WISC-III: POI). Academic scores were below expectation overall, when compared to her Verbal Comprehension Index score. Personality testing revealed mild depression and anxiety symptoms.

Testing conducted when Marjorie was in the sixth grade supported nonverbal learning disability and ADHD diagnoses. Specifically noted in the report summary were Marjorie's historical weaknesses in math and visual–spatial cognitive abilities, as well as difficulties recognizing social cues and establishing social relationships.

Current Testing. Marjorie chatted a great deal during the evaluation. In fact, it was a challenge to keep her focused on the tasks being presented to her because of her frequent conversational digressions. In replying to test questions, her verbalizations were often unnecessarily lengthy and complicated, even to fairly straightforward questions. She thanked me profusely at each break and at the end of each day, to a degree that was awkward and unusual, although she clearly did not perceive it this way.

Assessment of her math skills revealed how challenging it is for her. In one question related to being able to tell time—usually an extremely easy item for a high school student—Marjorie acknowledged that she was unable to tell time. She also demonstrated confusion about systems of measurement and, overall, had great difficulty setting up problems so that she could perform the calculations.

On the other hand, her vocabulary score on the WAIS-III was at the 98th percentile and comprehension was measured at the 99th percentile. With the latter, she demonstrated good understanding of issues related to social intelligence when measured through the use of language. This was in contrast to her score at the 50th percentile on picture arrangement, which measures common sense and social reasoning but in a visual–spatial sense. Marjorie's 91st percentile score on the information subtest, in conjunction with 98th percentile on vocabulary, revealed her exceptional fund of information. Marjorie's summary scores on the WAIS-III also fit with the previous diagnosis of a nonverbal learning disability.

Verbal IQ	114 (82nd percentile)
Performance IQ	91 (27th percentile)

Verbal Comprehension Index	126 (96th percentile)
Perceptual Organization	95 (37th percentile)

College Counseling: In conversations with Marjorie's parents, they expressed an awareness of her social challenges. In fact, Marjorie was involved in a social skills training group with other adolescents. Her mother described her loneliness because she had no friends at or outside of school, even though she felt "safe" and "accepted" there. They further acknowledged that Marjorie was a "homebody" who would probably prefer to go to college close to home, but they felt she'd become more independent if she attended a college away from her home environment, at a small residential college with good geographic diversity where most students stay on campus on the weekends.

The social skills counselor advised Marjorie and her parents that it would be best if she attended a college close to home at least for the first 2 years. The author also believed she could manage living on campus perhaps 4 nights a week, but would benefit from being able to come home when she needed to. Marjorie still suffered from anxiety when she felt uncomfortable and the difficulty she continued to have with reading social cues and language reciprocity was problematic. She had a strong desire to please and presented as very emotionally fragile. Her parents recognized that she strove mightily to please them, but believed her to be strong enough to cope with moving far away from home. As a consequence, Marjorie applied and was admitted to several colleges that were halfway across the country from her home. She chose a small liberal arts college after visiting several of these schools and had very high expectations for her upcoming college experience.

In the spring a meeting was held in the author's office with Marjorie, her mother, and her therapist. The author attempted to help Marjorie understand some of the challenges she would face, particularly the transition period during the early weeks of school. Academic, housing, and social issues were discussed, along with the resources that would be available to her on campus. At the conclusion of the meeting, Marjorie and her mother still appeared to have unrealistically high expectations, from the author's perspective.

Marjorie came home from college after 8 weeks. According to her mother, the school was "perfect" for her but was too far away from home. Even though Marjorie had been good about pursuing resources and acquiring accommodations, she felt overwhelmed and exhausted and became "sadder by the day." She was initially relieved to come home and be with her family again, but having to come home was also humiliating for her. In a subsequent meeting in the author's office, she struggled to keep her tears in check. While her mother emphasized the academic struggles Marjorie had in college, Marjorie expressed tremendous grief that she hadn't been able to make friends. Her disappointment in this aspect of college life appeared to be more devastating to her than the fact that she was getting C's in some of her classes.

It took Marjorie more than a year to recover from what she perceived as a "failure experience." She initially pursued purely extracurricular interests while living at home and she also resumed therapy. She gradually gained the strength and courage to reapply to college, this time to a small college near her home. She is presently living on campus and earning A and B grades. She continues to see her therapist and to come home frequently on weekends, but her mother reports that she is happy. She still has few friends and continues to be challenged socially, but she is now a junior and thinking about going on to graduate school once she graduates. She has better self-awareness and understanding of her strengths and weaknesses as well as her learning disability. It is unfortunate, however, that she went through such a painful experience along the way. This case exemplifies the difficult consequences that can occur when parents are in denial about their child's disability and unrealistic about the challenges their child with NVLD will encounter in the transition from high school to college. Each situation is unique and must be approached with that in mind; but there were plenty of warning signs in Marjorie's case suggesting that the path she took initially was ill-advised.

Summary

In this chapter a wide variety of issues related to the transition from high school to college for students with NVLD was discussed, including academic, social, personal, residential, and organizational problems that are typically challenging for this population. Concerns about leaving home, parents, and other support systems were also discussed since the underlying conflicts between desire for independence and feelings of dependency are so prominent for professionals working with students with NVLD at this time in their lives. While the number of learning-disabled students attending college has increased dramatically in recent years, very little has been written about the NVLD population specifically. Much of the information in this chapter, therefore, is offered as knowledge gained from experience practicing in the college-counseling field.

The importance of working with the family system, as well as with other professionals assisting students with NVLD, is stressed. Determining the level of support that will be necessary for students to succeed in college is addressed, including an informal instrument created by the author and a colleague to assess executive function competence. Three levels of support, and suggestions for evaluating what level of support a student will need, are described. Finally, a case study is presented—one which highlights the consequences of not recognizing the challenges an NVLD student is likely to face in the transition from high school to college.

Appendix A. Scale of Executive Function

Student: ____________________ Birthdate: _______ Gender: M F Today's Date: ______

Completed by (circle one): student parent tutor resource teacher Name: ______________

Instructions: The following are areas in which the student may be receiving assistance at home and at school. For each item indicate the level of independence the student has demonstrated over the past 2 months.

	Always	Most of the time	Sometimes	Rarely	Never
Sleep					
Independently goes to bed at appropriate time					
Independently wakes up and gets up on time					
Personal hygiene					
Bathes and washes hair regularly without reminders					
Combs hair, brushes teeth, and shaves without reminders					

(continued)

	Always	Most of the time	Sometimes	Rarely	Never
Independently chooses appropriate attire for each day's weather and activities					
Independently remembers to take prescribed medications					
Nutrition					
Can prepare simple breakfast, lunch, and snacks					
Independently makes good food choices					
Independently schedules meals appropriately					
Time management					
Appropriately limits use of electronic media (computer, TV, games, cell phone)					
Independently schedules time for homework and follows through					
Independently keeps track of daily assignments					
Independently plans steps to complete projects					
Independently plans time for step-by-step completion of projects					
Turns in long-term projects/assignments on time					
Feels confident of own ability to schedule and handle school assignments and chores					
Organization					
Independently turns completed homework to teachers on time					
Independently brings home or plans to obtain materials required to complete homework (textbooks, assignment sheets, art supplies, etc.)					
Reliably brings home announcements from school					

(continued)

	Always	Most of the time	Sometimes	Rarely	Never
Reliably returns completed forms to school					
Keeps track of personal items at school					
Independently locates personal items at home					
Independently maintains orderly backpack and binder					
Money management					
Can create workable a budget for personal expenses					
Can manage daily personal expenses within a budget					
Can independently balance a checkbook					
Reading					
Understands content of textbook material at first reading					
Can take notes from written material, identifying main ideas and supporting points					
Can retain information obtained from reading					
Reads for pleasure					
Writing					
Can organize own ideas for writing					
Uses correct grammar when writing					
Uses correct spelling (or spell-check) when writing					
Can independently write a 3–5-page research paper					
Note taking					
Understands information presented orally					
Can stay focused and listen for an entire class period					
Can listen, take notes, and identify key points and supporting ideas					
Can learn new material by reviewing own notes					
Can accurately copy notes from board or screen					

(continued)

	Always	Most of the time	Sometimes	Rarely	Never
Test taking					
Can effectively demonstrate acquired knowledge on each of the following:					
Multiple-choice test					
Short-answer test					
Fill-in-the-blank test					
Essay test					
True/false test					
Student currently uses the following academic accommodations					
Assistive technology for reading (e.g., Kurzweil)					
Preferential seating					
Reduced homework					
Quiet testing environment					
Up to 50% extra time on tests					
Reader for tests					
Use of a computer for all written assignments					
Use of computer for tests					
Scribe for tests					
Alternative test format					
Indicate any additional support student receives for activities of school or daily living					

References

Adreon, D. (2009). *Asperger's disorder. The college sourcebook for students with learning and developmental differences* (pp. 18–20). Massachusetts: Wintergreen Orchard House.

Babbitt, B., & White, C. (2002). "R U Ready?" Helping students assess their readiness for postsecondary education. *Teaching Exceptional Children, 35*, 62–66.

Brinckerhoff, L. (1994). Developing effective self-advocacy skills in college-bound students with learning disabilities. *Intervention in School and Clinic, 29*, 229–237.

Conley, D. (2007). Toward a more comprehensive conception of college readiness. Eugene, OR: Educational Policy Improvement Center. Retrieved July 8, 2008, from http://www.s4s.org/upload/Gates-College%20Readiness.pdf

Dalke, C., & Schmitt, S. (1987). Meeting the transition needs of college-bound students with learning disabilities. *Journal of Learning Disabilities, 20*(3), 176–180.

Davis, J., & Broitman, J. (2011). *Nonverbal learning disabilities in children: Bridging the gap between science and practice*. New York: Springer.

Durlak, C., Rose, E., & Bursuck, W. (1994). Preparing high school students with learning disabilities for the transition to postsecondary education: Teaching the skills of self-determination. *Journal of Learning Disabilities, 27*(1), 51–59.

Hamblet, E. (2009). Helping your students with disabilities during their college search. *Journal of College Admission*, Fall, 6–15.

Helmus, A. (2009). *Neuropsychological evaluation. The college sourcebook for students with learning and developmental differences* (pp. 23–25). Massachusetts: Wintergreen Orchard House.

Kravets, M., & Wax, I. (2010). *The K&W guide to colleges for students with learning disabilities or attention deficit/hyperactivity disorder (ADHD)* (10th ed.). Massachusetts: The Princeton Review, Inc.

Krebs, C. (2002). Self-advocacy skills: A portfolio approach. *Review, 33*, 160–163.

Lock, R., & Layton, C. (2001). Succeeding in postsecondary education through self-advocacy. *Teaching Exceptional Children, 34*(2), 66–71.

Luker, D., & May, T. (2009). *Learning disabilities. The college sourcebook for students with learning and developmental differences* (pp. 8–10). Massachusetts: Wintergreen Orchard House.

Mamlet, R., & Vandevelde, C. (2011). *College admission: From application to acceptance, step by step*. New York: Three Rivers.

Milsom, A., & Dietz, L. (2009). Defining college readiness for students with learning disabilities: A Delphi study. *Professional School Counseling, 12*(4), 315–323.

Rose, E., & Bursuck, W. (1990). Do services for students with learning disabilities in postsecondary education settings foster independence? Paper presented at the annual meeting of the Association on Handicapped Student Services Programs in Postsecondary Education, Nashville, TN.

Rourke, B. (1989). *Nonverbal learning disabilities: The syndrome and the model*. New York: Guilford.

Rubenstien, M. (2009). *Nonverbal learning disorder. The college sourcebook for students with learning and developmental differences* (pp. 14–17). Massachusetts: Wintergreen Orchard House.

Skinner, M. (2004). College students with learning disabilities speak out: What it takes to be successful in postsecondary education. *Journal of Postsecondary Education and Disability, 17*, 91–104.

Whitney, R. V. (2002). *Bridging the gap: Raising a child with nonverbal learning disorder*. New York: The Berkley Publishing Group.

http://www.commonapp.org

http://www.fairtest.org

http://www.petersons.com/college-search/college-admission-test-optional.aspx

Chapter 12
Social and Cultural Capital for Students with NVLD: The Transition to College

Catherine M. Brown and Bridget Leary

The interaction of multiple ecological systems such as the individual, family, and school will influence an adolescent's developmental trajectory into adulthood (Bronfenbrenner, 1974, 1986). Young adults with a foundation of positive traits in these domains will be best prepared for the transition to college and future independence. However, for some adolescents with nonverbal learning disorder (NVLD), the transition to independence can present challenges. Resilience traits that youth develop over time will have a significant effect on developmental outcomes (Rutter, 1987). For those who plan to attend college some predictive traits of? students who will be successful include a good academic self-concept, high educational aspirations, positive mental health, emotional maturity, independent living, and self-advocacy skills. These attributes will not only impact the initial transition to college but can later have a positive effect on retention, graduation, and employment outcomes for adults with NVLD (Brodeur, 2006; Smith, English, & Vasek, 2002; Wehmeyer & Palmer, 2003; Yu, Xiu-Zhu, Ai-Shu, & Zhang, 2008).

The dynamics between the child and the resources of the family also affect the adolescent's aptitude for the independence and self-determination that will be necessary in most college settings. On a personal level, the student must be able to take care of personal needs such as an ability to feed, shelter, and clothe oneself. The college student must be able to navigate through the community with developmentally appropriate abilities in the areas of personal safety, financial responsibilities, and social understanding. In the academic setting, a student must possess traits such as self-determination, independent decision-making, and technological savvy as well as be able to prioritize goals and communicate educational needs. These characteristics are even more important for students with NVLD.

C.M. Brown, Ph.D. (✉) • B. Leary
Accessibility Services, California State University, East Bay, 25800 Carlos Bee Blvd, Hayward, CA 94542-3095, USA
e-mail: katie.brown@csueastbay.edu

J. Broitman and J.M. Davis (eds.), *Treating NVLD in Children: Professional Collaborations for Positive Outcomes*, DOI 10.1007/978-1-4614-6179-1_12,

It is presumed that parents or guardians have substantial impact on the opportunities for their child's development and attainment of resources such as personal skills, education, environmental surroundings, and quality of life that will influence future trajectories. Thus, they have a certain amount of social and cultural capital to endow to their children (Furstenberg, 2006). However, parents of children with NVLD, regardless of the available resources to families, must also be willing to devote the time to cultivate those resources in the development of a resilient adolescent that is ready for college. While not all adolescents with NVLD will face significant obstacles, others may require strategic development in certain skill areas such as independent living, social, and organizational skills. These skills are essential for preparation for success in higher education settings. Parents or guardians who adequately prepare adolescents with NVLD for the increased independent decision-making needed in this setting can expect more positive outcomes in the transition to college and subsequent persistence through graduation than those without these skills (Brinckerhoff, Shaw, & McGuire, 1996; Brown, 2005; Clegg, 2011; Foley, 2006; Murray & Naranjo, 2008; Reed, Kennett, Lewis, & Lund-Lucas, 2011).

Furthermore, the climate of K-12 schools can have a significant impact on the individual's academic foundation. This will be the basis for the student's transition to college and future trajectory. In public education, the special education system employs teachers that are specifically credentialed to work with students with learning disabilities. Active parent participation in the Individual Education Plan (IEP) meetings and decision-making is critical. The interactive decisions school staff, students, and parents make throughout the K-12 years will set the tone for educational aspirations and affect future college eligibility (Dorow, 2011; Salter, 2010; Taymans, West, & Sullivan, 2000). Indeed, both the student and family should receive appropriate educational support in an inclusive school climate that embraces all diverse learners. Schools with a positive academic climate for students with NVLD will guide the student to attain their educational or vocational aspirations. However, it is evident that a supportive culture for students with NVLD can be lacking in some public schools (Bates & Davis, 2004; Bays & Crockett, 2007). Therefore, for some families the relationship with the school or district can be contentious (Black, 2010; Russo & Osborne, 2008; Shane, 2008) and can undermine foundations for success.

The school must provide education to both parents and students about the important legal and cultural differences between the K-12 and higher education settings prior to entering college. One of the most significant legal differences is that young adults with NVLD who want to receive accommodations are responsible for identifying themselves to the disability resource office on the college campus. Self-advocacy skills are the cornerstone to a successful transition in this area. In a survey of over seventy colleges, disability resource personnel reported that the biggest concern for transition from high school to college was self-advocacy (Janiga & Costenbader, 2002). Students must be able to seek out services for disabilities on campus, articulate their specific disability, and see to the implementation of their accommodations in the classroom in order for them to prove effective.

In other words, the individual resilience, family environment, and academic foundation are integral to the development of individual social and cultural capital (see below) that will influence the manner in which the youth transitions to and attains higher education. The individual can develop a foundation of social or cultural capital that can be leveraged to overcome obstacles in the transition to college or employment settings (Bates, 1997; Bourdieu, 1986; King, 2009; Pettit, Erath, Lansford, Dodge, & Bates, 2011; Smith, 2012). Social capital refers to the social resources that one can leverage in attaining goals. The adolescent's social status is a product of his or her familial environment. It may include socioeconomic status and a network of social environments or connections (Stanton-Salazar, 2011). Often the family system is a significant factor in an individual's aspirations and the opportunity for higher education. Cultural capital is the ability to navigate competently within a given societal setting. This includes a person's command of the language, social understanding, and behavioral expectations in various cultural situations. For the purposes of this chapter, social and cultural capital is addressed as it pertains to the ability to navigate the culture of higher education systems in particular.

In addition to the resources a person with NVLD can gain throughout development and interaction of these ecological systems, the environment to which the student is transitioning can also provide cultural capital to support the individual. In accordance with Title II of the Americans with Disabilities Act and Section 504 of the Rehabilitation Act, higher education settings are legally mandated to provide accommodations for individuals with disabilities to offer a college education that is as equally accessible to these individuals as it is to students without disabilities. College faculty and campus personnel who are well educated about diverse learners and related services for these students serve to contribute to an inclusive culture where individuals with disabilities will feel welcome (Ruiz, 2008), and thereby participate in the reciprocity of these ecological systems that will affect youth with NVLD.

Further, educational policy makers and administrators are aware that many students with learning disabilities may begin their higher education career with a disadvantage. Therefore, some campuses provide additional support services that are not required by law to assist with the transition, retention, and graduation of these students (Cowles & Keim, 1995; Scorgie, Kildal, & Wilgosh, 2010). These programs are generally supported by government grants or by supplemental fees in addition to regular tuition. These specialized programs assist with further development of their academic skills.

In order to realize future academic and employment aspirations for NVLD students, a well-formed strategy is necessary (Fast, 2003; Janiga & Costenbader, 2002). The student's own individual resilience traits, social support from the family, and formative school culture throughout this developmental period will prepare the young adult for this transition. This chapter will review the interplay between the ecological systems of individual, family, and school; the development of social capital; and the availability of college support programs which seek to realize the full educational or vocational potential of students with NVLD.

Individual Resilience

While it is important to address the learning challenges in academic domains for youth, it is equally important to address other developmental domains as they occur. Individual skills related to daily living, organization, emotional maturity, and mental health status will have an impact on the development of resilience. These traits will ultimately affect the success of the individual in new environments such as college (DaDeppo, 2009; Gerrard-Morris, 2008; Little, 1999; Vogel & Adelman, 1992).

Independent Living Skills

Independent living skills allow the individual to self-monitor and conduct daily life activities independently. These skills will increase the probability that students will take care of their health, be mindful of safety, be on time for class, and communicate various needs when parents are not available to monitor them. It is best to start developing independent living skills well before they are required for the transition to adulthood. Youth that come to college without such preparation are at risk for low academic achievement (DaDeppo, 2009; Dole, 2000; Vogel & Adelman, 1992).

Executive Functioning

Executive functioning includes attention, organization, time management, and ability to prioritize academic activities. Command of these skills will assist with planning time for studies, completing homework, and keeping academic materials organized. For example, attention problems affect organization as well as learning (Biederman et al., 2004; McKinney & Speece, 1986; Seidman, Biederman, Monuteaux, Doyle, & Faraone, 2001; Stadler, 1995). One's ability to prioritize is essential for attending to academic goals. The ability to attend to lectures or activities in the classroom can affect the pace of comprehension. Impulsivity, which often accompanies attention problems, can influence decision making in academic and social settings.

Social Skills

Social skills are critical to success in college, yet developing these skills is an area of difficulty for many students with NVLD (Gerrard-Morris, 2008; Harris, 1998).

Depending on the individual's level of communication skills, social interactions can present problems for the student with NVLD (Little, 1999). They may have difficulty with social understanding in the classroom such as determining if it is socially appropriate to ask questions in class or if it would be better to follow up after class via e-mail or office hours. Some students with NVLD lack awareness of social cues and may unwittingly put off others by dominating class time with additional comments or questions.

Cognitive aspects of learning disabilities such as attention, information processing speed, or comprehension can vary (Bireley, Languis, & Williamson, 1992; Wells, 2006). Sometimes these cognitive strengths or weaknesses affect the student's social behavior in the classroom. Some students with attention problems also exhibit impulsivity. This impulsivity trait can differ in its effect on the individual. Functional impulsivity traits such as enthusiasm may increase positive engagement in learning, whereas dysfunctional impulsivity traits such as disorganization may have negative learning outcomes (Brunas-Wagstaff, Bergquist, Morgan, & Wagstaff, 1996; Morgan & Norris, 2010). For example, students with very quick cognitive processing speeds or distractibility traits may prefer to shift attention between lecture, textbooks, laptop, or other electronic devices. However, multitasking with electronics in the classroom is typically not permitted and counterproductive to learning (Wood, Gentile, Archer, De Pasquale, & Nosko, 2012). Peers and faculty can easily misinterpret this behavior as off-task, aloof, or disrespectful. The student will require skills in social understanding to be aware of how his actions are perceived by others.

Communication

Challenges can include social communication protocols in the classroom, on-line classes, or over e-mail with faculty and students. Some may disengage from class discussions or participation in group activities if they are uncomfortable talking with peers due to social anxieties. In spite of the many hours they spend on computers, social interactions for online courses and e-mail communication can also result in confusion. Research on youth with similar social disabilities found that these youth were much less likely to use e-mail and social media for communication and socialization (Mazurek, Shattuck, Wagner, & Cooper, 2012). Relationships between student and faculty can be strained when students lack initiation and follow-up communication with instructors. Communication can also challenged when professors do not understand a student's specific communication styles such as tendencies to interpret language literally rather than figuratively, responding in a manner that is very direct, or presenting a socially flat affect (Little, 1999). Good social and communication skills are required for all students in higher education settings in order for the individual to receive maximum benefit from participation in campus activities.

Self-Advocacy Skills

It is necessary to be able to self-identify and have self-understanding of how NVLD specifically affects the individual to request relevant accommodations (Brinckerhoff, 1993; Merchant & Gajar, 1997; Scorgie et al., 2010). While it is true that youth with NVLD should focus on their learning strengths and not their learning weaknesses, it is also important for individuals to be able to articulate how they may need assistance. Often, young adults with disabilities come to college without self-advocacy skills (Janiga & Costenbader, 2002). Common obstacles to self-advocacy are a lack of self-understanding, not seeking out services for individuals with disabilities, and lack of self-determination to follow through with requests for accommodations. Families and educators in K-12 should prepare the adult child with self-advocacy skills to promote academic success in college (Lombardi, Gerdes, & Murray, 2011).

Hidden Disabilities and "New Start" Phenomenon

A common phenomenon with freshman students with invisible disabilities is that the student can experience a new start at college with the hope that they have outgrown the NVLD or have learned sufficient compensatory skills to mitigate the need for educational supports. Furthermore, self-advocating by asking for accommodations makes some students feel like they are not as mature as college students without disabilities (Hadley, 2006). This is also a result of the cultural perspective that college is a place where students learn to be adults (Graham-Smith & Lafayette, 2004). Consequently, they do not seek out the disability resource center on campus and self-identify. This is not recommended. Considering the increased academic rigor and self-discipline needed for college coursework, support from the disability resource office is essential during the transition from high school to college. Students should continue to receive academic accommodations such as a note-taker or alternative testing arrangements, to assist with this significant environmental transition. Parents and educational professionals in high school should encourage students to register with the college's disability resource center to access their legally mandated accommodations for coursework.

Self-Determination

Meeting with the resource counselor and receiving the documentation that assists with determining the appropriate accommodations for the individual's needs is only the first step. Even those students who register with the disability resource office may later shy away from requesting legal accommodations from faculty and underutilize the supports that they have used in the past (Cawthon & Cole, 2010). Again, it is the student's responsibility to ask for and implement the accommodation in their courses. Therefore, the student must initiate communication with the instructor and present the instructor with documentation of their legally determined accommodations. Further, the student must follow through with school policies such as acquiring approval signatures on any necessary paperwork to arrange various accommodations such as extra time and a location for taking the test in a space with minimal distraction. For students with NVLD that have challenges with communication or organization, following up on a multiple-step process can be overwhelming. The accommodation determination document can be ineffective if students do not follow through with the necessary steps to implement the accommodations. For these reasons, self-determination and advocacy skills are critical for success in college.

Mental Health

It is very common for students with NVLD to experience depression or anxiety, among other mental health issues (Little, 1999; Semrud-Clikeman, Walkowiak, Wilkinson, & Minne, 2010). A student with a significant history of depression or anxiety may find college unfulfilling, or overwhelming when moods are unstable. In addition, many students who experience significant depression also suffer from problems with concentration. This will ultimately affect their ability to learn. Alternatively, some students with mental health issues report that being enrolled in higher education provided stability and hope when all the other foundational elements in their lives such as personal finances, housing, relationships, etc. are in flux (Edward, 2005; Reynolds & Baird, 2010).

Medication

It is common for students with learning disabilities to take medication for attention, or psychosocial issues such as depression or anxiety. It is not uncommon for individuals with NVLD to experience emotional stressors in addition to the academic challenges. Transitioning to college and moving out of the parent's home to live in college housing can be a very overwhelming experience. The sheer number of new experiences can aggregate anxiety to unprecedented levels that can trigger depression and other psychosocial issues such as isolation or poor self-care. Frequent check-ins with counselors are recommended for students who take prescription medication to assist with monitoring the effectiveness of medication.

It is also common for students who transition to college to experiment with discontinuing medication as part of the "new start." Naturally, an adult may choose to discontinue taking medication at any time. However, it is important for the adult student with NVLD to consider carefully the best time to make this choice. It is not recommended to discontinue medication during this important transition time. Students are recommended to speak with their psychiatrists before discontinuing medication. Parents and counselors need to be proactive in addressing this issue.

Substance Experimentation

The new social freedoms that come with the young adult college lifestyle can be a time for experimentation. Students emerging from the special education system may have experienced years of stigma from previous academic settings or negative interactions with peers without disabilities (Harris, 2007). With the new adult status, limited parental monitoring, students with NVLD are at a higher risk for alcohol abuse, especially those with executive functioning challenges due to weaker planning and self-regulating skills (Blume, Marlatt, & Schmaling, 2000). Young adults may be inclined to self-medicate with alcohol or drugs to address feelings of anxiety, isolation, or low self-esteem. Individuals need to understand how medication will interact with alcohol or nonprescription substances. Therefore professionals and parents should be prepared to provide accurate information to guide the young adult whether or not signs of risk-taking behavior are present prior to enrollment in college.

Transition to Adulthood and Family Dynamics

Naturally, the diversity of students with a diagnosis of NVLD will come from families of diverse backgrounds. Academic self-concept, educational aspirations, independent living skills, adolescent interpersonal skills, and family relationships with school personnel will vary depending on differing cultural values (Duncan, 2003; Mandic, Rudd, Hehir, & Acevedo-Garcia, 2012; Taylor & House, 2010; Zeleke, 2004). Multicultural backgrounds, levels of parental educational attainment, socioeconomic status, and acculturation will all factor in to the adolescent's educational and personal development. Practitioners that work in traditional educational systems in American society may have a tendency to view these developmental issues through a Eurocentric or middle-class lens (Echemendía, 2006; Harry, 1994; Mandic et al., 2012; Poelma, 2002). It is important to be sensitive to these cultural norms when practitioners are assisting families and making educational recommendations.

Academic Self-Concept and Educational Aspirations

Students with NVLD will require social support from families to foster a positive academic self-concept. Parents that accurately educate their child about their specific strengths and challenges may be more likely to instill an enhanced understanding of the NVLD than when students learn about their LD from educational professionals (Cosden, Elliott, Noble, & Kelemen, 1999). Further, parents that value education provide a strong foundation for academic achievement and are linked to students' aspirations for higher education (Rothon, Goodwin, & Stansfeld, 2012; Wildhagen, 2009).

Development of Self-Advocacy and Self-Determination

Educators that work with students with NVLD will find that even though many of these students are very bright and have excellent GPAs that make them eligible for college, their delayed social, independent living skills, or emotional development can be more debilitating than the learning differences. Smith et al. (2002) found that nearly 40% of freshman with disabilities reported global negative self-assessments and dependency on parents to assist with educational decisions. One of the top ten difficulties that freshman students with LD experience is discontinued academic support from parents. Over 60% of students in this category do not receive assistance from parents with course selection and activities (Graham Smith, English, & Vasek, 2002). These findings suggest that many students are not prepared for academic independence.

Therefore, it is equally important to develop a strong foundation in these skills, as it is to develop strengths that compensate for learning challenges in order to increase the individual's social and cultural capital (Bates, 1997; Smith & Young, 2004).

Development of Independent Living Skills

Likely, a key area of focus for parent support for many young adults with NVLD has been to assist with executive functioning challenges such as attention, organization, prioritizing, and time management. Since completing or organizing tasks requires competency in executive functioning skills, many parents have a history of twelve consecutive, academic years of compensating for the child's challenges in this area. This scenario is understandably common. Progressive development of these independent living skills may not be easy for the student or family. This is especially true when other concurrent family life stressors such as the daily dynamics between the youth and the parent (Antshel & Joseph, 2006), health needs of other family members, or changes in parents' employment status are also a challenge. It can sometimes be easier for parents to perform the tasks for their child with the hope that the child will outgrow these underdeveloped skills.

Parents may have a difficult time allowing the adult child to take on some of the responsibilities that they have been handling over the youth's developmental life span. In doing so, some parents may inadvertently delay the development of these skills. Sometimes letting go of these responsibilities to organize and prioritize the child's academic activities may mean initial failure for the developing young adult. Children with NVLD may develop these skills at a slower rate than individuals without NVLD (Rourke, 2000; Speece, McKinney, & Appelbaum, 1985). However, these organizational and time management skills are critical for developing the youth's independent living skills. Letting go of this role will be one of the biggest challenges for both the student and the parent. Parents would benefit from transitioning from the parenting role in K-12 years to more of a "coaching" role as the student enters college (Maitland, 2011). In addition, due to these delays, some students may benefit from starting their postsecondary education at a 2-year college while they are working on these skills (Finn, 1999; Johnson, Zascavage, & Gerber, 2008; Scorgie et al., 2010).

The strategy to transition the adult child to a new environment is critical. However, this is often left unaddressed (NJCLD, 2007; Patwell & Herzog, 2000). If students with NVLD and their families have not acknowledged and prepared for the practical development of these skills these individuals may also be less mature than same-age peers. Students with underdeveloped independent living skills may require years to transition from familiar support to independence after graduation from high school. Research on students with learning disabilities indicates that only half live independently or complete postsecondary education 6 years after high school graduation (Lugas, Timmons, & Smith, 2010; Sanford, Newman, Wagner, Knokey, & Shaver, 2011). Families must make efforts towards developing the individual's compensatory strategies for underdeveloped independent living skills. To aid in this endeavor examples of independent living skills checklists provide practical guidance for parents (Adolescent Autonomy Checklist, 1987; Children's Administration Division of Children and Family Services, 2012). A parent can use these checklists to clarify ways in which the student is ready for college and areas that need to be addressed prior to the first year of transition to postsecondary school.

Typical accommodations that are offered in college do not address the organizational and social challenges that can affect students with NVLD. The young adult with NVLD may require some prompting through the educational accommodation process to understand it, complete the forms, and remember important timelines related to accommodations. If students are in the learning rather than the competency stage young adults may also benefit from using a coach to assist with the transition from dependence on parents to practicing self-advocacy and self-understanding of their LD (Bettinger & Baker, 2011; Klassen, Krawchuk, Lynch, & Rajani, 2008). Several colleges offer coaching services to address these issues. Naturally, these supports must be strategically decreased over time to increase independence.

Challenges with Previous Special Education Environments

Several factors can affect the culture of special education placements and school climate. An inclusive and positive environment in high school promotes understanding among school administrators, faculty, students, and families about NVLD and the appropriate recommendations for college preparation. However, some schools identify these students as being "at risk" and perpetuate a stigma about students with disabilities (Denhart, 2008; Moore et al., 2007). Although students with NVLD are not intellectually less capable than students without learning challenges, studies have shown that a high percentage of students in special education are not referred to college readiness programs such as Advancement Via Individual Determination (AVID) in high school (King, 2009).

Quality of the IEP and Transition Plan

The education that school personnel provide to students and families in the IEP meetings varies. It is important to have an accurate assessment of the levels of functioning. This comprehensive information can be found in the IEP and psychoeducational report. The summary of performance document that is completed prior to transitioning from high school to college addresses the specific strengths and challenges of the individual with NVLD. Typical challenges, such as executive functioning, cognitive processing, academic organizational skills, independent living skills, and social skills to address these challenges, should be clearly identified along with relevant goals (Kochhar-Bryant & Vreeburg, 2006). This is the time to assess current levels of functioning and the future supports needed for transition to college.

Some transition plans may demonstrate much integrity with consistent aims to document achievement of short-term benchmarks and the student's progress towards long-term aspirations. If families and students lack accurate information about NVLD they may mistakenly believe that their child is not college bound. Consequently, they may not encourage the child to enroll in college preparatory coursework in high school (Brown, 2005; Kortering, Braziel, & McClannon, 2010; Poelma, 2002) or waive the student's participation in college entrance testing such as the Scholastic Aptitude Test (SAT) (Kochhar-Bryant & Vreeburg, 2006; Poelma, 2002). Moreover, some students are not aware that they are receiving special education services, why they are eligible, or what kind of disability they have (Kawanishi, 2005; Wurm, 1999). Without this information, students with NVLD will not know how to advocate for themselves effectively.

Academic Preparation

When applying for college admission students with NVLD are often academically unprepared. They are often not exposed to the same curriculum as students without disabilities (Bryan, 1994; Schulman, 1984; Smith & Young, 2004) and are commonly missing preparation courses such as math, foreign language, and science (Boatman & Long, 2010; Gregg, 2007; Laird, 2009). Students who have not been adequately exposed to technical vocabulary and writing that is often used in science texts from elementary age through high school will have difficulty with the expectations of college-level courses (Ofiesh, 2007).

Transition to 4-Year Colleges and Special Admission

Students with NVLD who are missing course requirements and intend to apply to a 4-year university may request a special review for college admission. Some students may be accepted to college under special admission criteria and one or two college preparation courses may be waived for admittance. However, this review is affected by the students' academic patterns prior to college such as GPA and ability to complete attempted coursework (Demerjian, 1996; Howell, 2011).

After a student is accepted with special admittance status, the individual will often be required to take the college preparation courses as a remediation during their first year of college. Since students with disabilities are often at greater risk for college dropout, success during the first year of college will have an effect on future college retention and graduation. College students with disabilities who are found eligible under special admittance criteria will fare better academically if parents have been positive advocates throughout the educational process and have encouraged the development of academic self-determination traits (Hudson, 2008).

Math

Without math college preparation courses the individual will be admitted to the college conditionally and be required to take math remediation courses (Howell, 2011) and pay regular tuition fees, but will not receive a grade that will be factored into the student's GPA or credited towards the degree. For students who have a documented disability in math, many public colleges require that student make multiple attempts to pass math classes to meet state requirements. If the student is unsuccessful, some colleges may consider a substitute class for traditional math classes such as a course in logic.

Cognitive Learning Challenges Versus Math Anxiety

Challenges with math are common for some subtypes of NVLD, and it is important to understand that there are differing types of cognitive functions that affect the ability to do math. For example, some students experience executive functioning issues such as prioritizing the sequences of steps in problem solving. Some cognitive challenges are related to memory, and processing speed to retrieve information; some are due to the individual's challenges with visual spatial information on the page (Geary, 2004). Therefore, accommodations such as use of calculators or providing partial credit to students with LD should be the goal, rather than waiving a math requirement (Ofiesh, 2007). Other students experience emotional factors that will affect their ability to perform well in math. Some individuals with NVLD may have been misdiagnosed with a cognitive disability that affects performance in math when they may actually have math anxiety without a cognitive learning disability in math (Sanders, 2012). It also stands to reason that some students with cognitive challenges that affect their ability to understand math concepts may also experience anxiety when performing math computations, thereby significantly increasing the learning challenge. If coping mechanisms for math anxiety are not addressed, avoidance and procrastination may ultimately limit entrance eligibility to their preferred 4-year college.

Foreign Language

Some students with learning disabilities have been identified as students with a specific learning disability in foreign languages (FLLD). In these cases, universities may receive requests to waive the foreign language requirement towards degree completion. However, some researchers recommend that educators should consider development of individualized or diverse instruction of foreign languages (Miller, 2008) and focus on the importance of respecting diverse learners (Sparks, 2009). Further, others recommend strategies for collaboration between the speech and language specialists in high school and the disability resource office in college (Ganschow, Philips, & Schneider, 2001). To aid in completing the foreign language requirements, typical accommodations such as alternative testing methods and extra time on tests are recommended (Ofiesh, 2007). However, depending on individual cognitive strengths such as in the visual-motor area and memory, sign language may be an alternative for students who struggle in this area (Gómez, Molina, Benítez, & de Torres, 2007; Miller, 2008), although perhaps not so likely for typical for students with NVLD.

Challenges with Parent Involvement and School Climate

Depending on the type and the severity of the disability, the student and family may enter the college setting from a defensive standpoint if they have had a history of difficult or litigious negotiations during IEP meetings with the previous school district. Evidence of the student's increased academic independence requires less academic assistance. This inherently reduces the youth's frequency of special education service time and para-educational supports in the classroom. Reduction should signify a positive benchmark in the student's increased academic independence. However, parents can perceive these reduced supports negatively. This perception can sometime result in acrimonious legal negotiations between the school and the family to assess the validity of decreasing special education supports for an individual. This type of history with the public education system may have left parents and students with a negative perception of programs for individuals with disabilities.

Unrealistic Expectations

Preparing for these legal and cultural changes in high school and college settings for parents and students is critical (Foley, 2006; Kochhar-Bryant & Vreeburg, 2006). If legal differences between high school and higher education settings were not clarified prior to enrollment in college, families will have unrealistic expectations that students are entitled to the same laws and supports they received in K-12 settings. The legal responsibilities of resource counselors in college will differ considerably from the school psychologist's roles and resource teacher's responsibilities in secondary education settings.

Transition from Parent Involvement to Adult Independence

Family dynamics have a role in the development of the youth's individual competency (Summers, 2000). The transition from parent involvement in the special education process to the adolescent's independence in college will depend on the ability to self-advocate. The responsibility of ensuring that the students with NVLD receive accommodations shifts from the educational professionals in the high school setting to the young adult in higher education. Some families are not prepared for this change. Families should expect positive outcomes if they are proactive in their approach to teach these important skills to their child.

Cultural of Higher Education Environments

Role of College Resource Personnel

Once the student is registered with the disability resource office, students are typically assigned a resource counselor to determine the type of supports needed (Troiano, Liefeld, & Trachtenberg, 2010). The title of this professional varies among colleges and may be referred to as the learning specialist or the college disability resource counselor. The resource counselor in higher education settings will review documentation and make a determination of appropriate accommodations. The main role of the resource counselor in college is to ensure that students with NVLD receive appropriate legally mandated accommodations. The philosophy of these legal mandates is similar to the K-12 setting: to allow individuals with disabilities equal, not better, access to university coursework than the access that students without disabilities experience. The college counselor can also play a key role in making sure that the student understands the legal and philosophical differences between special education services in public education and accommodations under the ADA for higher education settings.

Although documentation of a disability is not required by law in order to receive services in college, any related documentation is still helpful for the resource counselor. A review of previous documentation and an interview with the student will indicate how to proceed, especially if the summary of performance (SOP) from high school is thorough (Kochhar-Bryant & Vreeburg, 2006). For a more detail exploration of the current laws regarding requirements for documentation see chapter 14 or Association on Higher Education and Disability (AHEAD) http://www.ahead.org/resources/documentation_guidance. It is important to pay careful attention to which academic areas are affected and how acutely; the functional impact of the specific subtype of NVLD; and the impact of any comorbid mental health diagnoses. Additional concerns may include how the student's knowledge will be evaluated in college such as, written essays multiple choice tests or availability of aides such as notes or calculators (Ofiesh, Hughes, & Scott, 2004). Although the IEP and report from high school are not typically requested, the student may wish to provide this documentation.

2-Year Colleges

Research on young adults with learning disabilities indicates that they are more likely to enroll in a 2-year college than a 4-year university (Sanford et al., 2011). This may be because of the availability of special support programs or college personnel that make them better equipped to support adult students with learning disabilities, thus making 2-year college campuses more accessible (Finn, 1999; Scorgie et al., 2010). For families that are uncertain of their child's level of independent functioning in the academic and social domains, initial transition to a community college may be the best choice. Students with future aspirations of attending a 4-year college will have an opportunity to complete remediation coursework at the community college and general education requirements to transfer to a 4-year college. Moreover, research suggests that students with learning disabilities that attend a community college prior to transferring to a 4-year university are more likely to graduate (Johnson et al., 2008).

Faculty Attitudes

While there is evidence to suggest that faculty and peers have a positive understanding of students with learning disabilities (Murray, Wren, & Keys, 2008), often college instructors have little to no experience teaching students with special learning or social needs. Special education instruction does not exist in higher education. Some faculty are more knowledgeable than others about cognitive processes involved in learning. Except for professors that specialize in the area of disabilities, there is limited institutional support for special learning differences. Many college personnel that encounter these students do not understand how and why they need to accommodate these students (Bourdieu, 1986; Malangko, 2009). Some educators have misconceptions about learning disabilities and may erroneously believe that individuals with NVLD are not intellectually capable of attaining a college education.

Some obstacles to equal access to course content on the college campus are due to negative faculty perceptions or lack of education about students with learning disabilities (Beilke & Yssel, 1999; Hedrick, Dizén, Collins, Evans, & Grayson, 2010). Further, the added stressor of adjusting to college can exacerbate existing mental health issues such as anxiety or depression for the student. This can lead to difficulty with concentration, irritability, emotional stability, and patience. In these cases, college personnel may be left with an unfavorable impression of the individual with NVLD, thereby discouraging faculty collaboration and perpetuating the stigma associated with disabilities. The student's lack of disclosure to faculty about the need for accommodations can add to this myth (Forrest, 2003). This is especially true for students with invisible disabilities, such as NVLD. If a student is uncomfortable with informing faculty about their diagnosis, they do not need to disclose what their specific disability is to the faculty, but may instead wish to address how specific accommodations can address the individual's unique learning challenges. For example, rather than informing the professor that a student has been diagnosed with NVLD, the student may inform an instructor that he or she experiences problems with concentration and how the approved accommodation for extended time on tests and a room with minimal distraction assists with any lapses in focus throughout an exam.

Alternatively, sometimes students may inadvertently contribute to negative faculty and student dynamics, often due to the student's poor social skills. Students with disabilities with insufficient education about the important differences between college and K-12 education laws often assume similar laws apply in both settings. This can develop into a false sense of entitlement and student may make demands for accommodations that do not meet the legal mandates or intent of the ADA law and Section 504 regulations in higher education settings. These accommodations are designed to provide the student with the same access to the curriculum and experiences as students without learning disabilities in order to provide them with equal, not better, access to coursework, or a less challenging curriculum.

Few campuses have prioritized inclusion of students with disabilities (King, 2009). Misguided faculty may equate academic freedom with the ability to sanction the modality of instruction rather than the essential course content (Scott, 1995). Some may speciously question an individual's intellectual ability to comprehend the course material or eligibility for college. Faculty with tenure or full professorship may be less likely than faculty with lower rankings to provide teaching accommodations (Skinner, 2007; Vogel, Leyser, Wyland, & Brulle, 1999). Faculty in the social sciences may be more willing to provide accommodations than faculty in other sciences (Nelson, Dodd, & Smith, 1990). It is up to individual campuses to facilitate inclusive campuses and ensure that faculty and students are aware of their relative rights and responsibilities. This can be accomplished through the disability resource office's outreach and education activities on campus.

Varying Institutional Philosophies

In higher education, there are differing philosophies about what college support personnel feel that they should do to assist students with additional organizational and social challenges for these students. It appears that professionals recognize the need for additional support, but the law in higher education settings does not mandate this type of support (Gomez, 2011). Further, even disability resource counselors that do provide some type of support services for these students generally agree that this level of support is often too time intensive. Most professionals agree that it is better to be proactive and teach self-advocacy, independent living, organizational, and social skills earlier in the child's developmental process rather than allow these challenges to turn into additional stressors in college (Gomez, 2011; Hadley, 2006).

Types of Support Programs

The ADA law ensures that students with disabilities receive "reasonable accommodations" for students with learning disabilities. Higher education settings do not typically provide additional support services such as one-on-one coaching or mentoring. However, some college administrators recognize the need for such services and offer these additional services with financial support generated by external program fees or government grants. These programs benefit both the student and the institution by providing increased accessibility, retention, graduation, and achievement for students with disabilities in higher education (Bates, 1997; Gugerty & Knutsen, 2000; Hagen et al., 1991; Kerka, 2002; Miller, Hinterlong, & Greene, 2010; Parker & Boutelle, 2009; Robinson & Gahagan, 2010; Rooney, 2012; Rothman, Maldonado, & Rothman, 2008). This next section will address these types of support services and related outcome research. Some programs are specific to students with NVLD, and others are programs for similar but unspecified types of learning disabilities.

TRIO Programs

Federal TRIO Student Support Services program grants specifically serve students with disabilities, low income, or first-generation college students throughout the United States. Prospective college students, school counselors, and parents can identify both 2-year and 4-year campuses that have been awarded funding for these programs by reviewing the TRIO website http://www2.ed.gov/programs/triostudsupp/awards.html. In addition, this information is typically available by reviewing the websites of colleges that families are considering. Federal TRIO Student with additional social and academic support services other than those required by law and have a positive effect on retention, grades, self-advocacy, self-esteem, and graduation rates (Boughton, 1996; Zhang & Chan, 2007). Students that participate in these support programs show significant gains compared to students with learning disabilities that do not participate in these support programs (Ruiz, 2008). Further, from the students' perspective, campuses with these types of programs are more welcoming to students with learning disabilities.

Service Learning

A review of the literature provides some evidence for types of effective programs for all students, including students with disabilities. Educational settings that use service learning programs can be beneficial to increase cultural and social understanding (Oster-Aaland, Sellnow, Nelson, & Pearson, 2004). Opportunities to provide volunteer service in the community and to apply practical and educational problem-solving techniques that address community issues have been shown to be effective for students with LD (Miller et al., 2010).

Coaching Programs

Although independence is the goal, some families may not have been as successful as they would like preparing their young adult for the transition to college. To respond to this need, coaching programs in higher education and other community based settings are designed to support individuals with disabilities with underdeveloped social, independent living, or academic organizational skills though this transition period. The role of the coach can also be described as a peer mentor and a "… dynamic, reciprocal, long-term formal, or informal, relationship that focuses on personal and/or professional development …" (Foster Heckman, Brown, & Roberts, 2007, p. 2). An authentic and consistent rapport between mentor and mentee in an educational setting can remove obstacles and increase equal access for students with disabilities through electronic types of communication or in person (Stumbo et al., 2010).

Ninety percent of students with a GPA under 2.0 who used coaching services demonstrated improved GPAs, increased retention outcomes, reduced negative self-talk, decreased stress, and increased self-understanding (Parker & Boutelle, 2009; Robinson & Gahagan, 2010). Further, collaboration between coaches and the resource counselor would be beneficial during this transition period. This collaboration can be facilitated with the student's authorization to share information between the coach and other parties. Most colleges have this authorization form readily available to facilitate such communications when necessary. Depending on the level of independent functioning, the student may benefit from a coach who will initially monitor student needs and assess progress in various domains during this critical time.

Residential Life on Campus

If youth with NVLD decide to attend a 4-year college, the decision to live at home or to live on campus can also be a critical transition consideration. Domestic organizational skills, buying books, using debit or credit cards, or socializing, hygiene practices, and relationships with roommates may be emerging skills for some freshmen. For young adults with NVLD who have delayed independent living and social skills, it may be beneficial to remain at home for the first year of college when possible. Objectivity and accurate assessments of the individual's level of independent functioning can be difficult for parents. If students live at home during the first year of college, parents should be mindful of transitioning their young adult to function independently. Some parents may still feel the need to monitor homework completion, facilitate social interaction, and continue to perform some daily tasks for their child. By doing this, an overly involved parent inadvertently delays the young adult's independent living skills.

If students decide to live on campus their first year, some colleges have programs that may provide coaching or mentoring to assist with the development of these skills. These programs may also address other skills needed for college life such as stress management, organization, social connections, and suggestions for good safety practices.

Vocational and Rehabilitation Programs

In addition, some state vocational rehabilitation programs provide financial assistance to students that participate in programs that specifically serve students with learning disabilities. For young adults with NVLD who are still exploring employment, college options, or life skills, some public universities have fee-based programs that provide "life coaching." This type of coaching can assist students with finding the right school or employment, socialization, and learning independent living skills. Preparation programs that teach strategies to improve self-esteem, self-advocacy, or performance in college coursework have shown positive results for retention and graduation (Gugerty & Knutsen, 2000). Students learn to increase their independence and set personal goals for success.

Evidence-Based or Specialized Programs for Students with Learning Disabilities

Adelphi University is noteworthy because it offers services specifically for students with NVLD. The Bridges to Adelphi Program in Garden City, New York, assists college students with NVLD with peer support and coaching. Coaches and learning specialists are graduate students with specialized training in working with students with NVLD and other disabilities.

Longview Community College's ABLE program in Kansas City, Missouri, provides both social–emotional and academic services. Emphasis is on self-advocacy and self-regulation. The ABLE program offers remediation coursework in reading, writing, communication, and math concepts. It has proven effective in supporting students with learning disabilities, traumatic brain injury, ASD, and other neurological disabilities (Gugerty & Knutsen, 2000).

The SUNY Albany program assists students with precollege or job placement. The program teaches independent living, self-advocacy, and study skills, as well as an introduction to college systems and accommodations. High school students who attended summer courses demonstrated success in college (Rothman et al., 2008).

Landmark College uses coaching programs to support students in obtaining an associate degree or bachelor's degree in liberal arts. The program reports student growth in independence, compensatory skills for learning challenges, and increased educational aspirations (Parker & Boutelle, 2009).

The program for advancement of learning (PAL) at Curry College in Massachusetts has been nationally recognized as an exemplary program with support and motivation as key factors to success (Ijiri et al., 1998; Rooney, 2012). The program provides services for students with learning disabilities whose first language is not English. Summer transition options as well as specialized courses for academic and social learning are available.

It is important for students and families to remember that these programs are only effective if the student utilizes the resources that are available in these programs. It is important to consider the individual's commitment and attendance in such programs. Youth with learning disabilities that participated in program activities consistently had higher GPAs and graduation rates than students with lower rates of attendance (Reed et al., 2009; Troiano et al., 2010).

Challenges in the Transition to Employment

Once a student graduates from college, continuing transition to independence will likely involve obtaining gainful employment. Research provides encouraging employment statistics as well as some areas of concern for individuals with learning disabilities. About 75% of students with LD are employed after college and most are employed in business and education settings. However, approximately half earn less than $50,000 annually and 36% of individuals with learning disabilities report that they receive support from others outside the workplace, such as family members for work tasks by (Madaus, 2006).

It is critical that students with NVLD understand that their specific and individual challenges will affect their career choice and how. The fit for a career depends on characteristics inherent in the individual, such as tenacity, ambition, and so on, as well as factors related to use of external resources, such as use of community supports that aid in the fit (Kerka, 2002). The combination of individual factors and programs is also important for adults with learning disabilities that wish to pursue careers in the field of medicine and law (Weinstein, Wolf, & Schreiber, 2008).

It is also recommended that individuals with NVLD do not wait until graduation to prepare for their first internship placement or position of employment. Individuals with NVLD may need to advocate for themselves creatively in the job market. It may be necessary to create a market demand for a specialized skill set that "carves out" tasks from an existing job description or several positions at one company that allow the individual to work in areas where skills are strong, leaving tasks that are more challenging for individuals with NVLD for other employees without NVLD and their relevant strengths (Griffin & Targett, 2006; Nietupski & Hamre-Nietupski, 2000). This type of strategy allows the individual with NVLD to creatively highlight his or her strengths as a candidate for an employer, rather than to limit oneself to a fit with a specific job description.

Further, some subtypes of NVLD require "soft" job skills preparation and coaching to transition young adults for interviews (Gulian, 1986). Individuals with NVLD sometimes require coaching in the area of social skills associated with the interview process, grooming, interview etiquette, and self-advocacy. Once employed, college staff or independent coaches can work with individuals with NVLD to transition students to employment settings.

Self-Advocacy and Employment

Individuals with NVLD may need assistance with the decision whether or not to disclose their disability. As with the desire for a fresh start in college, transfer to a nonacademic setting can sometimes retrigger old feelings of wanting a fresh start. In a new job, individuals may opt for not disclosing their disability. However if problems arise later, research indicates that employers view candidates more preferably when they disclose their invisible disability earlier rather than later (Roberts & Hoff Macan, 2006).

The knowledge that an employee has NVLD does not provide adequate information to build a working relationship with a supervisor. Specific individual challenges should be addressed in the workplace regardless of whether a supervisor is aware of a specific diagnosis or label. For example, focusing on individual characteristics, such as a need for clear written instructions on specific company procedures, is a specific modification to verbal instructions. This can set the employee up for success in the workplace. Simply informing an employer that the employee has a disability without suggestions for support with the employee's specific challenges does not assist with a strategy for success. In addition, the individual should remember to focus on informing supervisors and coworkers about their strengths, such as attention to detail or knowledge base in a particular area.

Career Support Programs

A number of public colleges collaborate with their respective state department of rehabilitation. These programs assist with the transition from college to employment for students with disabilities. For example, Life Development Institute in Arizona has programs specifically designed for students with NVLD. It assists in developing independent life skills, disability education, and transitional skills for the workplace in addition to academic skills (Bates, 1997; Kerka, 2002). In addition, current federal policies ensure that people with disabilities are considered for employment, particularly in government offices (National Council on Disability, 2010). Educational professionals and coaches that work with students with NVLD should be aware of this resource and include contact with these programs in their college activities and planning.

Summary

There is a significant need for program planning that supports the unique needs of students with NVLD. Current practices in special education in K-12 settings and IEP processes leave students without proper preparation of social, emotional, academic, and independent living skills for the transition to work or college. Family dynamics can also negatively influence the development of necessary skills. Parent over-involvement with the youth can inadvertently delay age-appropriate development of these skills. Delayed development of these skills leaves the young adult lacking in social and cultural capital, resulting in college dropout and lower rates of employment or salaries compared to adults without disabilities. Previous school placements can present critical obstacles to eligibility for some higher education settings. Families need concrete information on college preparation courses needed for college eligibility. Conscientious efforts from families and schools will prepare youth for the transition to adulthood with skills that can last a lifetime and positively affect the functional relationship of the individual with NVLD in various environments.

Recommendations

K-12 Special Education

Special education should assist with strategies to teach student self-advocacy, technological competency, and in-class support through peer mentoring or coaching, and preparation for independence rather than dependence on the type of supports available in K-12 is recommended (Kochhar-Bryant & Vreeburg, 2006). More strategic transition is needed in academic, social, and independent living skills (Adreon & Durocher, 2007). Moreover, students with disabilities should be encouraged to participate in student leadership roles starting in secondary schools and continue service in college (Swain, 1993; Wilson, Carvalho, & Alvarez, 2007).

Postsecondary Education

Accountability measures for disability resource centers should be in place to address university climate for students with disabilities. It behooves disability resource personnel to provide outreach and education to the entire college campus. It is the responsibility of the resource office on campus to make efforts to reduce stigma and facilitate accessible education. Yuen and Shaughnessy (2001) recommended that universities provide outreach to secondary schools to develop cultural capital on college campuses for students with disabilities. Fostering a culture of inclusion is essential. The effectiveness of the outreach and education will also depend on eliciting support from the campus' key personnel or specific programs that are dedicated to retention and graduation of students with LD. Outreach and education activities at each college should be a regular occurrence with a consistent message, rather than token "disability awareness days." Student groups on campus would benefit by collaborating with feeder schools to assist with the transition process.

Residential Community

Residential housing is a very significant aspect of the culture of the entire campus. Residential housing staff would benefit from regular educational activities provided by students with disabilities and support personnel. This requires collaboration in the form of shared philosophies about the inclusion of individuals with disabilities from administration, residential assistants, student housing activity coordinators, associated student groups, fraternities, and advertising student activities to people with diverse backgrounds.

Professional Development

All educational institutions have requirements that direct university staff to participate in "mandated reporter," "FERPA," harassment, and diversity trainings. Even campuses that celebrate ethnic and religious diversity do not inherently understand that students with learning, social, or communication differences are also a group that requires equal treatment to students that are neurotypical (Barnard-Brak, Davis, Tate, & Sulak, 2009). Campus personnel would benefit from participation in educational workshops about resources for working with students with NVLD. Education in this area facilitates a climate of inclusion that can help students with NVLD feel like they are welcome on campus. Research suggests that the social culture of a college campus can have more impact on college success than targeted support programs or services (Graham-Smith & Lafayette, 2004). A number of educational resources are available for postsecondary faculty such as *NLDline* that does not require additional workshop development efforts on the part of the institution.

Coaching/Mentoring Programs

Coaches will be able to serve students with NVLD or other disabilities when educators and support staff are informed about the specific characteristics of NVLD in addition to the purpose and parameters of coaching services. For the coach, building this rapport with instructors and employers is critical (Beyer & Kaehne, 2008). As mentioned earlier, this relationship is based on integrity, trust, and consistency in services. Educational partnerships between students with disabilities and college staff and faculty may be mutually beneficial, especially when the relationship is reciprocal and includes formal and informal rapport building opportunities such as defined mentor/mentee relationships and opportunities for social activities, respectively (Foster Heckman et al., 2007; Hadley, 2006).

Technology

Outreach must also include education on the use of assistive technology to inform educators not only how students with NVLD use technology but also to inform on how to make their course materials accessible for the various types of technology available. Many educators are not informed about the impact that accessibility has on students who use this technology from requesting alternative formats of texts, the length of time it takes for conversion, as well as working relationships with textbook publishers and additional time needed for the students to comprehend material in this alternative format. Math can be particularly challenging for alternative formats due to the symbols and some incompatibility with screen readers or on-line math courses. Some technologies such as talking calculators do not sync visual and auditory information well. Further, a limited number of higher education institutions or K-12 instructors have access to a technology advisory committee for guidance or professional development on how to make this technology accessible to students with disabilities. The culture of public education requires improvement in these efforts (Dalton, 2010; Fitchen et al., 2002; Obudo, 2008).

Although many students with NVLD will complete college successfully, many of them will be caught off guard when they begin to transition from college to career. Students with NVLD may need more time to transition to work settings. Career exploration needs to start earlier in their college career. It should include interview and soft job skills, experiences in service learning, volunteer work in field of interest, internships, and networking skills.

Research

NVLD

Research on NVLD is limited in comparison to research on learning disabilities in general. Given the possible subtypes of NVLD (Davis & Broitman, 2011), further investigation and replication studies are needed. Certainly, some general findings on students with general learning disabilities could similarly apply to individuals with NVLD such as in the area of self-concept, co-occurring mental health issues, educational aspirations, etc. Nevertheless, research specific to NVLD will ultimately affect applicability of subsequent development of unique types of supports to individuals, families, educators, and employers for adults with NVLD.

Programs

It is also true that research is especially lacking on support programs for NVLD. Many programs exist, but few have been independently evaluated with published findings, especially in higher education settings. More research is needed to update antiquated educational policies and practices related to the types of supports that are "appropriate" in the K-12 settings and "reasonable" in postsecondary settings to reflect research-based strategies. Research on institutional support for coaching programs, or special curriculums in conventional educational setting, is required (Herrera, Sipe, McClanahan, Arbreton, & Pepper, 2000; Kochhar-Bryant, Bassett, & Webb, 2009; Kochhar-Bryant & Vreeburg, 2006).

Transition from College to Career

Some state rehabilitation programs utilize systematic assessments for career preparation for NVLD. However, there is often a disconnect between the Individualized Plan for Employment regarding the individual student's strengths, their college major, and career goals. Often students will choose a major that is general such as Liberal Studies yet have aspirations to work in a field where experience that is more specific is required. Therefore, utilizing standardized assessments of career exploration, work readiness, and daily living skills is essential (Dipeolu, 2007; Rojewski, 1996). Additional research and publications are needed on skills, interventions, and programs that contribute to independent living and job satisfaction for adults with NVLD.

Conclusion

The development from adolescence to adulthood is a process that requires decisive monitoring from families and educational institutions for youth with aspirations of higher education and independence. Concerted efforts within these systems will ensure that adolescents with NVLD have the same opportunities to build social and cultural capital as do youth without learning disabilities. With these resources, adolescents with NVLD will be able to realize their highest potential.

References

Adolescent Autonomy Checklist. (1987). Family to Family Health Center. Retrieved July 4, 2012, from http://www.spannj.org/Family2Family/adolescent_autonomy_checklist.htm

Adreon, D., & Durocher, J. S. (2007). Evaluating the college transition needs of individuals with high-functioning autism spectrum disorders. *Intervention in School and Clinic, 42*, 271–279.

Antshel, K., & Joseph, G. R. (2006). Maternal stress in non-verbal learning disorder: A comparison with reading disorder. *Journal of Learning Disabilities, 39*(3), 194–205.

Association of Higher Education and Disability. (2011). Supporting Accommodation Requests: Guidance on Documentation Practices. Retrieved April 2012 from http:/www.ahead.org/resources/documentation_guidance.

Barnard-Brak, L., Davis, T., Tate, A., & Sulak, T. (2009). Attitudes as a predictor of college students requesting accommodations. *Journal of Vocational Rehabilitation, 31*(3), 189–198.

Bates, B. (1997). Transitions: Issues for the adult learner with learning disabilities. *LINKAGES, Linking Literacy & Learning Disabilities, 4*(1).

Bates, P., & Davis, F. A. (2004). Social capital, social inclusion and services for people with learning disabilities. *Disability & Society, 19*(3), 195–207.

Bays, D. A., & Crockett, J. B. (2007). Investigating instructional leadership for special education. *Exceptionality, 15*(3), 143–161.

Beilke, J. R., & Yssel, N. (1999). The chilly climate for students with disabilities in higher education. *College Student Journal, 33*(3), 364–371.

Bettinger, E. P., & Baker, R. (2011). *The effects of student coaching in college: An evaluation of a randomized experiment in student mentoring*. Cambridge, MA: National Bureau of Economic Research. NBER Working Paper No. 16881.

Beyer, S., & Kaehne, A. (2008). The transition of young people with learning disabilities to employment: What works? *Journal on Developmental Disabilities, 14*(1), 85–94.

Biederman, J., Monuteaux, M. C., Doyle, A. E., Seidman, L. J., Ferrero, F., Morgan, C., et al. (2004). Impact of executive function deficits and attention-deficit/hyperactivity disorder (ADHD) on academic outcomes in children. *Journal of Consulting and Clinical Psychology, 72*(5), 757–766.

Bireley, M., Languis, M., & Williamson, T. (1992). Physiological uniqueness: A new perspective on the learning disabled/gifted child. *Roeper Review, 15*(2), 101–107.

Black, D. O. (2010). Review of 'How to compromise with your school district without compromising your child: A field guide for getting effective services for children with special needs'. *Journal Of Autism And Developmental Disorders, 40*(6).

Blume, A. W., Marlatt, G., & Schmaling, K. B. (2000). Executive cognitive function and heavy drinking behavior among college students. *Psychology of Addictive Behaviors, 14*(3), 299–302.

Boatman, A., & Long, B. (2010). *Does remediation work for all students? How the effects of postsecondary remedial and developmental courses vary by level of academic preparation. An NCPR working paper*. New York, NY: Research on National Center for Postsecondary Education, National Center for Postsecondary Research.

Bourdieu, P. (1986). The forms of capital. In J. Richardson (Ed.), *Handbook of theory and research for the sociology of education* (pp. 241–248). New York: Greenwood.

Brinckerhoff, L. C. (1993). Self-advocacy: A critical skill for college students with learning disabilities. *Family & Community Health, 16*(3), 23–33.

Brinckerhoff, L. C., Shaw, S. F., & McGuire, J. M. (1996). Promoting access, accommodations, and independence for college students with learning disabilities. In J. R. Patton & E. A. Pollock (Eds.), *Learning disabilities: The challenges of adulthood* (pp. 71–92). Austin, TX, US: PRO-ED.

Brodeur, C. (2006). Building social competence in children with nonverbal learning disabilities: A preliminary study. *Dissertation Abstracts International, 67*.

Bronfenbrenner, U. (1974). Is early intervention effective? *Teachers College Record, 76*(2), 279–303.

Bronfenbrenner, U. (1986). Ecology of the family as a context for human development: Research perspectives. *Developmental Psychology, 22*(6), 723–742.

Brown, C. M. (2005). Parent home involvement and student achievement for Mexican-American and European American students with learning disabilities. *Dissertation Abstracts International Section A*, 66.

Brunas-Wagstaff, J., Bergquist, A., Morgan, K., & Wagstaff, G. F. (1996). Impulsivity, interference on perceptual tasks and hypothesis testing. *Personality and Individual Differences, 20*(4), 471–482.

Bryan, T. (1994). The social competence of students with learning disabilities over time: A response to Vaughn and Hogan. *Journal of Learning Disabilities, 27*(5), 304–308.

Cawthon, S. W., & Cole, E. V. (2010). Postsecondary students who have a learning disability: Student perspectives on accommodations access and obstacles. *Journal of Postsecondary Education and Disability, 23*(2), 112–128.

Children's Administration Division of Children and Family Services. (2012, June 13). Washington State Department of Social and Health Services. Retrieved July 4, 2012, from http://www.dshs.wa.gov/pdf/ms/forms/10_267.pdf

Clegg, S. (2011). Cultural capital and agency: Connecting critique and curriculum in higher education. *British Journal of Sociology of Education, 1*, 93–108.

Cosden, M., Elliott, K., Noble, S., & Kelemen, E. (1999). Self-understanding and self-esteem in children with learning disabilities. *Learning Disability Quarterly, 22*(4), 279–290.

Cowles, J. R., & Keim, M. C. (1995). The graduation rate, intellectual functioning level, and matriculation time of university students with learning disabilities. *College Student Journal, 2*, 145–149.

DaDeppo, L. W. (2009). Integration factors related to the academic success and intent to persist of college students with learning disabilities. *Learning Disabilities Research and Practice, 24*(3), 122–131.

Dalton, E. (2010). The relationship between assistive technology state standards for teachers, assistive technology implementation, and student performance in the context of evidence-based practice. *Dissertation Abstracts International Section A, 70.*

Davis, J. M., & Broitman, J. (2011). *Nonverbal learning disabilities in children: Bridging the gap between science and practice*. New York: Springer.

Demerjian, M. (1996). *Matriculation project: Prerequisite challenges*. Santa Clarita, CA: Office of Institutional Development.

Denhart, H. (2008). Deconstructing barriers: Perceptions of students labeled with learning disabilities in higher education. *Journal of Learning Disabilities, 41*(6), 483–497.

Dipeolu, A. O. (2007). Career instruments and high school students with learning disabilities: Support for the utility of three vocational measure. *Journal of Career Development, 34*(1), 59–78.

Dole, S. (2000). The implications of the risk and resilience literature for gifted students with learning disabilities. *Roeper Review, 23*(2), 91–96.

Dorow, R. (2011). Transition planning for postsecondary students with disabilities: Espoused versus actual transition planning. *Dissertation Abstracts International Section A*.

Duncan, N. (2003). Awkward customers? Parents and provision for special educational needs. *Disability & Society, 18*(3), 341–356.

Echemendía, R. J. (2006). Cultural perspectives in pediatric rehabilitation. In J. E. Farmer, J. Donder, & S. Warschausky (Eds.), *Treating neurodevelopmental disabilities: Clinical research and practice* (pp. 289–307). New York, NY: Guilford Press.

Edward, K. (2005). Resilience: A protector from depression. *Journal of the American Psychiatric Nurses Association, 11*(4), 241–243.

Fast, Y. (2003). *Employment for individuals with Asperger syndrome or non-verbal learning disability: Stories and strategies*. London, England: Jessica Kingsley Publishers.

Finn, L. L. (1999). Learning disabilities programs at community colleges and four-year colleges and universities. *Community College Journal of Research and Practice, 23*(7), 629–639.

Fitchen, C., Asuncion, J. V., Barile, M. F., Myrtis, E., Robillard, C., Judd, D., et al. (2002). Access to information and instructional technologies in higher education I: Disability service providers' perspective. *Journal of Postsecondary Education and Disability, 17*(2), 114–133.

Foley, N. E. (2006). Preparing for college: Improving the odds for students with learning disabilities. *College Student Journal, 40*(3), 641–645.

Forrest, K. (2003). Overcoming unintentional barriers with intentional strategies: Educating faculty about student disability. *Teaching of Psychology, 30*(3), 270–276.

Foster Heckman, E., Brown, S. E., & Roberts, K. D. (2007, November). *Mentoring partnership project: Exploring mentoring practices for students with disabilities in postsecondary education*. The George Washington University HEATH Resource Center. Retrieved July 27, 2011, from http://www.heath.gwu.edu/assets/24/heath_mentoring_partnership_project.pdf

Furstenberg, F. (2006). *Diverging Development: The not-so-invisible hand of social class in the United States. Paper presented at the Society for Research on Adolescents*. San Francisco: The Network on Transitions to Adulthood.

Ganschow, L., Philips, L., & Schneider, E. (2001). Closing the gap: Accommodating students with language learning disabilities in college. *Topics in Language Disorders, 21*(2), 17–37.

Geary, D. C. (2004). Mathematics and learning disabilities. *Journal of Learning Disabilities, 37*, 4–15.

Gerrard-Morris, A. (2008). Internalized socioemotional functioning of children and adolescents with nonverbal learning disability and Asperger's syndrome. *Dissertation Abstracts International, 68*.

Gomez, C. (2011). *Students with disabilities that impact behavior require more than accommodations*. Disability Compliance for Higher Education. Retrieved June 29, 2011, from http://www.disabilitycompliancefhttp://webany.net/Sites/wileyDHE-ada/sample-articles/disabilities-impact-behavior-require-more.aspx

Gómez, M., Molina, T., Benítez, P., & de Torres, J. (2007). Predicting proficiency in signed language interpreting: A preliminary study. *Interpreting, 9*(1), 71–93.

Graham Smith, S., English, R., & Vasek, D. (2002). Student and parent involvement in the transition process for college freshmen with learning disabilities. *College Student Journal, 36*(4), 491–503.

Graham-Smith, S., & Lafayette, S. (2004). Quality disability support for promoting belonging and academic success within the college community. *College Student Journal, 38*(1), 90–99.

Gregg, N. (2007). Underserved and unprepared: Postsecondary learning disabilities. *Learning Disabilities Research and Practice, 22*(4), 219–228.

Griffin, G., & Targett, P. (2006). Job carving and customized employment. In P. Wehman (Ed.), *Life beyond the classroom: Transition strategies for young people with disabilities* (4th ed., pp. 289–307). Baltimore, MD: Paul H Brookes Publishing.

Gugerty, J., & Knutsen, C. (2000). *Serving students with significant disabilities in two-year colleges: ABLE program, longview community college*. Lee's Summit, MO: Wisconsin University.

Gulian, E. (1986). The comparative efficiency of various rehearsal modes: A field experiment. *Human Learning, 5*(1), 45–57.

Hadley, W. M. (2006). L.D. Students' access to higher education: Self advocacy and support. *Journal of Developmental Education, 30*(2), 10–16.

Hagen, J. W., et al. (1991). *Implementing and evaluating a program for college students with learning disabilities*. Washington, DC: Distributed by ERIC Clearinghouse.

Harris, D. (1998). Non-verbal learning difficulties: More questions than answers. *Educational Psychology in Practice, 13*(4), 258–265.

Harris, J. (2007). The effect of labeling on the postsecondary student with learning disabilities: A phenomenological study. *Dissertation Abstracts International Section A, 68*.

Harry, B. (1994). Behavioral disorders in the context of families. In S. Ishii-Jordan & R. L. Peterson (Eds.), *Multicultural issues in the education of students with behavioral disorders* (pp. 149–161). Cambridge, MA, US: Brookline Books.

Hedrick, B., Dizén, M., Collins, K., Evans, J., & Grayson, T. (2010). Perceptions of college students with and without disabilities and effects of STEM and non-STEM enrollment on student engagement and institutional involvement. *Journal of Postsecondary Education & Disability, 23*(2), 129–136.

Herrera, C., Sipe, C., McClanahan, W., Arbreton, A. J., & Pepper, S. (2000). *Mentoring school-age children: Relationship development in community-based and school-based programs*. Philadelphia, PA: National Mentoring Partnership Public Policy Council.

Howell, J. S. (2011). What influences students' need for remediation in college? Evidence from California. *Journal of Higher Education, 82*(3), 292–318.

Hudson, W. (2008). The relationship between academic self-efficacy and resilience to grades of students admitted under special criteria. *Dissertation Abstracts International Section A, 68*.

Ijiri, L., Carroll, J., Fletcher, S., Hubbard, L., Manchester, J., & Van Someren, D. (1998). *A comprehensive model of a post-secondary learning disabilities program: The program for advancement of learning (PAL) at Curry college*. Washington, DC: ERIC Clearinghouse Languages and Linguistics.

Janiga, S., & Costenbader, V. (2002). The transition from high school to postsecondary education for students with learning disabilities: A survey of college service coordinators. *Journal of Learning Disabilities, 35*(5), 463–470.

Johnson, G., Zascavage, V., & Gerber, S. (2008). Junior college experience and students with learning: Implications for success at the four year university. *College Student Journal, 42*(4).

Kawanishi, K. T. (2005). Trends and issues in research on the self-perception of students with learning disabilities: Self-perception problems of students with LD and their relationships with others. *Japanese Journal of Special Education., 42*(6), 531–546.

Kerka, S. (2002). *Learning disabilities and career development. Practice application brief no. 20*. Columbus, OH: ERIC Clearinghouse on Adult, Career, and Vocational Education.

King, K. A. (2009). A review of programs that promote higher education access for underrepresented students. *Journal of Diversity in Higher Education, 2*(1), 1–15.

Klassen, R. M., Krawchuk, L. L., Lynch, S. L., & Rajani, S. (2008). Procrastination and motivation of undergraduates with learning disabilities: A mixed-methods inquiry. *Learning Disabilities Research and Practice, 23*(3), 137–147.

Kochhar-Bryant, C., Bassett, D. S., & Webb, K. W. (2009). *Transition to postsecondary education for students with disabilities*. Thousand Oaks, CA: Corwin Press.

Kochhar-Bryant, C. A., & Vreeburg, I. (2006). Access to post-high school services: Transition assessment and summary of performance. *Career Development and Exceptional Individuals, 29*(2), 70–89.

Kortering, L. J., Braziel, P. M., & McClannon, T. W. (2010). Career ambitions: A comparison of youth with and without SLD. *Remedial and Special Education, 31*(4), 230–240.

Laird, B. (2009). The trouble with transferring: It shouldn't be so difficult. *The Chronicle of Higher Education, 55*(29), B22.

Little, L. (1999). The misunderstood child: The child with a nonverbal learning disorder. *Journal of the Society of Pediatric Nurses, 4*(3), 113–121.

Lombardi, A., Gerdes, H., & Murray, C. (2011). Validating an assessment of individual actions, postsecondary supports, and social supports of college students with disabilities. *Journal of Student Affairs Research and Practice, 48*(1), 107–126.

Lugas, J., Timmons, C., & Smith, F. (2010). *Vocational rehabilitation services received by youth with autism: Are they associated with an employment outcome*? Retrieved October 2, 2011, from Institute for Community Inclusion.

Madaus, J. W. (2006). Employment outcomes of university graduates with learning disabilities. *Learning Disability Quarterly, 29*(1), 19–31.

Maitland, T. (2011). *Ready for take-off: Preparing your teen with ADHD or LD for college*. Washington, DC: Magination Press/American Psychological Association.

Malangko, M. C. (2009). Attitudes and willingness of California community college public safety (police, fire and emergency medical services) faculty to provide accommodations for students with learning disabilities. *Dissertation Abstracts International Section A: Humanities and Social Sciences, 69*(7-A), 2548.

Mandic, C., Rudd, R., Hehir, T., & Acevedo-Garcia, D. (2012). Readability of special education procedural safeguards. *The Journal of Special Education, 45*(4), 195–203.

Mazurek, M. O., Shattuck, P. T., Wagner, M., & Cooper, B. P. (2012). Prevalence and Correlates of Screen-Based Media Use among Youths with Autism Spectrum Disorders. *Journal Of Autism and Developmental Disorders, 42*(8), 1757–1767.

McKinney, J. D., & Speece, D. L. (1986). Academic consequences and longitudinal stability of behavioral subtypes of learning disabled children. *Journal of Educational Psychology, 78*(5), 365–372.

Merchant, D. J., & Gajar, A. (1997). A review of the literature on self advocacy components in transition programs for students with learning disabilities. *Journal of Vocational Rehabilitation, 8*(3), 223–231.

Miller, K. R. (2008). American sign language: Acceptance at the university level. *Language, Culture and Curriculum, 21*(3), 226–234.

Miller, C. R., Hinterlong, J., & Greene, A. (2010). Service learning and students with disabilities: Perspectives from a statewide model program in Florida. *School Social Work Journal, 34*(2), 71–89.

Moore, R. S., Moore, M., Grimes, P. W., Millea, M. J., Lehman, M., Pearson, A., et al. (2007). Developing an intervention bridging program for at-risk students before the traditional pre-freshman summer program. *College Student Journal, 40*(1), 151–159.

Morgan, K., & Norris, G. (2010). An exploration into the relevance of Dickman's functional and dysfunctional impulsivity dichotomy for understanding ADHD-type behaviors. *Individual Differences Research, 8*(1), 34–44.

Murray, C., & Naranjo, J. (2008). Poor, Black, learning disabled, and graduating: An investigation of factors and processes associated with school completion among high-risk urban youth. *Remedial & Special Education, 29*(3), 145–160.

Murray, C., Wren, C. T., & Keys, C. (2008). University faculty perceptions of students with learning disabilities: Correlates and group differences. *Learning Disability Quarterly, 31*(3), 95–113.

National Joint Committee on Learning Disabilities (NJCLD). (2007). The documentation disconnect for students with learning disabilities: Improving access to postsecondary disability services. *Learning Disability Quarterly, 30*(4), 265–274.

NCD. (2010). *Workforce infrastructure in support of people with disabilities: Matching human resources to service needs*. Washington, DC: National Council on Disability.

Nelson, J., Dodd, J., & Smith, D. (1990). Faculty willingness to accommodate students with learning disabilities: A comparison among academic divisions. *Journal of Learning Disabilities, 23*(3), 185–189.

Nietupski, J. A., & Hamre-Nietupski, S. (2000). A systematic process for carving supported employment positions for people with severe disabilities. *Journal of Developmental and Physical Disabilities, 12*(1), 103–119.

Obudo, F. (2008). Teaching mathematics to students with learning disabilities: A review of literature. Online submission. *ERIC*, EBSCO*host* (accessed December 28, 2012).

Ofiesh, N. S. (2007). Math, science, and foreign language: Evidence-based accommodation decision making at the postsecondary level. *Learning Disabilities Research and Practice, 22*(4), 237–245.

Ofiesh, N. S., Hughes, C., & Scott, S. S. (2004). Extended test time and postsecondary student with learning disabilities: A model for decision making. *Learning Disabilities Research and Practice, 19*(1), 57–70.

Oster-Aaland, L. K., Sellnow, T. L., Nelson, P. E., & Pearson, J. C. (2004). The status of service learning in departments of communication: A follow-up study. *Communication Education, 4*, 348–356.

Parker, D. R., & Boutelle, K. (2009). Executive function coaching for college students with learning disabilities and ADHD: A new approach for fostering self-determination. *Learning Disabilities Research and Practice, 24*(4), 204–215.

Patwell, M., & Herzog, A. (2000). Bridging the gap: A disability services perspective on transition. *Disability Studies Quarterly, 20*(4).

Pettit, G. S., Erath, S. A., Lansford, J. E., Dodge, K. A., & Bates, J. E. (2011). Dimensions of social capital and life adjustment in the transition to early adulthood. *International Journal of Behavioral Development, 35*(6), 482–489.

Poelma, J. (2002). Do parent educational aspirations affect the educational aspirations of adolescents with learning disabilities? *Dissertation Abstracts International, 62*.

Reed, M. J., Kennett, D. J., Lewis, T., & Lund-Lucas, E. (2011). The relative benefits found for students with and without learning disabilities taking a first-year university preparation course. *Active Learning in Higher Education, 12*(2), 133–142.

Reed, M. J., Kennett, D. J., Lewis, T., Lund-Lucas, E., Stallberg, C., & Newbold, I. L. (2009). The relative effects of university success courses and individualized interventions for students with learning disabilities. *Higher Education Research and Development, 26*(4), 385–400.

Reynolds, J. R., & Baird, C. L. (2010). Is there a downside to shooting for the stars? Unrealized educational expectations and symptoms of depression. *American Sociological Review, 75*(1), 151–172.

Roberts, L. L., & Hoff Macan, T. (2006). Disability disclosure effects on employment interview ratings of applicants with nonvisible disabilities. *Rehabilitation Psychology, 51*(3), 239–246.

Robinson, C., & Gahagan, J. (2010). Coaching students to academic success and engagement on campus. *About Campus, 15*(4), 26–29.

Rojewski, J. W. (1996). Educational and occupational aspirations of high school seniors with learning disabilities. *Exceptional Children, 62*(5), 463–476.

Rooney, G. (2012). *Providing support services for college students with learning disabilities who are not native english speakers*: *The challenge of the LD/ESOL student*. ERIC, EBSCOhost. Retrieved June 29, 2012.

Rothman, T., Maldonado, J. M., & Rothman, H. (2008). Building self-confidence and future career success through a pre-college transition program for individuals with disabilities. *Journal of Vocational Rehabilitation, 28*(2), 73–83.

Rothon, C., Goodwin, L., & Stansfeld, S. (2012). Family social support, community "social capital" and adolescents' mental health and educational outcomes: A longitudinal study in England. *Social Psychiatry and Psychiatric Epidemiology, 47*(5), 697–709.

Rourke, B. P. (2000). Neuropsychological and psychosocial subtyping: A review of investigations within the University of Windsor laboratory. *Canadian Psychology/Psychologie Canadienne, 41*(4), 34–51.

Ruiz, E. A. (2008). TRIO student support services: First-generation, low-income, and disabled students. UCLA community college bibliography. *Community College Journal of Research and Practice, 32*(8), 629–635.

Russo, C. J., & Osborne, A. (2008). *Essential concepts and school-based cases in special education law*. Thousand Oaks, CA: Corwin Press.

Rutter, M. (1987). Psychosocial resilience and protective mechanisms. *The American Journal of Orthopsychiatry, 57*(3), 316–331.

Salter, S. (2010). An exploratory study of secondary educator knowledge of disability legislation and its relationship to planning for the transition from secondary to postsecondary education settings. *Dissertation Abstracts International Section A, 70.*

Sanders, A. L. (2012). Malingering by college students on evaluations for mathematics learning disabilities. *Dissertation Abstracts International*, *72*.

Sanford, C., Newman, L., Wagner, M., Knokey, A.-M., & Shaver, D. (2011). *The post-high school outcomes of young adults with disabilities up to 6 years after high school. Key Findings from the National Longitudinal Transition Study-2 (NLTS2) (NCSER 2011-3004).* Menlo Park, CA: SRI International.

Schulman, S. S. (1984). Psychotherapeutic issues for the learning disabled adult. *Professional Psychology: Research and Practice, 15*(6), 856–867.

Scorgie, K. K., Kildal, L., & Wilgosh, L. (2010). Post-secondary students with disabilities: Issues related to empowerment and self-determination. *Developmental Disabilities Bulletin, 38*(1–2), 133–145.

Scott, J. (1995). Academic freedom as an ethical practice. *Academe, 81*(4), 44–48.

Seidman, L. J., Biederman, J., Monuteaux, M. C., Doyle, A. E., & Faraone, S. V. (2001). Learning disabilities and executive dysfunction in boys with attention-deficit/hyperactivity disorder. *Neuropsychology, 15*(4), 544–556.

Semrud-Clikeman, M., Walkowiak, J., Wilkinson, A., & Minne, E. (2010). Direct and indirect measures of social perception, behavior, and emotional functioning in children with Asperger's disorder, nonverbal learning disability, or ADHD. *Journal of Abnormal Child Psychology, 38*(4), 509–519.

Shane, J. (2008). The impact of special education mediation which reaches agreement on the ongoing relationships between the parents of a child with special needs and school personnel involved with the child. *Dissertation Abstracts International Section A, 65.*

Skinner, M. E. (2007). Faculty willingness to provide accommodations and course alternatives to postsecondary students with learning disabilities. *International Journal of Special Education, 22*(2), 32–45.

Smith, K. Y. (2012). The impact of parental involvement on student achievement. *Dissertation Abstracts International Section A, 72.*

Smith, S. G., English, R., & Vasek, D. (2002). Student and parent involvement in the transition process for college freshmen with learning disabilities. *College Student Journal, 34*(4), 491–503.

Smith, J. J., & Young, K. (2004). Issues in transition from school to postsecondary education: Focus on students with learning disabilities. In E. M. Levinson (Ed.), *Transition from school to post-school life for individuals with disabilities: Assessment from an educational and school psychological perspective* (pp. 217–249). Springfield, IL: Charles C. Thomas Publisher.

Sparks, R. L. (2009). If you don't know where you're going, you'll wind up somewhere else: The case of "foreign language learning disability". *Foreign Language Annals, 42*(1), 7–26.

Speece, D. L., McKinney, J. D., & Appelbaum, M. I. (1985). Classification and validation of behavioral subtypes of learning-disabled children. *Journal of Educational Psychology, 77*(1), 67–77.

Stadler, M. A. (1995). Role of attention in implicit learning. *Journal of Experimental Psychology: Learning, Memory, and Cognition, 21*(3), 674–685.

Stanton-Salazar, R. D. (2011). A social capital framework for the study of institutional agents and their role in the empowerment of low-status students and youth. *Youth & Society, 43*(3), 1066–1109. doi:10.1177/0044118X10382877

Stumbo, N. J., Martin, J. K., Noststrom, D., Rolfe, T., Burgstahler, S., Whiney, J., et al. (2010). Evidence-based practices in mentoring students with disabilities: Four case studies. *Journal of Science Education for Students with Disabilities, 14*(1), 33–54.

Summers, P. P. (2000). The roots of leadership. *Psychology, 37*(1), 27–36.

Swain, J. (1993). A vocational special college: Preparing students for a participatory democracy? *Disability, Handicap & Society, 8*(3), 295–309.

Taylor, J., & House, B. (2010). An exploration of identity, motivations and concerns of non-traditional students at different stages of higher education. *Psychology Teaching Review, 1*, 46–57.

Taymans, J. M., West, L. L., & Sullivan, M. (2000). *Unlocking potential: College and other choices for people with LD and AD/HD*. Bethesda, MD US: Woodbine House.

Troiano, P. F., Liefeld, J. A., & Trachtenberg, J. V. (2010). Academic support and college success for postsecondary students with learning disabilities. *Journal of College Reading and Learning, 40*(2), 35–44.

Vogel, S. A., & Adelman, P. B. (1992). The success of college students with learning disabilities: Factors related to educational attainment. *Journal of Learning Disabilities, 25*(7), 430–441.

Vogel, S., Leyser, Y., Wyland, S., & Brulle, A. (1999). Students with learning disabilities in higher education: Faculty attitude and practices. *Learning Disabilities Research and Practice, 14*(3), 173–186.

Wehmeyer, M. L., & Palmer, S. B. (2003). Adult outcomes for students with cognitive disabilities three-years after high school: The impact of self-determination. *Education and Training in Developmental Disabilities, 38*(2), 131–144.

Weinstein, C., Wolf, L. E., & Schreiber, H. (2008). The professional student with a learning disorder: Focus on medicine and law. In L. E. Wolf, H. E. Schreiber, & J. Wasserstein (Eds.), *Adult learning disorders: Contemporary issue* (pp. 159–190). New York: Psychology Press.

Wells, J. W. (2006). Exploring relative cognitive strengths among rigorously selected private school students with ADHD. *Dissertation Abstracts International, 66.*

Wildhagen, T. (2009). Why does cultural capital matter for high school academic performance? An empirical assessment of teacher-selection and self-selection mechanisms as explanations of the cultural capital effect. *The Sociological Quarterly, 1*, 173–200.

Wilson, M. G., Carvalho, M., & Alvarez, A. E. (2007). Consortia for future leadership: Student perspectives. *Journal of Applied Rehabilitation Counseling, 38*(3), 25–30.

Wood, E. Z., Gentile, P., Archer, K., De Pasquale, D., & Nosko, A. (2012). Examining the impact of off-task multi-tasking with technology on real-time classroom learning. *Computers in Education, 58*(1), 365–374.

Wurm, T. (1999). Students' understanding of learning disabilities and their acceptability ratings of special education placements. *Dissertation Abstracts International Section A, 59.*

Yu, H., Xiu-Zhu, Z., Ai-Shu, L., & Zhang, Y. (2008). Characteristics of social information processing in children with nonverbal learning disabilities. *Chinese Mental Health Journal, 22*(11), 787–790. 795.

Yuen, J. L., & Shaughnessy, B. (2001). Cultural empowerment: Tools to engage and retain postsecondary students with disabilities. *Journal of Vocational Rehabilitation, 16*(3–4), 199–207.

Zeleke, S. (2004). Differences in self-concept among children with mathematics disabilities and their average and high achieving peers. *International Journal of Disability, Development and Education, 3*, 253–269.

Zhang, Y., & Chan, T. (2007). *An interim report on the Student Support Services program: 2002–03 and 2003–04, with select data from 1998–2002*. US Department Office of Postsecondary Education (ED) Washington, DC, & American Institutes for Research (CRESS), Kensington, MD.

Chapter 13
Employment and Vocational Rehabilitation Services for Individuals with NVLD

Lynn Koch

Introduction

Although limited research addresses the impact of nonverbal learning disabilities (NVLD) on employment, the challenges that individuals with NVLD encounter in educational contexts are also likely to be encountered in work settings. Despite the fact that individuals with NVLD have the potential to work in occupations of their choosing, the negative impact of this disorder on multiple functional domains (e.g., neuropsychological, academic, adaptive, social) can lead to unemployment or underemployment. Exacerbating the problem, long-term exposure to the negative attitudes, and actions of others (e.g., stigmatization, prejudice, bullying, teasing) can result in a restriction of early social and vocational experiences, career decision-making difficulties, negative self-appraisals, and poor worker self-concepts (Kosciulek, 2004). The negative attitudes and actions that children and adolescents with NVLD encounter in the classroom are likely to be encountered to an even greater degree by adults with NVLD in the workplace (Koch, Rumrill, & Conyers, 2012). In fact, Kosciulek's observation that "social attitudes toward disability may be as important as the disability itself in that the negative attitude of others plays a part in shaping the life role of the individual with a disability" (p. 41) certainly holds true for individuals with NVLD. Consequently, approaches to eradicating employment barriers must target both the individual's functional limitations and work environment barriers such as negative attitudes and discrimination.

The purpose of this chapter is to introduce the state–federal vocational rehabilitation (VR) program as a resource for individuals with NVLD who desire assistance with overcoming all of the above barriers to meaningful employment. In the following paragraphs, we (a) describe vocational implications of NVLD, (b) provide an overview of

L. Koch, Ph.D., C.R.C. (✉)
Rehabilitation Education and Research Program, University of Arkansas,
106 Graduate Education Building, Fayetteville, AR 72701, USA
e-mail: lckoch@uark.edu

J. Broitman and J.M. Davis (eds.), *Treating NVLD in Children: Professional Collaborations for Positive Outcomes*, DOI 10.1007/978-1-4614-6179-1_13,

the federal–state vocational rehabilitation (VR) program, and (c) examine the VR process and specific VR services that could benefit individuals with NVLD in terms of maximizing their vocational potential and achieving their self-determined employment goals.

Vocational Implications of NVLD

Occupations in the twenty-first-century American labor market are characterized by team work, and as mentioned in the introduction, the functional limitations associated with NVLD can be even more problematic in employment contexts where the failure to understand and adhere to workplace norms is often less tolerated than it is in educational settings. In the following paragraphs, some of the work-related challenges that individuals with NVLD may encounter in areas of social, cognitive, and physical functioning on the job are described.

Exhibiting the necessary social skills to function effectively as members of work teams (e.g., demonstrating good listening skills, communicating empathy for others, correctly interpreting body language and innuendo) can be especially challenging for individuals with NVLD (Telzrow & Koch, 2003). Understanding the unspoken cultural norms of the workplace and gaining acceptance by coworkers into the organizational culture can also be problematic. The idiosyncrasies of individuals with NVLD can create discomfort in others. For example, workers may feel uncomfortable if the individual with NVLD violates their personal space. They may view the individual with NVLD as pompous or arrogant due to his or her pedantic conversational skills. Supervisors may lose their patience with the worker with NVLD who appears to lack understanding about unspoken social norms and exhibits poor social awareness of others' perceptions of him or her. Supervisors and coworkers may then respond by avoiding, teasing, ignoring, or otherwise harassing the employee with NVLD. These reactions are likely to create an environment where the worker with NVLD feels unwelcome or, in the extreme, feels unsafe. Research on the effects of these types of workplace incivilities on individual workers has documented the outcomes of reduced job satisfaction and job satisfactoriness, employee turnover, and negative mental and physical health problems (Cortina, Magley, Williams, & Langhout, 2001). For employees with NVLD, who may already be prone to symptoms of anxiety and depression, workplace incivility can have detrimental consequences.

Because of their neuropsychological and physical deficits, individuals with NVLD may experience difficulties with carrying out a variety of cognitive and physical tasks (Telzrow & Koch, 2003). In particular, they are likely to encounter challenges in performing job tasks that require the use of gross motor skills, fine motor skills, and eye–hand coordination. Occupations that require proficient tactile perception or visual perception skills (e.g., dental technician, seamstress, jeweler) are likely to present significant challenges to individuals with NVLD. Likewise, limitations in mathematical abilities can interfere with the successful completion of job tasks in occupations that require arithmetic operations (e.g., accountant, bookkeeper, carpenter). In contrast, individuals with NVLD may perform well in occupations that emphasize basic reading and spelling (e.g., editor, technical writer, proofreader) because their verbal skills are relatively superior as compared to their perceptual-performance abilities, and they tend to have well-developed verbal fluency and reading skills.

The State–Federal Vocational Rehabilitation Program

The state–federal vocational rehabilitation (VR) program is administered by the US Department of Education's Office of Special Education and Rehabilitative Services (OSERS) under the legal authority of Title I of the Rehabilitation Act of 1973 and its amendments. OSERS administers the state–federal VR program through the Rehabilitation Services Administration (RSA). The mission of RSA is "to provide leadership and resources to assist state and other agencies in providing vocational rehabilitation (VR), independent living (IL) and other services to individuals with disabilities to maximize their employment, independence and integration into the community and the competitive labor market" (http://rsa.ed.gov/). RSA provides grants to states to:

> Support a wide range of services designed to help individuals with disabilities
>
> prepare for and engage in gainful employment consistent with their strengths
>
> resources, priorities, concerns, abilities, capabilities, interests, and informed choice (http://www2.ed.gov/programs/rsabvrs/index.html)

RSA distributes and monitors funds to state VR agencies in the provision of employment-related services for individuals with disabilities, giving priority to individuals who are significantly disabled (http://www2.ed.gov/about/offices/list/osers/rsa/indes.html). These funds are allocated based on a formula that takes into account the population size and per capita income to cover the cost of direct VR services and program administration, and they are administered under an approved state plan by VR agencies designated by each state.

State VR agencies provide services in a manner consistent with the principles that (a) individuals with disabilities are presumed to be capable of engaging in gainful employment and VR services can improve their ability to become employed; (b) opportunities must be provided to individuals with disabilities to obtain employment in integrated settings; (c) VR applicants and eligible consumers are active and full partners in the VR process who make meaningful and informed choices about all aspects of VR service delivery including assessments, employment outcomes, VR services, VR service providers, and methods for securing services; and (d) involvement of family members in the VR process if the VR consumer requests, desires, or needs such supports (29 U.S.C. §701 *et seq.*).

VR services are provided by VR counselors and case managers. These individuals are specialized professionals who assist people with disabilities to achieve their career goals in the most integrated settings possible through the application of the counseling process (Commission on Rehabilitation Counselor Certification, 2011). The specific techniques that VR counselors use to facilitate consumer goal achievement include assessment and appraisal; diagnosis and treatment planning; career counseling; individual and group counseling, case management, referral, and service coordination; interventions to remove environmental, employment, and attitudinal barriers; consultation with employers and other parties; job analysis, job development, and placement services; job accommodations planning; and consultation about rehabilitation technology (Commission on Rehabilitation Counselor Certification, 2011).

The Vocational Rehabilitation Process

The VR process includes the phases of eligibility determination, evaluation of vocational needs, VR planning, VR plan implementation, and termination of VR services (job placement). Although many VR consumers will move through the process in stepwise sequential phases, VR service providers and policymakers are beginning to recognize that some individuals with disabilities, like those with NVLD, will require a more flexible sequencing of services (e.g., job placement followed by an evaluation of service and support needs as opposed to the reverse; Rubin & Roessler, 2008). As such, the VR process is highly individualized, dynamic, and creative (Kosciulek, 2004).

The VR process is characterized by four central factors: (a) the VR counselor–consumer working alliance, (b) informed choice, (c) self-determination, and (d) empowerment (Chan, Shaw, McMahon, Koch, & Strauser, 1997; Kosciulek, 2004; Wehmeyer, 2003). The *working alliance* refers to the equal partnership between the VR counselor and consumer who collaborate in (a) assessing the individual's vocational strengths, preferences, employment goals, barriers to goal achievement, and service needs and (b) developing and implementing an individualized plan of action that will result in employment for the consumer that is meaningful, consistent with his or her desires, and based on his or her informed choice (Kosciulek, 2004). *Informed choice* is defined as consumer choice of services, service providers, service procurement, and employment goals. The VR counselor facilitates informed choice by educating the consumer about his or her options and providing consumers with the resources and tools to learn how to make choices. *Self-determination* is the "right and capacity of people to exert control over their lives" (Wehmeyer, 2003, p. 68). It is an important construct in vocational rehabilitation because it is a right that has historically been denied to people with disabilities and because of a continuously growing body of research evidence indicating that self-determination leads to better VR outcomes. *Empowerment* is "the process by which people who have been rendered powerless or marginalized develop the skills to take control of their lives and their environment" (Kosciulek, 2004, p. 45). Empowerment is the "operative term" in service delivery, and at each phase of the VR process, the VR counselor is committed to maximizing opportunities for the consumer to exert control and authority over what occurs. In the VR planning process, empowerment also means that "people with disabilities have the same degree of control over their lives and the conditions that affect them as generally possessed by people without disabilities. It entails the transfer of power and control over their lives from external entities, such as VR counselors, to the individuals themselves" (Kosciulek, 2004, p. 45).

In the VR planning process, VR counselors often work with youths with disabilities who are as young as 14 as part of a formalized transition team to develop and implement individualized plans for the transition from secondary education to community living and postsecondary outcomes (e.g., employment, independent living, postsecondary education) (Flexor, Simmons, Luft, & Baer, 2005; Koch, 1999). The purpose of transition planning is to coordinate services and delineate transition team members' responsibilities for assisting the student with a disability to make successful transitions into adult roles. In addition to the student, parents or guardians, and VR counselor, other members of the transition team may include special education teachers, school psychologists, school counselors, vocational education teachers, adult service agency representatives (e.g., residential, vocational, child welfare), advocates, attorneys, employers, and other community representatives (29 U.S.C. §701 *et seq.*).

The VR counselor's role on the transition team is to facilitate the career development and employment preparation of the student with a disability. Transition services that may be provided by the VR counselor include career exploration and counseling, psychosocial adjustment counseling, consultation to other transition team members about the vocational implications of disability, classroom and job accommodations planning, work adjustment counseling, coordination of services and supports for career planning and preparation, job development, placement and placement follow-up, job analysis, job restructuring, and follow-along support (29 U.S.C. §701 *et seq.*).

VR Program Eligibility Determination and Vocational Needs Assessment

As mandated by the Rehabilitation Act of 1973 and its amendments, a person is eligible for VR services if he or she:

1. Has a physical or mental impairment which for such individual constitutes or results in a substantial impediment to employment
2. Can benefit in terms of an employment outcome from vocational rehabilitation services provided pursuant to title I, III, or VI (29 U.S.C. §701 *et seq.*)

In some cases, state VR agencies may be unable to serve all persons who apply for services, and when this occurs, they are required to have a state plan which specifies the order in which individuals are to be served, with the requirement that individuals with the most severe disabilities be served first.

Eligibility decisions are made on a case-by-case basis by conducting a preliminary assessment that includes an initial interview, medical evaluation, and review of existing records documenting disability (e.g., school records, pervious professional assessments, medical records). The initial interview is conducted by a VR counselor or technician who gathers information from the VR applicant about the consumer's reasons for applying for VR services, disability and health status, socioeconomic background, functional limitations, educational history, work experiences, career goals, and VR expectations (Koch & Rumrill, 2005; Rubin & Roessler, 2008). Other evaluations (e.g., psychological evaluation) may also be arranged if needed to facilitate eligibility determination. An eligibility decision must be made within 60 days after initial application for services (29 U.S.C. §701 *et seq.*).

For VR applicants with NVLD, eligibility determination and rehabilitation needs assessment involves a "comprehensive understanding of the individual's vocational strengths and functional deficits so that employment goals and remedial services can be planned accordingly" (Telzrow & Koch, 2003, p. 14). In referring students with NVLD for VR services, school psychologists can assist with expediting eligibility determination and identification of VR service needs by providing information about the student's (a) functional deficits and how these may interfere with job performance, (b) functional strengths that could facilitate job performance, (c) compensatory strategies that could be targeted in VR planning to improve the individual's employability, and (d) recommendations for specific services that may assist the individual in achieving his or her employment goal (Hartlage & Telzrow, 1984; Telzrow & Koch, 2003). If any gaps in this information are present, the VR counselor may arrange for a neuropsychological evaluation to "formulate diagnostic hypotheses and to recommend rehabilitation interventions or further assessment based on these tentative diagnoses" (Telzrow & Koch, 2003, p. 14).

Comprehensive Assessment and Development of Individualized Plan for Employment

In addition to gathering assessment information for eligibility determination purposes, the VR counselor also conducts a comprehensive assessment to identify VR needs. During this phase of the VR process, the VR counselor and consumer work together to (a) choose an employment goal and (b) determine services that the consumer will need to achieve his or her goal. Additional diagnostic information (e.g., learning assessments, vocational evaluations, medical evaluations, psychological evaluations) may be gathered at this point to assist with planning and developing an Individualized Plan for Employment (IPE). The IPE is "the central document of the VR process and is based on the findings of the assessment and is consistent with the informed choice of the consumer" (Brabham, Mandeville, & Koch, 1998, p. 42). The IPE includes several mandatory components (29 U.S.C. §701 *et seq.*). First, a specific employment outcome chosen by the VR consumer is identified that is consistent with her or his unique strengths, resources, abilities, and interests. Descriptions of the specific VR services that are needed by the individual to achieve the employment outcome are then described in the IPE. Time lines are delineated for the achievement of the employment outcome and for the initiation of each service identified on the IPE. The IPE also includes a description of the entity (e.g., service provider) chosen by the VR consumer or, as appropriate, his or her representative (e.g., legal guardian) who will provide each VR service and the methods to be used to procure services as well as the VR consumer's responsibilities in participating in the services designated on the IPE. The IPE must stipulate that all goods and services are provided in the most integrated settings possible and must indicate the extent to which other comparable goods and services are provided.

Job Development, Placement, and Follow-Up

Once the VR consumer has completed the services outlined on the IPE, job seeking efforts are initiated. The amount and type of job seeking assistance that is provided or procured by the VR counselor is dependent on each individual consumer's needs. Some individuals will be able to conduct their own independent job searches with little assistance from the VR counselor whereas others will require more intensive and direct assistance from their VR counselor and/or other designated placement professionals. Examples of the types of assistance that can be provided include job seeking skills training (JSST), direct placement assistance, and supported employment. In the next section, we describe characteristics of JSST and supported employment because these are two services that could be particularly beneficial to consumers with NVLD given the barriers to employment they often encounter.

When VR consumers have been employed for a minimum of 90 days in competitive employment in an integrated work setting doing work that is compatible with their abilities, interests, and choices, the case is closed as successfully rehabilitated (Brabham et al., 1998). However, VR consumers can still be eligible for post-employment services if these are needed to maintain, regain, or advance in their employment. Furthermore, extended services (ongoing support services) may be provided to individuals with the most significant disabilities in a supported employment context (to be described in greater detail in a later section of this chapter).

Vocational Rehabilitation Services for Individuals with NVLD

Vocational rehabilitation (VR) services are any services described in the IPE to assist the individual to achieve her or his employment outcome. The VR counselor and consumer collaboratively determine what the individual's specific service needs are as they develop the IPE. Table 13.1 includes a comprehensive list of vocational rehabilitation services provided under Title I of the Rehabilitation Act.

Although the IPE is individualized to the unique strengths, needs, and preferences of each consumer, VR services that may be especially beneficial to individuals

Table 13.1 Vocational rehabilitation services as mandated by the Rehabilitation Act of 1973

1. An assessment for determining eligibility and vocational rehabilitation needs by qualified personnel, including, if appropriate, an assessment by personnel skilled in rehabilitation technology
2. Counseling and guidance, including information and support services to assist an individual in exercising informed choice consistent with the provisions of Section 102(d)
3. Referral and other services to secure needed services from other agencies through agreements developed under Section 101(a)(11), if such services are not available under this title
4. Job-related services, including job search and placement assistance, job retention services, follow-up services, and follow-along services
5. Vocational and other training services, including the provision of personal and vocational adjustment services, books, tools, and other training materials, except that no training services provided at an institution of higher education shall be paid for with funds under this title unless maximum efforts have been made by the designated state unit and the individual to secure grant assistance, in whole or in part, from other sources to pay for such training
6. To the extent that financial support is not readily available from a source (such as through health insurance of the individual or through comparable services and benefits consistent with Section 101(a) (8)(A)), other than the designated state unit, diagnosis and treatment of physical and mental impairments, including:
   (a) Corrective surgery or therapeutic treatment necessary to correct or substantially modify a physical or mental condition that constitutes a substantial impediment to employment, but is of such a nature that such correction or modification may reasonably be expected to eliminate or reduce such impediment to employment within a reasonable length of time
   (b) Necessary hospitalization in connection with surgery or treatment
   (c) Prosthetic and orthotic devices
   (d) Eyeglasses and visual services as prescribed by qualified personnel who meet state licensure laws and who are selected by the individual
   (e) Special services (including transplantation and dialysis), artificial kidneys, and supplies necessary for the treatment of individuals with end-stage renal disease
   (f) Diagnosis and treatment for mental and emotional disorders by qualified personnel who meet state licensure laws
7. Maintenance for additional costs incurred while participating in an assessment for determining eligibility and vocational rehabilitation needs or while receiving services under an individualized plan for employment
8. Transportation, including adequate training in the use of public transportation vehicles and systems, that is provided in connection with the provision of any other service described in this section and needed by the individual to achieve an employment outcome
9. On-the-job or other related personal assistance services provided while an individual is receiving other services described in this section
10. Interpreter services provided by qualified personnel for individuals who are deaf or hard of hearing, and reader services for individuals who are determined to be blind, after an examination by qualified personnel who meet state licensure laws
11. Rehabilitation teaching services, and orientation and mobility services, for individuals who are blind
12. Occupational licenses, tools, equipment, and initial stocks and supplies

(continued)

Table 13.1 (continued)

13. Technical assistance and other consultation services to conduct market analyses, develop business plans, and otherwise provide resources, to the extent such resources are authorized to be provided through the statewide workforce investment system, to eligible individuals who are pursuing self-employment or telecommuting or establishing a small business operation as an employment outcome
14. Rehabilitation technology, including telecommunications, sensory, and other technological aids and devices
15. Transition services for students with disabilities that facilitate the achievement of the employment outcome identified in the individualized plan for employment
16. Supported employment services
17. Services to the family of an individual with a disability necessary to assist the individual to achieve an employment outcome
18. Specific post-employment services necessary to assist an individual with a disability to retain, regain, or advance in employment (29 U.S.C. §701 *et seq.*)

with NVLD include vocational evaluation, work adjustment training, and supported employment. These are described in greater detail in the following paragraphs.

Vocational Evaluation

Vocational evaluations are administered by vocational evaluators to "assess the individual's abilities, aptitudes, interests, and behaviors in order to determine career development and community integration goals and the services needed to achieve them" (Rubin & Roessler, 2008, p. 101). Vocational evaluations are particularly useful for planning purposes when the individual has limited work experiences. Thus, they are likely to be an important career development resource for youths with NVLD in identifying appropriate employment alternatives and services and supports needed to achieve employment objectives. Information that is gathered in a vocational evaluation includes vocational interests, aptitudes, current work skills and behaviors, and the person's ability to develop additional work skills and behaviors. Information from a variety of assessment approaches is compiled into a vocational evaluation report that synthesizes and summarizes the observations and results and provides recommendations regarding feasible employment goals, potential job accommodations, and rehabilitation services to facilitate achievement of employment goals. In addition to the assessment interview and paper-and-pencil vocational interest inventories, vocational evaluations also include work samples. Work samples are evaluation approaches used to assess the individual's performance of actual or simulated job tasks (Rubin & Roessler, 2008). Work samples are standardized "mock-ups" of common job tasks organized into a system that measures performance of a wide range of job tasks. They provide information on an individual's current level of functioning on a specific job task or clusters of job tasks and are useful in identifying potential job accommodations to facilitate execution of job tasks.

Standardized work sample systems that are commonly used in vocational evaluations with VR consumers include the VALPAR Component Work Samples Series (VCWS), Micro-TOWER Evaluation System, and the McCarron-Dial Evaluation System (MDS). The VCWS contains 19 standardized work samples that each resemble a work-like task (e.g., electrical circuitry and print reading, eye–hand–foot coordination, money handling, drafting) and is administered using standardized instructions and scoring. Scores are compared to industrial performance standards to determine the evaluee's potential to successfully meet entry-level requirements in occupations that make demands similar to those of the work sample. Based on the evaluee's occupational interests, specific work samples can be selected for administration that best represent the skills required in these occupations. The Micro-TOWER system of vocational evaluation contains 13 work samples to measure aptitudes required in a variety of skilled and semiskilled occupations. The work samples are organized into in five areas (motor, clerical perception, verbal, spatial, numerical), and the entire battery can be administered in a 2–5-day period to groups of 5–12 evaluees. The MDS is used for both clinical and vocational assessment purposes to evaluate individuals with neuropsychological disabilities (Chan, Lynch, Dial, Wong, & Kates, 1993). The MDS is individually administered to identify strengths and weaknesses in verbal–spatial–cognitive, sensory–motor, and emotional-coping domains. It is a well-researched evaluation system that consists of a battery of standardized tests and behavioral measures. It provides normative data for each of the functional domains and can be used to assist individuals with transition planning and job placement.

Situational assessments rely on direct observations to evaluate the individual's performance of real or simulated work tasks in a specific work or community setting over an extended period of time (Flexor et al., 2005; Rubin & Roessler, 2008). Situational assessments are typically conducted by vocational evaluators or work adjustment specialists who are specially trained to use systematic behavioral observation skills and techniques to gather and report assessment information that can then be used to assist the evaluee with career planning. Evaluators observe and assess the evaluee's general work behaviors and performance on specific job tasks; ability to perform the specific cognitive, physical, and emotional demands of employment; and interactions with coworkers, supervisors, and customers. School environments are excellent sites for situational assessments because opportunities for performing real work tasks (e.g., clerical, janitorial, food service) abound. Evaluators and work adjustment specialists conducting situational assessments focus their observations on such behaviors as getting along with coworkers, accepting criticism, following directions, punctuality, and attendance (Flexor et al., 2005). Based on their observations, they can then identify potentially problematic behaviors, reasonable accommodations, and rehabilitation interventions to remediate those behaviors in order to enhance the individual's employability. One of those strategies, work adjustment training, is explained below.

Work Adjustment Training

Work adjustment services are implemented to evaluate and teach the behaviors necessary to perform work roles (Rubin & Roessler, 2008; Telzrow & Koch, 2003). These behaviors include interpreting and responding appropriately to social cues, managing one's behavior in work settings, responding appropriately to supervision, dealing effectively with problems on the job, self-assessing one's job performance, and understanding and adhering to work rules and norms. Work adjustment services include an evaluation of work adjustment training needs, identification of target behaviors, development and implementation of a work adjustment plan, and continual measurement of target behaviors. Target behaviors can be categorized in the domains of job responsibility, task performance, and social–vocational competence. For individuals with NVLD, target behaviors in these domains are likely to include problem-solving to address deficits in cognitive functioning, social skills training to improve interpersonal functioning, and cognitive–behavioral interventions to manage emotional disorders.

So that individuals can readily transfer what they learn to actual employment settings, work adjustment training involves the performance of authentic work activities in settings that are comparable to work settings. School environments offer ample opportunities for youths with NVLD to develop work adjustment skills that will be crucial to their future success as employees. Students can participate in authentic work activities (e.g., clerical, janitorial, food service) that are similar to those found in actual employment settings. These experiences will also enable them to develop general employment skills (e.g., punctuality, following directions, responding appropriately to feedback, social skills) that are transferrable to any occupation. Because school environments are familiar to students and ample support is available to help them develop the necessary skills and attributes for future success as employees, these environments are often less threatening than community-based situational assessments for the student with NVLD who has limited or negative work experiences (Telzrow & Koch, 2003).

Job Seeking Skills Training

Even when equipped with the necessary training, knowledge, and skills to qualify for employment, the functional limitations associated with NVLD in the areas of social interactions and pragmatic language skills may present barriers to acquiring positions compatible with the strengths, abilities, and preferences of individuals who have this disorder. Because job seeking activities such as contacting employers to inquire about potential job openings and responding to interview questions with brief and relevant information could be challenging for individuals with NVLD, job seeking skills training (JSST) in a nonthreatening environment is a VR service that could be especially beneficial to removing these barriers to employment. JSST focuses on (a) the strengths and assets that the individual has to offer employers and

(b) breaking down the varied tasks of finding a job into manageable steps. Whether provided on a one-on-one basis or in a group format, the key components of JSST include:

(a) Identification of multiple sources of job leads
(b) Information on employment rights and responsibilities
(c) Instruction on what employers look for in prospective employees
(d) Instruction on organizing and managing the job search
(e) Practice in completing job application blanks
(f) Job interview training
(g) Supervised practice in job seeking skills
(h) Support during the job seeking process
(i) Orientation to the accommodations request process and examples of reasonable accommodations
(j) Reentry into the job seeking group should the person be laid off or terminated (Rubin & Roessler, 2008, p. 426)

Scripts, role play scenarios, and immediate constructive feedback from both the JSST facilitator and other job seekers are provided to assist the individual with NVLD to develop the competencies and self-confidence to conduct a successful job search. In addition to providing skills training, the VR counselor or JSST trainer is familiar with employers in the local market and can act as an intermediary, serving both consumers and employers (Rubin & Roessler, 2008).

Accommodations Planning

Because individuals with NVLD are likely to need job accommodations to maintain employment, another key service that VR counselors can provide them is assistance with accommodations planning (Koch, 2000). The three steps that are carried out in the accommodations planning process include (a) obtaining accurate information about one's employment rights as mandated in Title I of the Americans with Disabilities Act (ADA) of 1990 and the ADA Amendments Act (ADAAA) of 2008, (b) identifying barriers to employment and accommodation strategies, (c) requesting accommodations from the employer, and (d) collaborating with the employer to implement accommodations to eliminate or reduce barriers to employment (Roessler & Rumrill, 1995).

In completing the first step, the VR counselor assesses the consumer's awareness of his or her rights and, based on this assessment, provides needed information and resources about the ADAAA. In completing the second step, the VR counselor may arrange for a job analysis to gather detailed information about a specific position with a local employer to identify essential functions of the position that may need to be modified in order for the employee with NVLD to succeed in the position. "Information is gathered about both the work performed (e.g., specific job tasks, work materials, products developed or services provide) and required worker characteristics (e.g., general educational development, specific vocational preparation, aptitudes, temperaments, interest areas, physical demands, environmental conditions)" (Koch, 2000, p. 6). The job is evaluated in terms of the specific tasks required of the worker, and the VR counselor and consumer can then identify accommodations that may be needed to successfully carry out each task. The VR counselor then assists the consumer with developing appropriate communication skills to request accommodations from employers through activities such as role plays, workshops, and videotaping (step 3). In the final step, the VR counselor consults, as needed, with the employer to facilitate successful implementation of the accommodations and evaluate the effectiveness of implemented accommodations.

A common misconception of employers is that accommodations are prohibitively costly, and a key role the VR counselor plays in educating both the consumer and the employer is to correct this misconception—the reality is that most accommodations cost little or nothing to implement. For example, a reasonable accommodation for a worker with NVLD who has difficulty interacting with coworkers might be the provision of a mentor to help the employee learn the social norms of the organization. As another example, a reasonable accommodation for an employee with NVLD who has difficulty working effectively with supervisors might be something as simple as providing clear expectations and consequences for failure to meet those expectations. Finally, for the individual with NVLD who has difficulty with mathematical computations, provision of a calculator could constitute a reasonable accommodation (https://askjan.org/media/lear.htm).

Supported Employment and Postsecondary Education Supports

Supported employment is a job placement, training, and retention intervention that prepares people with disabilities for competitive employment in integrated, community-based work settings (Koch, 1999; Rubin & Roessler, 2008; Telzrow & Koch, 2003). Supported employment services are designed to (a) determine the individual's abilities and support needs in the workplace, (b) locate and obtain employment compatible with his or her interests and abilities, (c) identify and provide workplace supports to enhance job performance, and (d) proactively problem-solve issues that could present barriers to job retention.

Supported employment services are typically provided by a job coach or employment specialist, who may provide these services either on or off the job site. The job coach supervises and evaluates the employee's job performance, assists the employee and employer with designing and implementing reasonable accommodations for the employee, and helps the employee to develop independence and natural supports (e.g., coworkers) on the job (Koch, 1999; Rubin & Roessler, 2008; Telzrow & Koch, 2003). The job coach can be an especially helpful resource to the employee with NVLD by identifying and remediating problems that can surface on the job such as interacting inappropriately with coworkers, misinterpreting and responding inappropriately to social cues, responding inappropriately to supervision, inability to conduct adequate self-assessments of one's job performance, and unintentionally violating unspoken work rules and norms.

As the supported employee adapts to the demands of the workplace and begins to develop natural supports on the job, the job coach gradually reduces the amount of support that he or she provides on the job site. However, the job coach can resume service provision when novel situations (e.g., personnel changes, alterations in job requirements, promotions or transfers, introduction of new technology) arise that present new challenges to the employee (Telzrow & Koch, 2003). This aspect of job coaching is especially beneficial to employees with NVLD who may have difficulties with adapting to change.

For individuals with NVLD who plan to pursue postsecondary education, colleges and universities have resource centers or offices that assist students with disabilities to obtain accommodations (e.g., note taking services, extended time for taking tests, alternative testing environments) needed to successfully complete their courses and achieve their academic goals. However, due to the large number of functional domains affected by NVLD, these students may require more intensive supports (e.g., stress management, adjustment counseling, peer support, problem-solving training, psychological services, career counseling, social skills training (Telzrow & Koch, 2003)) than are typically provided by such programs, and the VR counselor can assist the student with obtaining these supports as part of their IPE.

Conclusions

The purpose of this chapter was to introduce readers to the state–federal VR program as a resource to be considered for students with NVLD who are transitioning into adult roles such as employee. Each state in the US has a designated VR program with satellite offices to provide VR services to consumers with disabilities. These services can be provided to qualified individuals as early as the age of 14, and VR counselors are instrumental members of the transition team who, through the process of consumer-directed individualized planning, help to facilitate successful employment outcomes for youths with NVLD.

References

Brabham, R., Mandeville, K. A., & Koch, L. (1998). The state-federal vocational rehabilitation program. In R. M. Parker & E. M. Szymanski (Eds.), *Rehabilitation counseling: Basics and beyond* (3rd ed., pp. 41–70). Austin, TX: Pro Ed.

Chan, F., Lynch, R. T., Dial, J. G., Wong, D. W., & Kates, D. (1993). Applications of the McCarron-Dial system in vocational evaluation: An overview of its operational framework and empirical findings. *Vocational Evaluation and Work Adjustment Bulletin, 24*(2), 57–65.

Chan, F., Shaw, L. R., McMahon, B. T., Koch, L., & Strauser, D. (1997). A model for enhancing rehabilitation counselor-consumer working relationships. *Rehabilitation Counseling Bulletin, 41*, 122–137.

Commission on Rehabilitation Counselor Certification. (2011). *CRC/CRCC scope of practice*. Downloaded on November 18, 2011, from http://www.crccertification.com/pages/crc_ccrc_scope_of_practice/56.php

Cortina, L. M., Magley, V. J., Williams, J. H., & Langhout, R. D. (2001). Incivility in the workplace: Incidence and impact. *Journal of Occupational Health Psychology, 6*, 64–80.

Flexor, R. W., Simmons, T. J., Luft, P., & Baer, R. M. (2005). *Transition planning for secondary students with disabilities* (2nd ed.). Upper Saddle River, NJ: Merrill Prentice Hall.

Hartlage, L. C., & Telzrow, C. F. (1984). Rehabilitation of persons with learning disabilities. *Journal of Rehabilitation, 50*, 31–34.

Koch, L. C. (1999). Career development interventions for transition-age youths with disabilities. *Work, 13*, 3–11.

Koch, L. C. (2000). Assessment and Planning in the Americans with Disabilities Act era: Strategies for consumer self-advocacy and employer collaboration. *Journal of Vocational Rehabilitation, 14*, 103–108.

Koch, L. C., & Rumrill, P. D. (2005). Interpersonal communication skills for case managers. In F. Chang, M. J. Leahy, & J. L. Saunders (Eds.), *Case management for rehabilitation health professionals: Volume 1* (2nd ed.). Osage Beach, MO: Aspen Professional Services.

Koch, L. C., Rumrill, P. D., & Conyers, L. M. (2012). The nature and needs of people with emerging disabilities. In M. Bishop, P. Rumrill, & P. Toriello (Eds.), *New directions in rehabilitation counseling: Creative responses to professional, clinical, and educational challenges* (pp. 115–139). Springfield, IL: Charles C. Thomas.

Kosciulek, J. (2004). Empowering people with disabilities through vocational rehabilitation counseling. *American Rehabilitation, 28*, 40–47.

Rehabilitation Act of 1973, 29 U.S.C. §701 *et seq*.

Roessler, R. T., & Rumrill, P. D. (1995). Promoting reasonable accommodations: An essential postemployment service. *Journal of Applied Rehabilitation Counseling, 26*, 3–7.

Rubin, S. E., & Roessler, R. T. (2008). *Foundations of the vocational rehabilitation process* (6th ed.). Austin, TX: Pro-Ed.

Telzrow, C., & Koch, L. (2003). Nonverbal learning disability: Vocational implications and rehabilitation treatment approaches. *Journal of Applied Rehabilitation Counseling, 34*(2), 9–16.

Wehmeyer, M. L. (2003). Self-determination, vocational rehabilitation, and workplace supports. *Journal of Vocational Rehabilitation, 19*, 67–69.

Chapter 14
Clinical Practice and the Law for NVLD

Margaret Semrud-Clikeman and Jennifer Wheeler Maedgen

Neuropsychologists, school psychologists, school counselors, and educational therapists are particularly well suited to perform disability and education-related evaluations. One of the key roles of these clinicians is to provide recommendations to the K-12 and college educational system for their clients. Generally these recommendations serve as the foundation for academic accommodations within special education and general education that are appropriate for the child. Qualifying a child with a nonverbal learning disability (NVLD) for these services can often be difficult as NVLD is not an accepted category within the Individuals with Disabilities Education Act (IDEA) unless the child has concomitant learning or attentional problems. Approximately 20 years ago, it was debated whether a social learning disability would constitute a type of learning disability that should receive services. Although it was suggested that a social learning disability category be added to the revision of IDEA in 2004, no action was taken. For adults with NVLD it is unlikely that they will qualify for assistance under the Americans with Disabilities Act (ADA) unless there is a concomitant *Diagnostic and Statistical Manual* (DSM) recognized disorder (Foote, 2000).

For these reasons, it is important for the astute clinician to be aware of the laws affecting disability in education in order to obtain the best and most appropriate services for their clients. The process of gaining this knowledge can be difficult. The legislation mandating services is often conflicting and changes dramatically depending on relevant court decisions as well as differences in obtaining services in the secondary and postsecondary settings (Gordon, Lewandowski, Murphy, & Dempsey, 2002; Ranseen & Parks, 2005). The definitions that are used in the law for disability

M. Semrud-Clikeman, Ph.D. (✉)
Department of Pediatrics, University of Minnesota Medical School, MMC 486 Mayo, 8486A, 420 Delaware St. SE, Minneapolis, MN 55455, USA
e-mail: semru002@umn.edu

J.W. Maedgen
University of Texas, Austin, TX, USA

J. Broitman and J.M. Davis (eds.), *Treating NVLD in Children: Professional Collaborations for Positive Outcomes*, DOI 10.1007/978-1-4614-6179-1_14,

determination often do not match well with clinical diagnostic procedures or methods. In the case of clients with a sole diagnosis of NVLD, it is unlikely, given the state of relevant legislation and case law, that client will receive accommodations unless there is an accompanying learning disability in mathematics or an attentional problem. Because most nonschool-based clinicians are not exposed to information about the main laws governing special education services, these clinicians may find themselves confused when their recommendations are not incorporated within the secondary school environment and/or the client is not considered eligible for academic accommodations in college. The purpose of this chapter is to briefly summarize the major laws that affect accommodation provision in K-12 and college settings. To this end, these laws and the accompanying legislation will be briefly reviewed. The chapter will also discuss issues related to the transition from high school to college, with a particular focus on NVLD, and provide basic consultation suggestions for working with schools.

Relevant Laws

Four major pieces of legislation exist which directly affect the provision of services to people with physical, cognitive, and mental health disabilities. The first group of legislative action includes Section 504 of the Rehabilitation Act of 1973, the Americans with Disabilities Act of 1990 (ADA) and, most recently, the ADA Amendments Act of 2008 (ADAAA). These laws mandate the provision of reasonable accommodations to individuals with disabilities in higher education and the workforce. While these laws also apply to the secondary school environment, they are often overshadowed by IDEA, which ties state funding to the provision of services related to a free and appropriate education for children with disabilities in the least restrictive environment. This law was reauthorized in 2004 (P.L. 108-446) (IDEA, 2004) and included additional legislation for the diagnosis of learning disabilities requiring empirically validated treatments (Holdnack & Weiss, 2006).

Individuals with Disabilities Education Act

The IDEA (IDEA, 1990, 1997, 2000) was originally passed by Congress as the Education for All Handicapped Children Act in 1975 (EACHA) (EACHA, 1975). Two important cases provided precedent for the passage of the EACHA and eventually the IDEA: *Pennsylvania Association for Retarded Children (PARC) v. Commonwealth of Pennsylvania* (1971) and *Mills v. Board of Education of District of Columbia* (1972). These cases set the stage for teaching children with mental retardation and those with significant behavioral, emotional, and learning disabilities. They also led to the development of the child-find requirement, a mandate requiring states to locate and identify school-age children who may have educational

Table 14.1 Federal classifications of disabilities in IDEA 2004

1. Deafness/hearing impairment
2. Blindness/visual impairment
3. Deafness/blindness
4. Mental retardation
5. Specific learning disability
6. Speech/language impairment
7. Autism
8. Traumatic brain injury
9. Other health impairment
10. Emotional disturbance
11. Orthopedic impairment

needs. The cases also required the schools to develop a written program for the individual child's learning and set limits on suspensions and expulsions.

Ultimately, these cases led to the passage of the Education for All Handicapped Children Act (EACHA), which established that children with disabilities were entitled to special education and associated services designed to meet individual student needs (Altshuler & Kopels, 2003). The EACHA became IDEA in 1990. The reauthorization of IDEA in 1997 included new requirements and adopted and renewed several categories of classifications of disabilities (see Table 14.1). In this revision, children with attention deficit hyperactivity disorder (ADHD) were included under the category of "other health impairment" only if their difficulties adversely affected their academic performance (Altshuler & Kopels, 2003). Because there are frequent changes to the law and the interpretation of the law, clinicians need to keep updated as to the evolution of IDEA, 2004 and should access Web sites published by the Office of Special Education and Rehabilitative Services (OSERS) or interested parties such as the National Association of School Psychologists at www.nasponline.org/advocacy/RTI%20Final%20Aust@202005.pdf.

Revisions of IDEA (IDEA, 2004) also mandated that empirically validated assessment and intervention methods were required to determine whether children qualified for learning disabilities placement while retaining the basic premise of the original EACHA and IDEA 1990. One of the major changes for children with learning disabilities relates to how eligibility is determined. Documentation of interventions implemented within the regular classroom is now necessary prior to placement in a program (Skalski & Klotz, 2005). If the child does not make progress, then further evaluation is recommended (Semrud-Clikeman, 2005).

While this procedure, also known as response to intervention (RTI), is meant to provide interventions to a child prior to identification as having a learning disability, it has been mostly applied to children with reading disabilities and not those with a mathematics learning disabilities or NVLD. For children with NVLD and mathematical learning disabilities it may be helpful to adopt a model developed by Fuchs, Mock, Morgan, and Young (2003), which meets the requirements under IDEA. In this model RTI has two levels; the first is to provide the classroom teacher with instructional suggestions and the second is to utilize small group instruction after the child has had a comprehensive evaluation to determine the child's individual needs. Some initial work has proven helpful for remediating the mathematics and visual-spatial difficulties frequently seen in children with NVLD, but more research is needed to demonstrate that RTI is helpful for other academic issues experienced by children with this diagnosis (Fuchs et al., 2004). There is no data on RTI and possible executive function or social problems seen in children with NVLD (Semrud-Clikeman, Walkowiak, Wilkinson, & Christopher, 2010; Semrud-Clikeman, Walkowiak, Wilkinson, & Minne, 2010).

Aspects of IDEA

Six important aspects to IDEA have evolved over the course of the legislation through practice and case law. These six aspects form the basis of IDEA and are crucial to any understanding of how to deliver services. They include zero reject, nondiscriminatory evaluation, a free and appropriate education, least restrictive environment, due process, and parent/child education.

Zero Reject. Zero reject requires that every child, regardless of severity of disability, must be educated. Children with cultural and linguistic differences are also protected under this aspect of IDEA from over identification for special education. Under this mandate, a child who is a non-English speaker must be tested in his/her native language. Moreover, the evaluation needs to be multifaceted and be the result of several measures, both formal and informal, that can pinpoint the child's strengths and weaknesses.

Free and Appropriate Education. A key part of IDEA is that children with disabilities are provided a free and appropriate education (FAPE). Under this aspect, additional services such as occupational therapy, physical therapy, speech and language services, counseling, adaptive physical education, and assistive technology are considered mandatory if needed for the child to profit from the services provided.

Least Restrictive Environment and Individual Educational Plan. One issue under FAPE is how to determine what services and setting are appropriate. Two key components have been developed to make such a determination—the least restrictive environment (LRE) and the Individual Education Plan (IEP). The goal of LRE is for the child to remain in his/her regular classroom setting for as much of the day as possible, as opposed to the most restrictive setting, which could be a residential treatment facility. Determining the setting is dependent on the child's needs, but in most cases residential treatment is reserved only for the most severely affected children and for a prescribed amount of time.

The second key element, the IEP, documents the school district's responsibilities toward an individual child and outlines the services necessary for the child to benefit from education. Generally, the IEP is constructed by a team of individuals who are familiar with the child. It may include the special education teacher, regular education teacher(s), a school administrator or district representative, the parent(s), any consultant or advocate the parents want to attend, and the student (if appropriate). The IEP delineates goals and objectives as well as who is responsible for each goal and an estimated timeline for completing the goal. Case law has established that the intent behind IDEA is to provide a reasonable opportunity to learn and does not need to be the "best" possible program (Hendrik Hudson District Board of Education v. Rowley, 1982). Thus, if the IEP is found to contain the necessary requirements as defined by IDEA, then it is generally regarded as an appropriate education.

Due Process. Due process is a procedure that involves a hearing to be conducted when disputes about identification, assessment, placement, or provision of FAPE cannot be resolved (Jacob & Hartshorne, 2003). In some states, a mediation hearing can be held to assist in reaching an agreement between the parent and the school. While the decision from the hearing is final, either party can appeal the decision to the state educational agency (SEA). If the SEA agrees to hear the case, then an impartial review is conducted with a decision published. Finally, the parent can pursue civil action if the disagreement is not resolved.

Parent and Student Involvement. The final aspect mandates parent and student involvement in the development of programs. Funding is provided to assist with parent education, and programs are available for infants, toddlers, and preschool children with special needs and their families. Young adults up to 21 years of age (as long as they have not graduated from high school) can also be provided compensatory education including vocational and transitional services.

Section 504 and the ADA/ADAAA

Section 504 is part of the Rehabilitation Act of 1973 and protects the rights of individuals with disabilities in facilities that receive federal financial assistance. It differs from IDEA as it does not provide additional funding for these provisions and the assistance is contained within the general education classroom. The children who qualify under Section 504 do not receive services under IDEA generally because the disability does not fall under one of the recognized categories covered by the law. However, under Section 504 a disability is defined as a person who is experiencing significant problems in the activities of daily living and is *substantially limited* by their disorder.

A 504 plan has several elements including a description of the concern, the basis for determining whether a disabling condition exists, a description of how major life activities are affected, any necessary medications, the recommended modifications, a list of participants, and a review/reassessment date. Section 504 also allows for determination of building and program accessibility. Thus, if a child uses a wheelchair, then the bathrooms and physical education rooms must be accessible to him or her. Table 14.2 details the differences between IDEA and Section 504 in the primary and secondary education setting.

Table 14.2 A comparison of ADA, IDEA, and Section 504

ADA	IDEA	504
Type and purpose		
A civil rights law to prohibit discrimination solely on the basis of disability in employment, public services, and accommodations	An education act to provide federal financial assistance to State and local education agencies to guarantee special education and related services to eligible children with disabilities	A civil rights law to prohibit discrimination on the basis of disability in programs and activities, public and private, that receive federal financial assistance
Who is protected?		
Any individual with a disability who (1) has a physical or mental impairment that substantially limits one or more life activities or (2) has a record of such impairment or (3) is regarded as having such an impairment. Further, the person must be qualified for the program, service, or job	Children ages 3–21 who are determined by a multidisciplinary team to be eligible within one or more of 13 specific disability categories and who need special education and related services. Categories include autism, deafness, deaf-blindness, hearing impairments, mental retardation, multiple disabilities, orthopedic impairments, other health impairments, serious emotional disturbance, specific learning disabilities, speech or language impairments, traumatic brain injury, and visual impairments	Any person who (1) has a physical or mental impairment that substantially limits one or more major life activities, (2) has a record of such an impairment, or (3) is regarded as having such an impairment. Major life activities include walking, seeing, hearing, speaking, breathing, learning, working, caring for oneself, and performing manual tasks
Provides for a free, appropriate public education (FAPE)		
Not directly. However, (1) ADA protections apply to nonsectarian private schools, but not to organization or private schools, or entities controlled by religious organization; (2) ADA provided additional protection in combination with actions brought under Section 504. Reasonable accommodations are required for eligible students with a disability to perform essential functions of the job. This applies to any part of the special education program that may be community based and involve job training/placement	Yes. A FAPE is defined to mean special education and related services. Special education means "specially designed instruction at no cost to the parents, to meet the unique needs of the child with a disability ...." Related services are provided if students require them in order to benefit from specially designed instruction. States are required to ensure the provision of "full educational opportunity" to all children with disabilities. IDEA requires the development of an individualized education program (IEP) document with specific content and a required number of participants at an IEP meeting	Yes. An "appropriate" education means an education comparable to that provided to students without disabilities. This may be defined as regular or special education services. Students can receive related services under Section 504 even if they are not provided any special education. Section 504 does require development of a plan, although this written document is not mandated. The individualized education program (IEP) of IDEA may be used for the Section 504 written plan. Many experts recommend that a group of persons knowledgeable about the students convene and specify the agreed-upon services

Funding to implement services		
No, but limited tax credits may be available for removing architectural or transportation barriers. Also, many federal agencies provide grant funds to support training and to provide technical assistance to public and private institutions	Yes. IDEA provides federal funds under parts B and C to assist states and local education agencies in meeting IDEA requirements to serve infants, toddlers, and youth with disabilities	No. State and local jurisdictions have responsibility. IDEA funds may not be used to serve children found eligible under Section 504
Procedural safeguards		
The ADA does not specify procedural safeguards related to special education; it does detail the administrative requirements complaint procedures, and consequences for noncompliance related to both services and employment	IDEA requires written notice to parents regarding identification, evaluation, and/or placement. Further, written notice must be made prior to any change in placement. The Act delineates the required components of the written notices	Section 504 requires notice to parents regarding identification, evaluation, and/or placements. Written notice is recommended. Notice must be made only before a "significant change" in placement. Following IDEA procedural safeguards is one way to comply with Section 504 mandates
Evaluation and placement procedures		
The ADA does not specify evaluation and placement procedures: it does specify provision of reasonable accommodations for eligible activities and settings. Reasonable accommodations may include, but are not limited to, redesigning equipment, assigning aides, providing written communication in alternative formats, modifying tests, redesigning services to accessibility locations, altering existing facilities, and building new facilities	A comprehensive evaluation is required. A multidisciplinary team evaluates the child, and parental consent is required before evaluation. IDEA requires that reevaluations be conducted at least every 3 years. For evaluation and placement decisions, IDEA requires that more than one single procedure or information source be used; that information from all sources be documented and carefully considered; that the eligibility decision be made by a group of persons who know about the student, the evaluation data, and placement options; and that the placement decision serves the student in the least restrictive environment. An IEP meeting is required before any change in placement	Unlike IDEA, Section 504 requires only notice, not consent, for evaluation. It is recommended that district obtain parental consent. Like IDEA evaluation and placement procedures under Section 504 require that information be obtained from a variety of sources of the area of concern; that all data are documented and considered; and that decisions are made by a group of persons knowledgeable about the student, evaluation data, and placement options. Section 504 requires that students be educated with their nondisabled peers to the maximum extent appropriate. Section 504 does not require a meeting for any change in placement

(continued)

Table 14.2 (continued)

ADA	IDEA	504
Due process		
The ADA does not delineate specific due process procedures. People with disabilities have the same remedies that are available under the Title VII of the Civil Rights Act of 1964, as amended in 1991. Thus, individuals who are discriminated against may file a complaint with the relevant federal agency or due in federal court. Enforcement agencies encourage informal mediation and voluntary compliance	IDEA delineates specific requirements for local education agencies to provide impartial hearings for parents who disagree with the identification, evaluation, or placement of a child	Section 504 requires local education agencies to provide impartial hearings for parents who disagree with the identification, evaluation, or placement of a student. It requires that parents have an opportunity to participate in the hearing process and to be represented by counsel. Beyond this, due process details are left to the discretion of the local education agency. It is recommended that districts develop policy guidelines and procedures

The Americans with Disabilities Act of 1990 (ADA), the Individuals with Disabilities Education Act (IDEA), and Section 504 of the Rehabilitation Act of 1973 represent three attempts to improve the living conditions of those with disabilities

Reprinted with permission from the DREDF Disability Rights Education & Defense Fund Web site

DREDF

DISABILITY RIGHTS EDUCATION & DEFENSE FUND

Related to Section 504 is the ADA, which was signed into law on July 26, 1990 and amended (ADAAA) in 2008. Although its definitions and regulations are somewhat similar to those of Section 504, these laws are much broader in scope in that they apply to all public entities whether or not they receive federal financial assistance. In addition, they are generally applied to adults while Section 504 is applied to children and adolescents.

The definition of a disability under Section 504 and ADA/ADAAA is a "mental or physical impairment that substantially limits one or more major life activities." A person qualifies for assistance under Section 504 and ADA/ADAAA if he/she has:

(a) A mental or physical impairment (i.e., diagnosis)
(b) Substantial limitations related to that impairment
(c) The affected activities are central to daily life

Thus, the laws afford protection from discrimination to individuals who, by virtue of this definition, currently have a disability, have a record of having a disability, or are regarded as having a disability whether or not they actually have one. The goal of this latter prong was to protect individuals from discrimination based on stereotypical assumptions (Goodman-Delahunty, 2000). A main tenet of these laws is that they apply to individuals who are *otherwise qualified* to perform the necessary duties (or in education, meet the academic standards) with reasonable accommodations. Thus, the goal of accommodations is to provide equal opportunity or to essentially "level the playing field" for the person with a disability in order to allow that person to demonstrate his/her knowledge.

The ADA Amendments Act (ADAAA) was passed in 2008 with the purpose of clarifying congressional intent regarding the ADA (AHEAD). In particular, there was concern that several Supreme Court rulings had the untoward effect of narrowing the ADA's scope by focusing more on whether an individual met the definition of a disability versus whether or not discrimination occurred or there was a reasonable request for accommodations [Association of Higher Education and Disability (AHEAD); "What the ADA Amendments and Higher Education Mean," 2009]. While the definition of a disability remains the same under the ADAAA, its passage is important in that it broadened the scope of coverage under the law by rejecting holdings in several Supreme Court decisions viewed as too restrictive (Regulations to Implement the Equal Employment Provisions of the Americans with Disabilities Act, as Amended, 2011). Below are several issues that arise in determining eligibility under Section 504 and the ADA/ADAAA in the postsecondary setting.

Average Person Standard. One of the aspects of Section 504 and the ADA that has been subject to many court cases is the average person standard. This standard requires that in order to be considered substantially limited under the law, an individual's disability must be significant compared to the average person (Maedgen & Semrud-Clikeman, 2007). This means that a diagnosis, by itself, is not sufficient to qualify for accommodations under Section 504 and ADA/ADAAA. Rather, the focus is on functional limitations. This emphasis can present confusion for individuals seeking accommodations at the postsecondary level, particularly if they received services under IDEA for a qualifying diagnosis.

As an example, consider an individual who received services for a mathematics learning disability throughout her K-12 experience and is now seeking accommodations at the university level. Her most recent assessment revealed mathematics difficulties relative to her ability level, but her scores were within the average range of functioning. When she applied for services at a university, she was denied accommodations based on the lack of evidence of functional impairment. In this case, while the diagnosis may still have been appropriate, the student's seemingly successful compensatory skills belied the need for academic accommodations. As noted, the focus of Section 504 and ADA/ADAAA is on whether or not substantial limitations arise *as a result of* a diagnosis, not the diagnosis in and of itself. Because the relevant laws are civil rights legislation, the purpose of accommodations is to allow equal opportunity not to guarantee academic success or a certain outcome.

However, as a correlate to the above example, it is important to note that the "average person standard" does not always equate to the "average score on tests" (Mapou, 2008). If the individual displayed reading scores within the average range, but notable deficits in some of the underlying processes underlying reading skills (e.g., fluency and automaticity), accommodations may be appropriate. This was specifically spelled out in the decision in *Bartlett v. the New York State Board of Law Examiners* (2001) in which the plaintiff had originally been denied accommodations on the bar examination, despite having a documented reading disability, because her scores were within the average range and she had a history of academic success. The court overturned this on appeal, noting that Ms. Bartlett did not read in the same way as the average person and was in fact substantially limited in the way she did so.

The results of this case may be applied to our earlier described student who had compensated for her mathematics learning disability. While she still showed a deficit compared to her ability level, a sole measure of mathematics performance (which was in the average range) was not sufficient to provide her with accommodations. However, if the neuropsychologist had included measures of mathematics fluency and performance under time pressures as well as organizational and planning measures (all aspects that are frequently seen in people with NVLD), the student may have qualified for services. Thus, it is important to thoroughly document impairment in order for accommodations to be considered (see Mapou's (2008) excellent discussion of this topic for more information). Relatedly, the recently released ADAAA regulations note that the focus should be on how the individual is limited relative to "most people in the general population" versus what outcomes the individual has achieved (Regulations to Implement the Equal Employment Provisions of the Americans with Disabilities Act, as Amended, 2011).

Mitigating Measures. Prior to the ADAAA, another issue related to the determination of whether or not an individual had a disability under the ADA was whether or not the use of mitigating measures should be considered. The term mitigating measures refers to aids or devices that may ameliorate or lessen the effects of a disability. Several Supreme Court cases in the late 1990s allowed for their consideration with the result that many individuals were deemed ineligible for protection under the law because they used devices or took medication that minimized the functional impact of their condition(s) (*Albertsons v. Kirkingburg*, 1999; *Sutton v. United*

Airlines, 1999). The ADAAA rejects this interpretation and directs that the positive effects of such measures should be ignored in determining whether an impairment is substantially limiting (Regulations to Implement the Equal Employment Provisions of the Americans with Disabilities Act, as Amended, 2011).[1] This is of particular importance in determining whether an individual is protected under the law *as an individual with a disability*, but does not change much with respect to the determination of eligibility for services at the university level where the focus is functional impact and appropriate accommodations.

An example of this is a young adult with ADHD who is being treated with medication. If the medication is successful in assisting the student to the extent that he/she no longer experiences any limitations in functioning, then accommodations are likely to be unnecessary in the university setting. However, if the side effects from the medication are disabling, they may well warrant accommodations (Goodman-Delahunty, 2000). Treatments or medications themselves often impose additional functional limitations (e.g., difficulty sleeping, concentration problems), for which accommodations are appropriate (Wilens, 2004).

Relevance. A third issue relating to the interpretation of Section 504/ADA/ADAAA and the provision of accommodations is the issue of *relevance*, which has primarily been discussed with respect to professional licensing examinations, but is also likely appropriate for accommodation decisions in graduation requirements and programmatic issues at the graduate level (Ballard & Elwork, 2003; Ranseen & Parks, 2005). One of the debated issues is whether a person with a documented disability and clear limitations associated with it should be granted accommodations on professional hurdles, such as licensing examinations, when their limitations would pose a significant problem in performing the profession and/or their weaknesses may be ones that the examinations are designed to detect. Such weaknesses may include mathematics difficulties in professions that are heavily mathematically based (e.g., accounting), visual-spatial problems in fields dependent on these skills (e.g., architecture, engineering), and social deficits in areas dependent on social interaction and professional boundaries (e.g., clinical psychology). It is important for the clinician and the client to be prepared for accommodations to be denied when the essential elements or integrity of an exam or course rests on the very skills that prevent the client from performing adequately. For example, extended test-taking time would not be appropriate on examinations for which speed was the factor being tested. Similarly, multiple-excused absences or written in lieu of oral work would not be appropriate in courses in which the primary focus is class participation and debate. The ability of institutions to enforce academic standards and to deny accommodation requests that would fundamentally alter these was reiterated in the ADAAA (AHEAD, 2011a, 2011b).

Because of the differences in legislation and the distinction between a diagnosis and a disability warranting accommodations, it is important for the clinician to assist the client and his/her parents in preparing for the transition from high school to college. The feedback session during which the results of the assessment are discussed is an important time to talk about the differences between IDEA and the

---

[1] An exception to this is eyeglasses and contact lenses, which can still be considered.

laws that pertain to services at the postsecondary level. The transition to university/college life can be difficult to navigate for a well-adjusted adolescent, but for one with disabilities, it can be quite difficult. Asking for help and assistance may be particularly difficult for the adolescent with NVLD as well as knowing when the person is struggling. The clinician can assist in identifying trigger points that may pose problems for the students as well as assisting in determining methods for obtaining needed assistance. Table 14.2 describes several of these differences; ones of particular importance to nonschool-based clinicians and school personnel involved in transition planning are discussed in greater detail below.

Under Section 504 and in the K-12 setting, parents, teachers, doctors, or concerned parties can refer for a review of documentation and determination whether further assessment is needed. The assessment can be review of the records, use of standardized tests, and other data within the cumulative file and is not necessarily a formal neuropsychological, psychological, or psychoeducational evaluation; a requirement which is different from IDEA. There are students who may qualify for accommodations based on the finding that their condition is substantially limiting and meets the definition of a disability under Section 504 and the ADA/ADAAA. For many clients with NVLD, Section 504 may be the only route that needed accommodations can be obtained in the K-12 system since the diagnosis is not listed as a covered category under IDEA. The social disabilities that are frequently seen with the diagnosis, coupled with executive function deficits, particularly in planning and organization, are often appropriate for accommodations if they interfere with functioning. Because eligibility decisions are dependent on the severity and degree of functional impact, a comprehensive neuropsychological and/or psychoeducational evaluation which assesses factors such as attention, memory, and executive processes can be of tremendous relevance in determining whether or not the diagnosis is actually *disabling* and what types of academic accommodations are appropriate.

In contrast, a university student with a diagnosis of NVLD who is not experiencing significant academic or emotional difficulty may find it problematic to obtain services through ADA/ADAAA. In order to ascertain what services may be available to the student, the parents and student should visit the university disability service office as part of their college decision-making process. During that visit it is quite appropriate to request an earlier review of their documentation in order to know what, if any, accommodations may be provided. It is also important to recognize that if accommodations are approved, letters that detail these need to be requested each semester and it is the student's responsibility to deliver them to their professors. If the appropriate disability support office is not contacted each semester, the accommodations may not be provided.

In the K-12 setting, if a student has an IEP a triennial evaluation is required. This does not have to be a comprehensive evaluation but some additional and/or updated assessment of some sort. If a student has an IEP or a Section 504 plan, an annual update is also required which may or may not have some additional testing. When advancing to college, a student's coherent narrative of his or her experience of their disability, and the effective and ineffective accommodations previously utilized may be sufficient for establishing disability and a need for accommodation (http://www.ahead.org/resources/documentation_guidance). However, if the student is unable to convey a connection between the disability and the accommodations requested, and/or has not had a complete recent reevaluation for their IEP, additional or updated documentation on adult level tests may also be needed to demonstrate that the student meets disability status under ADA and continues to need accommodations in the college setting. The responsibility and cost of providing such documentation lies with the student. Such documentation must be comprehensive and current and conducted by a licensed professional. Although the time frame varies, it is generally helpful to have been conducted within 3 years from the time of application for accommodations and must clearly document the functional impact of the student's disability within the academic setting. The clinician must not only document that there is a disability but also supply sufficient information about functional limitations and link any recommended accommodations to these. For example, it would be very reasonable to recommend extended test-taking time for a student who is limited by slow reading, processing, and/or motor skills. Such an accommodation may be less appropriate for a student with an attentional disorder without corresponding reading or processing deficits whose difficulties during exams can be accommodated by taking tests in a reduced distraction environment.

In the majority of cases, documentation for NVLD in the higher education setting should include clinical interviews, psychoeducational measures, and behavioral rating scales as appropriate. As a general guide, the AHEAD's "seven essential elements of quality disability documentation" are presented in Table 14.3 (AHEAD, 2011a, 2011b).

College students are required to also deliver and discuss letters of accommodation with their instructors (Disability Compliance for Higher Education, 2007). While it is not required that they reveal the diagnosis, sufficient information must be presented so that the student and the faculty member can work out the logistical details of providing the accommodation in the classroom. Two issues frequently arise that may particularly apply to college students with NVLD. First, the student may lose the letters or forget to provide them to their professors. Clinicians can assist students diagnosed with NVLD with recommendations on how to follow-through with the delivery of letters through the use of memory aids or written reminders. In addition, many students with NVLD (and other disorders) may be reluctant to share this information with their professors and for fear that doing so will label them. In this case, the clinician needs to work through these issues with the client and assist in helping the student in ways to approach the professor. Role-playing various scenarios may be especially helpful. Clinicians who are working with college students in therapy should also consider having their clients sign a two-way release allowing them to work with the student's disability case manager directly. Clinicians can then appropriately work with their clients regarding how to best use their accommodations in the college setting.

Neuropsychological and/or Psychoeducational Evaluations

Most neuropsychologists and nonschool-based clinicians have very little training in special education law or in the ADA/ADAAA as it applies to college students. As discussed, there are significant differences between these two laws and these differences directly affect assessment and report writing. These aspects are particularly important for children/young adults with NVLD as this disorder continues to not be widely recognized by IDEA and for children in the K-12 system; Section 504 is the most likely vehicle for accommodations. For this reason the documentation section of the report is crucial in order to secure these accommodations. Another way to improve the success of the evaluation is to schedule a meeting with school personnel (with parent permission) to gather information as well as to garner administrative support. A conversation with the teachers involved in the student's education can pinpoint areas of concern as well.

Tied to the documentation is the writing of the recommendations for classroom modifications. Useful recommendations are those which can be adapted in general education classrooms with relative ease. The recommendations that are specific in nature are much more helpful than those which are more general. For example, a useful recommendation for a child with NVLD who is experiencing difficulty in mathematics due to visual-spatial difficulties would be to have him/her complete mathematics problems on graph paper so that the columns are aligned. An additional intervention that stresses planning strategy instruction has also been found to improve performance in mathematics (Iseman & Naglieri, 2011).

When making recommendations for accommodation in the college of university setting, the clinicians need to become very familiar with the specific school's guidelines for documentation as well as the standards illustrated in Table 14.3. It is also important for the clinician not to mislead parents and students into thinking that by qualifying for a diagnosis they will receive accommodations. Becoming familiar with the local college and university staff of the disability service office can help not only in referring the parent and student to a specific person but also to assist with follow-through of needed recommendations. In addition, college personnel refer to outside parties when students are seeking an evaluation and they are more likely to refer to someone they know and who has conducted useful evaluations than to other professionals.

One model that can be helpful as a guide for useful neuropsychological assessments is that of Robert Mapou (2004, 2008). The core features of the model include (1) an evaluation of intellectual ability; (2) assessment of academic skills (reading, writing, and mathematics) and analysis of how ability/achievement discrepancies relate to everyday functioning; (3) a thorough neuropsychological history, assessing medical, developmental, educational, occupational, family, and social realms; (4) evaluation of executive functions and modality-specific skills (e.g., learning, memory, language, visuospatial functions, attention, problem solving); and (5) personality and emotional assessment to help rule out other disorders as the primary cause of learning problems. For assessment of NVLD, the addition of motor and sensory skills is recommended also (Mapou, 2008). Assessed deficits in the areas of academic and behavioral functioning need to be related to the academic setting and consequent need for accommodations. For example, a neuropsychological evaluation of a student with NVLD may reveal weaknesses in reading comprehension, working memory, and planning and organization. In the college setting, these may relate to difficulties keeping up with the volume of reading, completing tests under

Table 14.3 Seven essential elements of quality disability documentation (AHEAD, 2011a, 2011b)

1. *Credentials of the evaluation*—Documentation should be provided by a licensed or otherwise credentialed professional who has gone through appropriate and comprehensive training, has relevant experience, and does not have a personal relationship with the individual being evaluated. There should be a match between the credentials of the person doing the evaluation and the condition being reported (e.g., an orthopedic limitation might be documented by a physician, but not a licensed psychologist)
2. *Diagnostic statement of disability*—Documentation should include a clear diagnostic statement that describes how the condition was diagnosed, provides information on the functional impact, and details the typical progression or prognosis of the condition
3. *Description of diagnostic methodology*—Documentation should include a description of the diagnostic criteria, evaluation methods, procedures, tests, and dates of administration, as well as a clinical narrative, observation, and specific results. Diagnostic methods should be congruent with the particular disability and current professional practices in the field. Summary data and specific test scores (with the norming population identified) should be included also
4. *Description of functional limitations*—Documentation should include information on how the disabling condition currently affects the individual. Such information is helpful in establishing the presence of a disability and identifying possible accommodations. A combination of the results of formal evaluation procedures, clinical narrative, and the individual's self-report is the most comprehensive approach to documenting impact. The documentation should be thorough enough to demonstrate whether and how a major life activity is substantially affected by providing information on the severity, frequency, and pervasiveness of the condition(s)
5. *A description of the expected progression or stability of the disability*—Information on how the individual's condition is expected to change over time and on any known or suspected triggers to periods of exacerbation is helpful in determining appropriate accommodations and planning timelines for reevaluation
6. *History of current and past accommodations, academic services, and treatment*—Documentation should include a description of accommodations used in the past and current support services or treatment modalities (e.g., medications), including their effectiveness in ameliorating any functional impacts of the disability. It is also helpful to document any side effects associated with medication regimens as these may warrant particular accommodations
7. *Recommendations for accommodations, adaptive devices, assistive services, compensatory strategies, and/or collateral support services*—Documentation should include recommendations for accommodations that are based on the individual's functional limitations. Recommended accommodations should be logically related to functional limitations; if connections are not obvious, a clear explanation of their usefulness should be provided. While the postsecondary institution does not have an obligation to provide accommodations recommended by others, those that are congruent with the individual's disability and fit with the universities' programs and services may be helpful

Adapted and reprinted with permission from the Association of Higher Education and Disability (AHEAD, 2011a, 2011b)

standard time conditions, and in completing homework in a timely and appropriate manner. Linking these learning challenges to the need for accommodations, the evaluator might recommend extended test-taking time, taking tests in a quiet area, and the use of a smart phone that provides advance notice of due dates. Such an evaluation is also likely to uncover the presence of any co-occurring conditions (e.g., depression) that additionally affect learning and should be taken into account when determining appropriate support in the academic setting.

Conclusion

The goal of this chapter was to discuss the laws affecting disability accommodations in education for children and adults with NVLD and to provide recommendations as to how to best utilize the framework of IDEA, Section 504, and the ADA/ADAAA to obtain appropriate services. Qualifications and accommodations differ depending on the setting as well as on the law that is most appropriate for the case. For children and young adults with NVLD who do not evidence significant mathematical learning disabilities, services under Section 504 or ADA/ADAAA may be appropriate if documentation of significant problems with executive functioning and/or social functioning can be provided. Clinicians who perform such evaluations need to be conversant with these laws and the requirements of the laws when preparing the assessment and report. It is crucial that the report not only documents the areas of difficulty but also specifies how these areas negatively impact the child/young adult's functioning in order for the client to qualify for services.

Parents also need to be aware of the differences in the law from the K-12 setting to the university setting and prepare for these prior to the student entering college. There are Web sites that may be helpful in selecting appropriate college/universities (www.petersons.com/college-search.aspx) and books (e.g., K & W Guide to Colleges for Students with Learning Disabilities, 10th Edition). Laws concerning accommodations are changing and it is strongly recommended to consult the specific university. Also it is recommended to access the website http:/www.ahead.org/resources/documentation_guidance. All of these resources can be used to make the transition from high school and living at home to the university and living on one's own. For some clients with NVLD, this transition may be difficult. Making sure that all accommodations and support are in place prior to entry can go a long way to making the college experience a success.

References

Albertsons, Inc. v. Kirkingburg, 527 U.S. 555 (1999).

Altshuler, S. J., & Kopels, S. (2003). Advocating in schools for children with disabilities: What's new with IDEA? *Social Work, 48*, 320–329.

Association of Higher Education and Disability. (2011). *ADA Amendments Act of 2008 policy implications for accommodating students with disabilities*. Retrieved March 24, 2011 from http://www.ahead.org/resources/government-relations

Association of Higher Education and Disability. (2011). *Seven essential elements of quality disability documentation*. Retrieved March 24, 2011 from http://www.ahead.org/resources/best-practices-resources/elements

Association of Higher Education and Disability. (2011). Supporting Accommodation Requests: Guidance on Documentation Practices. Retrieved April 2012 from http:/www.ahead.org/resources/documentation_guidance.

Ballard, R. S., & Elwork, A. (2003). Learning disability and professional licensing examinations: What accommodations are reasonable under the ADA? *The Journal of Psychiatry & Law, 31*, 43–66.

Bartlett v. New York State Board of Law Examiners, 2001 U.S. Dist. LEXIS 11926 (S.D.N.Y. August 15, 2001).

Disability Compliance in Higher Education (2007). Palm Beach Gardens, FL: LRP Publications.

Education for All Handicapped Children Act of 1975, 20 U.S.C. Section 401 (1975).

Foote, W. E. (2000). A model for psychological consultation in cases involving the Americans with Disabilities Act. *Professional Psychology, Research and Practice, 31*, 190–196.

Fuchs, L. S., Fuchs, D., Prentice, K., Hamlett, C. L., Finelli, R., & Courey, S. J. (2004). Enhancing mathematical problem solving among third-grade students with schema-based instruction. *Journal of Educational Psychology, 96*, 635–746.

Fuchs, D., Mock, D., Morgan, P., & Young, C. (2003). Responsiveness-to-intervention: Definitions, evidence and implications for the learning disabilities construct. *Learning Disabilities Research and Practice, 18*, 157–171.

Goodman-Delahunty, J. (2000). Psychological impairment under the Americans with Disabilities Act: Legal guidelines. *Professional Psychology, Research and Practice, 31*, 197–205.

Gordon, M., Lewandowski, L., Murphy, K., & Dempsey, K. (2002). ADA-based accommodations in higher education: A survey of clinicians about documentation requirements and diagnostic standards. *Journal of Learning Disabilities, 35*(4), 357–363.

Hendrik Hudson District Board of Education v. Rowley. (1982). *458 U.S. 176, 207 fn. 28.*

Holdnack, J. A., & Weiss, L. G. (2006). IDEA 2004: Anticipated implications for clinical practice-integrating assessment and intervention. *Psychology in the Schools, 43*, 871–882.

IDEA. (1990). *Individuals with Disabilities Education Act*. 20 U.S.C. 1400 et seq.

IDEA. (1997). *Individuals with Disabilities Education Act*. 20 U.S.C. 1400 et seq.

IDEA. (2000). *2nd Annual Report to Congress on the Implementation of the Individuals with Disabilities Education Act*. Washington, DC: U.S. Dept. of Education.

IDEA. (2004). *Individuals with Disabilities Education Improvement Act of 2004*. Washington, DC: U.S. Dept. of Education.

Iseman, J. S., & Naglieri, J. A. (2011). A cognitive strategy instruction to improve math calculation for children with ADHD and LD: A randomized controlled study. *Journal of Learning Disabilities, 44*, 167–183.

Jacob, S., & Hartshorne, T. S. (2003). *Ethics and law for school psychologists*. Hoboken, NJ: Wiley.

Maedgen, J. W., & Semrud-Clikeman, M. (2007). Bridging neuropsychological practice and educational intervention. In S. J. Hunter & J. Donders (Eds.), *Pediatric neuropsychological practice: A critical review of science and practice*. London: Cambridge Press.

Mapou, R. L. (2004). Assessment of learning disabilities. In J. Ricker (Ed.), *Differential diagnosis in adult neuropsychological assessment* (pp. 370–420). New York: Springer.

Mapou, R. L. (2008). Learning disabilities in adults. In J. E. Morgan & J. H. Ricker (Eds.), *Textbook of clinical neuropsychology* (pp. 696–728). New York: Psychology Press.

Mills v. Board of Education for District of Columbia, 348F. Suppl. 866 (1972).

Pennsylvania Association for Retarded Citizens (P.A.R.C.) v. Commonwealth of Pennsylvania, 334F. Supp. 1257 (D.C. E.D. Pa. 1971), 343F. Supp. 279 (D.C. E.D. Pa. 1972).

Ranseen, J. D., & Parks, G. S. (2005). Test accommodations for post-secondary students: The quandary resulting from ADA's disability definition. *Psychology, Public Policy, and Law, 11*, 83–108.

Regulations to Implement the Equal Employment Provisions of the Americans with Disabilities Act, as Amended, 76 Fed. Reg. 16978 (March, 25, 2011) (to be codified at 29 C.F.R. pt. 1630).

Semrud-Clikeman, M. (2005). Neuropsychological aspects for evaluating LD. *Journal of Learning Disabilities, 38*, 563–568.

Semrud-Clikeman, M., Walkowiak, J., Wilkinson, A., & Christopher, G. (2010). Neuropsychological findings in nonverbal learning disabilities. *Developmental Neuropsychology, 35*, 582–600.

Semrud-Clikeman, M., Walkowiak, J., Wilkinson, A., & Minne, E. (2010). Behavior and social perception in children with Asperger's disorder, nonverbal learning disability, or ADHD. *Journal of Abnormal Child Psychology, 38*, 509–519.

Skalski, S., & Klotz, M. B. (2005). NASP comments on the proposed IDEA regulations. *Communiqué, 34*, 6–7.

Sutton v. United Air Lines, Inc., 537 U.S. 491. (1999). What the ADA amendments and higher education acts mean for law schools (2009). *The American University Journal of Gender, Social Policy & the Law, 18*(1), 13–40.

Wilens, T. (2004). *Straight talk about psychiatric medications for kids* (2nd ed.). New York: Guilford.

Chapter 15
Overview of the Current Research on NVLD

Jodene Goldenring Fine

For psychologists practicing in the field, the research on NVLD might appear to be as easy to untangle as the proverbial Gordian knot. So much has been written from so many perspectives that one might find one's self wondering how to begin. The purpose of this chapter will be, first, to loosen the strings a little by showing how the literature as a whole evolved, then to provide some guidelines about how one might assess the utility of research articles available, and finally to offer some of the more reliable findings in the literature and to raise some questions still unresolved.

It is impossible to think about NVLD research without acknowledging the substantial contributions of one individual and his laboratory: Byron Rourke. While Myklebust (1975) initially coined the term "nonverbal learning disabilities" to describe children with high verbal ability and difficulty negotiating the nonverbal aspects of their environment, Rourke embarked on a lifelong journey to describe and treat these children. He and his colleagues made the first attempt to methodically define NVLD behaviorally and to propose a neurological model to explain how the observed symptoms might arise.

Rourke's early studies from the 1970s and 1980s compared children with learning disabilities in reading to those with problems performing in mathematics (e.g., Rourke & Finlayson, 1978; Rourke & Strang, 1978, 1983; Strang & Rourke, 1983), a legacy that has persisted into the twenty-first century (for a review, see Fine, Semrud-Clikeman, Bledsoe, & Musielak in press). Many of these studies were small and descriptive. From them, Rourke and his colleagues began to establish a set of behavioral criteria, including specific assets and deficits, which described children with intact language and poor arithmetic skills. In later years, Rourke and his colleagues used larger samples to validate neuropsychological markers that could be used to identify children with NVLD (e.g., Harnadek & Rourke, 1994).

J.G. Fine, Ph.D. (✉)
Michigan State University, East Lansing, MI, USA
e-mail: jodene.fine@gmail.com

J. Broitman and J.M. Davis (eds.), *Treating NVLD in Children: Professional Collaborations for Positive Outcomes*, DOI 10.1007/978-1-4614-6179-1_15,

These studies helped to define a set of an operational research and clinical diagnostic criteria although controversy remains as to their utility (Ris & Nortz, 2008).

As Rourke was shaping his behavioral model, he was also developing a neurological explanation for NVLD symptoms, known as the "white matter model" (Rourke, 1989, 1995). White matter refers to long myelinated axons, which serve to connect and integrate regions of the brain. Rourke based his model on the work of Goldberg and Costa (1981), who suggested that the white matter connectivity in the right hemisphere is more abundant, multimodal, and widely distributed throughout the cortex compared to the left hemisphere. Rourke hypothesized that any disease or developmental process that disrupted white matter would affect the right hemisphere disproportionately, and that those functions requiring intermodal integration would be most affected (Rourke, 1995). To validate the model, Rourke turned to special populations of persons with genetic or acquired neurological disorders. NVLD was posed as a heuristic model to explain the neurological and psychosocial functioning of these patients (McDonald, 2002).

As a body of research, NVLD work tends to be divided between neurological/medical explorations into the white matter model and research addressing the learning and psychosocial characteristics of children with nonverbal learning problems. The white matter model research has largely been accomplished using groups that are easily identifiable because they have distinct, verifiable genetic or neurological conditions, and the purpose of the work has seemed to seek neurological evidence for NVLD symptoms. On the other hand, the work on NVLD as a learning or developmental disorder is more difficult to understand due to considerable variation in how research groups are defined, the size and heterogeneity of comorbid conditions within research groups, and the typically small sample sizes utilized (Fine et al., in press).

Reading NVLD Research

Ranging from clinical case studies to large-sample empirical work, the research literature as a whole varies widely in methods and results. Much of the work has been carried out qualitatively, with little or no clearly communicated replicable explanation of how the NVLD groups have been identified (Fine et al., in press). Thus, much of the commonly accepted knowledge about NVLD derives from clinical impressions. While clinical impressions are a very important step in formulating the behavioral phenotype, quantitative empirically derived information about how children with NVLD can be differentiated from their typical developing peers and from children with other disorders is important to both the internal and external validation of the syndrome (Pennington, 2009a), neither of which has been soundly established.

Diagnostic Criteria. Of those studies that have utilized a quantitative method of identifying children with NVLD, many have favored the neuropsychological test criteria proposed and refined by Rourke's laboratory in several seminal papers

(Drummond, Ahmad, & Rourke, 2005; Harnadek & Rourke, 1994; Pelletier, Ahmad, & Rourke, 2001). The criteria are flexible in that some but not all of the assets and deficits associated with NVLD are required. Criteria are ranked in order of importance based on their discriminatory value (from Drummond et al., 2005; Pelletier et al., 2001):

First 5 or 7 ± of 8 below:

- Target Test 1 SD below mean
- Finger agnosia/dysgraphia/astereognosis composite > 1 SD below mean and fewer than two errors on tactile perception
- Two of WISC Vocabulary, Similarities, and Information subtests are highest of the Verbal Scale
- Two of WISC Block Design, Object Assembly, and Coding are lowest of Performance Scale
- WRAT Reading > Arithmetic (8 points)
- Tactile Performance Test Right > Left > Both
- Grip strength within 1 SD of mean and Grooved Peg > 1 SD below mean
- WISC VIQ > PIQ (10 points)

Note that the WISC Verbal IQ-Performance IQ split is the lowest item on the list, indicating its weaker discriminatory value in comparison to the items above.

Most researchers have not used the full neuropsychological criteria, but many have incorporated aspects of it. The most common methods of identification have included a Verbal IQ (VIQ) > Performance IQ (PIQ) split in the presence of poor math and at least average single-word-reading skills (Fine et al., in press). The size of the VIQ-PIQ splits used has ranged from 9 to 15 standard score points. As a marker for NVLD that can be generalized to the population, a VIQ-PIQ split of this size may not be useful, since 35.8% of the standardization population had a 12-point split on the WISC-III (Wechsler, 1991). Most of the extant studies utilized the WISC-III or an older version of the Wechsler intelligence tests; thus it is unknown how children with NVLD might look on the current WISC-IV or other intellectual assessments.

Sample Characteristics. When reading the NVLD research, it is very important to carefully check the sample size, sample description, exclusion criteria (if certain types of participants were not allowed in the study), diagnostic criteria (how participants were included), and the variables utilized to describe study outcomes. For example, one often-repeated concern regarding children with NVLD is that they are more prone to suicide. Parents have suffered considerable anxiety over this expectation. A review of the literature, however, finds that no study has shown this to be true. Rather, this “feature” of NVLD was based on a conjecture derived from one paper published in 1989 that described a single-case study (Rourke, Young, & Leenaars, 1989). In subsequent research, three studies have indicated that children with NVLD are no more, and in some cases, less prone to internalizing disorders than children with reading disability (Antshel & Joseph, 2006; Forrest, 2004; Yu, Buka, McCormick, Fitzmaurice, & Indurkhya, 2006). Two have suggested that the incidence of internalizing disorders was higher among children with NVLD (Pelletier et al., 2001; Petti, Voelker, Shore, & Hayman-Abello, 2002), and one has suggested higher rates of familial history of bipolar in the NVLD population (Antshel & Khan, 2008). None of these studies evaluated suicide attempts. Thus, the true incidence of suicide attempts in the NVLD population is unknown, and the premise that such children are more prone to disturbance of mood than are children with other learning disabilities is not well established.

Sample description is very important to consider when reading the NVLD research. Rourke and others (Klin, Volkmar, Sparrow, Cicchetti, & Rourke, 1995; Rourke & Tsatsanis, 2000) have suggested that NVLD might be considered to be a heuristic model for understanding some children with Asperger's syndrome. Likewise, NVLD has been used to characterize some features of several genetic and acquired disorders. While some studies have focused solely on distinguishing one particular group or another from otherwise typically developing children (e.g., Ris et al., 2007), many studies have included in the NVLD sample children who have neurological involvement such as hydrocephalus, Turner's syndrome, and Asperger's syndrome along with children who have no such apparent diagnoses. It is difficult to determine which observed characteristics should be attributed to the "NVLD group" and which to comorbid disorders.

Heterogeneity and Subtypes. It is possible that the heterogeneity seen in NVLD (Davis & Broitman, 2011; Grodzinsky, Forbes, & Bernstein, 2010) is partly due to differences between research criteria and those utilized diagnostically in the field. When making a clinical diagnosis, one looks for characteristics that align with NVLD expectations, even though any particular symptom may be associated with a variety of processing problems. For example, children with ADHD might display some of the mathematics (Forrest, 2004), social (Fine, Semrud-Clikeman, Butcher, & Walkowiak, 2008), and executive functioning (Schafer & Semrud-Clikeman, 2008) issues we have come to associate with NVLD.

This diagnostic overlap has led some to question the validity of NVLD, particularly with regard to the core symptoms of the disorder, since it could be conceptualized alternately as a primary deficit in mathematics, or social skills, or fine-motor control (Pennington, 2009b). Rourke strongly supported a unitary construct for NVLD, although subtypes have been proposed (Davis & Broitman, 2011; Grodzinsky et al., 2010) largely on the basis of clinical rather than empirical validation (Fine & Semrud-Clikeman, 2010). However, one recent study found qualitative evidence for at least three types of NVLD children (Grodzinsky et al., 2010). Because the incidence of NVLD is considered to be a small portion of LD overall, some have suggested that NVLD subtypes may lack utility (Ris & Nortz, 2008). Alternately, the observed heterogeneity of children with NVLD might lead one to consider whether these children might be better described by other disorders, but who also happen to have an NVLD presentation, as Rourke suggested when he proposed NVLD as a way to describe the neuropsychological profiles of children with right-hemisphere white matter problems, regardless of etiology (Rourke, Van der Vlugt, & Rourke, 2002).

White Matter Model Research

Rourke described his white matter model as "an attempt to capture and explain the syndrome of nonverbal learning disabilities (NLD) in those types of neurological disease wherein this behavioral phenotype is, to a greater or lesser extent, evident" (Rourke et al., 2002, p. 223). He arranged the neurological diseases along the lines of four levels ranging from Level 1, displaying virtually all of the assets and deficits of the proposed NVLD phenotype, to Level 4, "research evidence is ambiguous" (from Rourke et al., 2002, p. 224). Disorders for which the NVLD phenotype was considered to be most consistent include agenesis of the corpus callosum, Asperger's disorder, velocardiofacial syndrome, Williams syndrome, de Lange syndrome, hydrocephalus, and Turner's syndrome. A collection of evidence, consisting largely of case studies in the tradition of the medical model appeared in books, chapters, and peer-reviewed journals.

Since Rourke's initial studies, many researchers have used the NVLD model to explore the phenotypes of these various disorders using larger samples and modern neuroimaging techniques. One of the most commonly encountered Level 1 genetic disorders is velocardiofacial syndrome (VCFS). Research on VCFS is used below as an illustration of how researchers are seeking validation of the white matter model among special groups.

With regard to the NVLD phenotype, VCFS is among most well-studied groups. Also known as 22p11.2 deletion or DiGeorge syndrome, it is one of the most common genetic disorders, occurring in 1 out of 4,500 births (Devriendt, Fryns, Mortier, Van Thienen, & Keymolen, 1998). In addition to facial, cardiologic, and immune function abnormalities, children with VCFS are at high risk for psychosocial and learning disabilities (Kobrynski & Sullivan, 2007). Although many characteristics of VCFS are consistent with Rourke's model of assets and deficits of NVLD, some are not. For example, unlike those with NVLD, children with VCFS are reported to be notably language-delayed despite good single-word decoding skills (Woodin et al., 2001), while early, even precocious, language is associated with NVLD (Rourke, 1989). Children with VCFS are at high risk for schizophrenia, an outcome that has not been associated with NVLD. Consistent with NVLD, studies have indicated that patients with VCFS have higher verbal than nonverbal IQ scores and poor arithmetic relative to word decoding skills (Moss et al., 1999; Woodin et al., 2001).

A deeper look into the mathematics of children with VCFS indicates that these children have preserved math-fact retrieval, but difficulty with number comparison, strategy, and solving word problems (De Smedt et al., 2007). Rourke makes little mention of math-fact retrieval, but does suggest that "rote" memorization is an area of relative strength for children with NVLD (Rourke, Rourke, & van der Vlugt, 2002). Math-fact retrieval has been observed to be a semantic as opposed to a visuospatial task behaviorally (Geary, 2004), and neuroimaging evidence has suggested that the neural circuitries involved in math-fact retrieval and nonverbal numeracy are distinct (Dehaene, Piazza, Pinel, & Cohen, 2005). Thus, the common profile for VCFS mathematics learning appears to be consistent with NVLD academic expectations.

The neuroimaging research on VCFS has tended to support the white matter model in that several studies have reported a reduction of white matter volumes and disturbances of white matter in the brains of patients relative to controls. Findings have indicated differences bilaterally in frontal regions, the superior longitudinal fasciculus, and occipital regions in adults (van Amelsvoort et al., 2001), and reduced overall volume of white more than gray matter in children (Eliez, Schmitt, White, & Reiss, 2000). In a diffusion tensor imaging study (DTI), which highlights the integrity of the white matter tracts, widespread reduced anisotropy was observed (Barnea-Goraly et al., 2003), indicating reductions in density, myelination, and/or fiber organization. Contrary to expectations of the "right-hemisphere" syndrome associated with NVLD (Semrud-Clikeman & Hynd, 1990), left hemisphere tracts showed more differences than right in this study. There were differences in areas associated with psychomotor and tactile skills (pre- and post-central gyri) and in regions expected to be involved in visuospatial and arithmetical reasoning (fronto-parietal) in the DTI anisotropy. Temporal-parietal regions were observed to be different in patients with VCFS, a finding that may be related to the high risk of schizophrenia in this population (Barnea-Goraly et al., 2003). While there appears to be some support for Rourke's white matter model in the work on VCFS, the findings are not conclusive, as is often the case with neuroimaging.

A Note About Neuroimaging Findings. Neuroimaging studies tend to use small samples of convenience. Because the work is relatively new and there is considerable individual variation in brains, differences in equipment, and in analytic techniques, clinicians are well advised to be conservative in their estimation of the reliability of this type of research. Moreover, it is important to be cautious about assuming that reported group neuroimaging differences are related to specific behavioral characteristics. For example, in the VCFS research described above (Barnea-Goraly et al., 2003; Eliez et al., 2000; van Amelsvoort et al., 2001), all of the studies used well-described and well-defined clinical groups, and matched control groups. Morphometric differences were observed between patients and controls, but behavioral measures were not used to tie these differences to observable characteristics in the samples. This problem is highlighted by research suggesting that even when group differences are observed, individuals within the groups may vary considerably, as is discussed below.

Utility of White Matter Model Research. Some have called into question whether the NVLD heuristic can be reasonably applied to certain populations predicted by Rourke's white matter model. In their study of children with a severe form of spina bifida known as myelomeningocele (MM), Yeates and colleagues (2003) suggested that NVLD characteristics seen within the group may not apply to individuals. About 85% of children with MM also have hydrocephalus, which is known to cause disruption to white matter in the brain, including axonal degeneration and disruption of the myelination process. As a group, these children demonstrate verbal better than nonverbal IQ, sensory and motor deficits, poor visuospatial and visuoconstructional skills, poor mathematics, difficulty with pragmatic language, and preserved word-reading and spelling skills. Yeates et al. (2003) studied 32 children with MM and their unaffected siblings, looking at the incidence of NVLD assets and deficits in these children. The authors found that although group differences were observed, the variability in the MM group was considerably higher than in the sibling group. Not all children in the MM group demonstrated the pattern of assets and deficits associated with NVLD. The authors called into question the utility of applying the NVLD heuristic to all children with MM.

Although the white matter model is important for thinking about possible neural substrates for NVLD, it offers little in the way of identifying the incidence of NVLD or the likelihood of developing NVLD for any particular child (Ris & Nortz, 2008), even when a disorder thought to be associated with the NVLD phenotype is present. Most of the youngsters who are identified with NVLD are otherwise typical school children who come to the attention of schools and parents because of learning problems. There has been a rise in awareness of NVLD, and of subsequent referrals to professionals for assessment and treatment (Grodzinsky et al., 2010). One of the most difficult challenges has been to find reliable ways to identify these children for treatment, and to understand their characteristics against the background of their typical peers.

Research on NVLD as a Developmental Disorder

More than 80 publications on NVLD have been made available since the 1970s. Although many of these were disseminated by Rourke's research laboratory, other researchers have added significantly to the work. Despite the attention given to this syndrome, consensus has been elusive (for a critical review see Fine et al., in press). Below is a short review of some of the findings based on empirical research focused on children with NVLD compared to those who are developing typically or who have verbally based learning problems. Note that there is more research available than is discussed here. Studies with strong research characteristics were chosen to be featured here, and many well-cited studies not discussed may be omitted due to concerns about the sample characteristics, diagnostic criteria, size of the study sample, and/or lack of statistical power.

Sensorimotor. Data from Rourke's lab (Pelletier et al., 2001) predicted that children with NVLD would have early grapho-motor problems that resolve, a finding which has been supported by data from additional studies. In a small study with 20 adolescents with NVLD and 15 with RD, the Rey Complex Figure did not discriminate between the groups (Semrud-Clikeman & Glass, 2008). Several studies have found nonmotor tests of visual perception, particularly using the Judgment of Line Orientation Test (JLO: Benton, Varney, & Hamsher, 1978) (e.g., Ris et al., 2007), to be a strong indicator of group membership.

Memory. Until recently, this has been an underexplored area of NVLD. In their study utilizing well-defined inclusion criteria for children with visuospatial processing symptoms, Mammarella and colleagues (2010) found support for spatial memory deficits, specifically sequential-spatial recall, in children with symptoms of NVLD compared to controls.

Language. Children with NVLD are expected to have difficulty with pragmatic language and comprehension. Language pragmatics has not been studied in this population. A few small studies have indicated that children with NLVD may have reduced ability for spatial and emotional inferencing (Humphries, Cardy, Worling, & Peets, 2004), and narrative comprehension, but not factual information (Worling, Humphries, & Tannock, 1999).

Problem Solving. Difficulties with novel problem solving have been associated with the NVLD profile. Pelletier's (2001) NVLD classification study found that WISC-III Block Design performance was a strong indicator of NVLD. The Children's Category Test has also been found as a strong predictor of NVLD (Ris et al., 2007).

Academics. Low scores on mathematics calculation tests have been a consistent rule-in for NVLD in the research. Thus, this indicator is strong for NVLD because most children included in NVLD groups have demonstrated mathematics difficulty. Mathematics reasoning has not been well studied, and one study suggested that this skill is intact for children with NVLD (Forrest, 2004). Preserved single-word reading is also a common inclusion criteria in NVLD research. However, there is no empirical group-based research on reading comprehension in NVLD.

Psychopathology. As mentioned above, much has been reported regarding the increased risk of psychopathology in NVLD, but research has not supported this suggestion. Increased internalizing disorders have not consistently been identified in either children or adults with NVLD compared to those with other learning disorders (for a review, see Fine et al., in press).

Social Perception. The literature on social perception in children with NVLD suggests that their ability to perceive humor (Semrud-Clikeman & Glass, 2008), facial affect (Bloom & Heath, 2010; Petti et al., 2002), and language prosody (Ris et al., 2007) was not distinguishable from other learning disabled groups. A subset of children with NVLD who have social problems may be more visible because they are more often clinic-referred.

In summary, the research on NVLD that focuses on how such children differ from typically developing children and those with verbal learning disabilities is not conclusive. There is much to be done, particularly in the area of social and academic functioning as well as memory and other executive functions. Moreover, the influence of attention, not discussed here, has been shown to be an important factor in all of these areas of functioning as well. However, the research does support the construct of NVLD. There are children with learning problems whose characteristics are distinct from children with RD in several key aspects, including visual perception, novel nonverbal problem solving, mathematics skill, and some aspects of language.

Conclusion

NVLD has been conceptualized from many different perspectives: clinical, medical, and academic. The body of research has ranged widely in terms of how study samples have been defined as well as the instruments used to measure the characteristics of this population. Because of this, clinicians are wise to give thought as to how our conceptions about NVLD have been inherited. When looking to the literature, carefully consider how the NVLD group was defined for a study, and whether the findings can be reasonably applied to the population with which you are working. Researchers are encouraged to explore the many areas still needing attention, including establishing the boundaries of NVLD with AS, ADHD, and mathematics disability, and better defining the reliably consistent neuropsychological and learning characteristics of children with NVLD.

References

Antshel, K. M., & Joseph, G. R. (2006). Maternal stress in nonverbal learning disorder: A comparison with reading disorder. *Journal of Learning Disabilities, 39*(3), 194–205.

Antshel, K. M., & Khan, F. M. (2008). Is there an increased familial prevalence of psychopathology in children with nonverbal learning disorders? *Journal of Learning Disabilities, 41*(3), 208–217. doi:10.1177/0022219408317546.

Barnea-Goraly, N., Menon, V., Krasnow, B., Ko, A., Reiss, A., & Eliez, S. (2003). Investigation of white matter structure in velocardiofacial syndrome: A diffusion tensor imaging study. *The American Journal of Psychiatry, 160*(10), 1863.

Benton, A. L., Varney, N. R., & Hamsher, K. (1978). Visuospatial judgment: A clinical test. *Archives of Neurology, 35*, 364–367.

Bloom, E., & Heath, N. (2010). Recognition, expression, and understanding facial expressions of emotion in adolescents with nonverbal and general learning disabilities. *Journal of Learning Disabilities, 43*(2), 180–192. doi:10.1177/0022219409345014.

Davis, J. M., & Broitman, J. (2011). *Nonverbal learning disabilities in children: Bridging the gap between science and practice*. New York: Springer.

De Smedt, B., Swillen, A., Devriendt, K., Fryns, J. P., Verschaffel, L., & Ghesquière, P. (2007). Mathematical disabilities in children with velo-cardio-facial syndrome. *Neuropsychologia, 45*(5), 885–895.

Dehaene, S., Piazza, M., Pinel, P., & Cohen, L. (2005). Three parietal circuits for number processing. In J. I. D. Campbell (Ed.), *Handbook of mathematical cognition* (pp. 433–453). New York: Psychology Press.

Devriendt, K., Fryns, J. P., Mortier, G., Van Thienen, M., & Keymolen, K. (1998). The annual incidence of DiGeorge/velocardiofacial syndrome. *Journal of Medical Genetics, 35*(9), 789.

Drummond, C. R., Ahmad, S. A., & Rourke, B. P. (2005). Rules for the classification of younger children with nonverbal learning disabilities and basic phonological processing disabilities. *Archives of Clinical Neuropsychology, 20*, 171–182.

Eliez, S., Schmitt, J. E., White, C. D., & Reiss, A. L. (2000). Children and adolescents with velocardiofacial syndrome: A volumetric MRI study. *The American Journal of Psychiatry, 157*(3), 409.

Fine, J. G., & Semrud-Clikeman, M. (2010). Nonverbal learning disabilities: Assessment and intervention. In A. Davis (Ed.), *The handbook of neuropsychology*. New York: Springer.

Fine, J. G., Semrud-Clikeman, M., Bledsoe, J., & Musielak, K. (in press). A critical review of the NLD literature as a developmental disorder. *Child Neuropsychology*.

Fine, J. G., Semrud-Clikeman, M., Butcher, B., & Walkowiak, J. (2008). Brief report: Attention effect on a measure of social perception. *Journal of Autism and Developmental Disorders, 38*(9), 1797–1802. doi:10.1007/s10803-008-0570-x.

Forrest, B. (2004). The utility of math difficulties, internalized psychopathology, and visual-spatial deficits to identify children with the nonverbal learning disability syndrome: Evidence for a visualspatial disability. *Child Neuropsychology (Neuropsychology, Development and Cognition: Section C), 10*(2), 129–146.

Geary, D. C. (2004). Mathematics and learning disabilities. *Journal of Learning Disabilities, 37*(1), 4.

Goldberg, E., & Costa, L. D. (1981). Hemisphere differences in the acquisition and use of descriptive systems. *Brain and Language, 14*, 144–173.

Grodzinsky, G. M., Forbes, P. W., & Bernstein, J. H. (2010). A practice-based approach to group identification in nonverbal learning disorders. *Child Neuropsychology, 16*(5), 433–460.

Harnadek, M. C. S., & Rourke, B. P. (1994). Principal identifying features of the syndrome of nonverbal learning disabilities in children. *Journal of Learning Disabilities, 27*(3), 144–154.

Humphries, T., Cardy, J. O., Worling, D. E., & Peets, K. (2004). Narrative comprehension and retelling abilities of children with nonverbal learning disabilities. *Brain and Cognition, 56*, 77–88.

Klin, A., Volkmar, F. R., Sparrow, S. S., Cicchetti, B. P., & Rourke, B. P. (1995). Validity and neuropsychological characterization of Asperger syndrome: Convergence with nonverbal learning disabilities syndrome. *Journal of Child Psychology and Psychiatry, 36*(7), 1127–1140.

Kobrynski, L. J., & Sullivan, K. E. (2007). Velocardiofacial syndrome, DiGeorge syndrome: The chromosome 22q11. 2 deletion syndromes. *Lancet, 370*(9596), 1443–1452.

Mammarella, I. C., Lucangeli, D., & Cornoldi, C. (2010). Spatial working memory and arithmetic deficits in childrne with nonverbal learning difficulties. *Journal of Learning Disabilities, 43*(5), 455–468.

McDonald, B. (2002). Recent developments in the application of the nonverbal learning disabilities model. *Current Psychiatry Reports, 4*(5), 323–330. doi:10.1007/s11920-002-0079-5.

Moss, E. M., Batshaw, M. L., Solot, C. B., Gerdes, M., McDonald-McGinn, D. M., Driscoll, D. A., et al. (1999). Psychoeducational profile of the 22q11. 2 microdeletion: A complex pattern. *The Journal of Pediatrics, 134*(2), 193–198.

Myklebust, H. R. (1975). *Progress in learning disabilities* (Vol. 3). New York: Grune & Stratton.

Pelletier, P. M., Ahmad, S. A., & Rourke, B. P. (2001). Classification rules for basic phonological processing disabilities and nonverbal learning disabilities: Formulation and external validity. *Child Neuropsychology, 7*(2), 84–98.

Pennington, B. F. (2009a). Issues in syndrome validation. In *Diagnosing learning disorders: A neuropsychological framework* (2nd ed., pp. 23–41). New York: The Guildford Press.

Pennington, B. F. (2009b). Nonverbal learning disability. In *Diagnosing learning disorders: A neuropsychological framework* (2nd ed., pp. 242–248). New York: The Guildford Press.

Petti, V. L., Voelker, S. L., Shore, D. L., & Hayman-Abello, S. E. (2002). Perception of nonverbal emotional cues by children with nonverbal learning disabilities. *Journal of Developmental and Physical Disabilities, 15*(1), 23–36.

Ris, D. M., Ammerman, R. T., Waller, N., Walz, N., Oppenheimer, S., Brown, T. M., et al. (2007). Taxonicity of nonverbal learning disabilities. *Journal of the International Neuropsychological Society, 13*, 50–58.

Ris, D. M., & Nortz, M. (2008). Nonverbal learning disorder. In J. E. Morgan & J. H. Ricker (Eds.), *Textbook of clinical neuropsychology: Studies on neuropsychology, neurology and cognition* (pp. 346–359). New York: Elsevier Psychology Press.

Rourke, B. P. (1989). *Nonverbal learning disabilities: The syndrome and the model.* New York: Guilford Press.

Rourke, B. P. (1995). The NLD syndrome and the white matter model. In B. P. Rourke (Ed.), *Syndrome of nonverbal learning disabilities: Neurodevelopmental manifestations*. New York: Guilford Press.

Rourke, B. P., & Finlayson, M. A. J. (1978). Neuropsychological significance of variations in patterns of academic performance: Verbal and visual-spatial abilities. *Journal of Abnormal Child Psychology, 6*(1), 121–133.

Rourke, B. P., Rourke, S., & van der Vlugt, H. (2002). *Practice of child-clinical neuropsychology*. Lisse, The Netherlands: Swets & Zeitlinger.

Rourke, B. P., & Strang, J. D. (1978). Neuropsychological significance of variations in patterns of academic performance: Motor, psychomotor and tactile-perceptual abilities. *Journal of Pediatric Psychology, 3*(2), 62–66.

Rourke, B. P., & Strang, J. D. (1983). Subtypes of reading and arithmetical disabilities: A neuropsychological analysis. In M. Rutter (Ed.), *Developmental neuropsychiatry*. Guildford: New York.

Rourke, B. P., & Tsatsanis, K. (2000). Nonverbal learning disabilities and Asperger syndrome. In A. Klin, F. R. Volkmar, & S. S. Sparrow (Eds.), *Asperger syndrome* (pp. 231–253). New York: The Guilford Press.

Rourke, B. P., Van der Vlugt, H., & Rourke, S. B. (2002). *Practice of child-clinical neuropsychology: An introduction* (Vol. 6). Taylor & Francis. Lisse, The Netherlands..

Rourke, B. P., Young, G. C., & Leenaars, A. A. (1989). A childhood learning disability that predisposes those afflicted to adolescent and adult depression and suicide risk. *Journal of Learning Disabilities, 22*, 169–175. doi:10.1177/002221948902200305.

Schafer, V., & Semrud-Clikeman, M. (2008). Neuropsychological functioning in subgroups of children with and without social perception deficits and/or hyperactivity-impulsivity. *Journal of Attention Disorders, 12*(2), 177–190.

Semrud-Clikeman, M., & Glass, K. L. (2008). Comprehension of humor in children with nonverbal learning disabilities, reading disabilities, and without learning disabilities. *Annals of Dyslexia, 58*(2), 163–180.

Semrud-Clikeman, M., & Hynd, G. W. (1990). Right hemispheric dysfunction in nonverbal learning disabilities: Social, academic, and adaptive functioning in adults and children. *Psychological Bulletin, 107*(2), 196–209.

Strang, J. D., & Rourke, B. P. (1983). Concept-formation/non-verbal reasoning abilities of children who exhibit specific academic problems in arithmetic. *Journal of Clinical Child Psychology, 12*(1), 33–39.

van Amelsvoort, T., Daly, E., Robertson, D., Suckling, J., Ng, V., Critchley, H., et al. (2001). Structural brain abnormalities associated with deletion at chromosome 22q11: Quantitative neuroimaging study of adults with velo-cardio-facial syndrome. *The British Journal of Psychiatry, 178*(5), 412.

Wechsler, D. (1991). *WISC-III manual*. San Antonio: The Psychological Corporation.

Woodin, M., Wang, P. P., Aleman, D., McDonald-McGinn, D., Zackai, E., & Moss, E. (2001). Neuropsychological profile of children and adolescents with the 22q11.2 microdeletion. *Genetics in Medicine, 3*(1), 34–39.

Worling, D. E., Humphries, T., & Tannock, R. (1999). Spatial and emotional aspects of language inferencing in nonverbal learning disabilities. *Brain and Language, 70*, 220–239.

Yeates, K. O., Loss, N., Colvin, A. N., & Enrile, B. G. (2003). Do children with myelomeningocele and hydrocephalus display nonverbal learning disabilities? An empirical approach to classification. *Journal of International Neuropsychological Society, 9*(4), 653–662.

Yu, J. W., Buka, S., McCormick, M. C., Fitzmaurice, G. M., & Indurkhya, A. (2006). Behavioral problems and the effects of early intervention on eight-year-old children with learning disabilities. *Maternal and Child Health Journal, 10*(4), 329–338.

Chapter 16
Dealing with NVLD: A Family's Perspective

Brett Mills

Family Support

I have grown up with NVLD. It has not been easy, but I am proud to say that I have achieved academically and pursued my passions. Anyone with NVLD can learn to work with (and even surpass) the barriers that they face if they receive caring guidance along the way. If you are guiding a student with NVLD, the best way to help is to listen. Understanding a student's perspective makes it easier to interject new ideas into their world. My parents were great listeners, and their dedication allowed me to be diagnosed by fourth grade. Education is important to my parents, and they did not want my learning disability to limit my future. They provided me with as many resources as they could. Through a process based in communication, my parents gave me every chance to lead a successful independent life.

My parents admit when they are wrong. They were not born experts in NVLD; they saw when things were beyond their abilities and sought advice. They sent me to a myriad of specialists before they received a conclusive diagnosis. I started seeing specialists when I was 6 years old but did not learn that I had NVLD till I was 10. There were 4 years of searching before we found an explanation for my behavior.

I needed to be an active participant in my own learning. My parents wanted me to understand why I was being asked to complete tasks that I found to be unpleasant. They made me feel like I was in the driver's seat (even when I wasn't). They helped me see learning as collecting resources so I could make my own choices. I never felt that my parents were ashamed of me or that I had to fit their vision of a perfect child. I didn't work hard because my parents or school needed me to. I worked hard for myself.

B. Mills (✉)
C/O Dr. Broitman, 2940 Forest Avenue, Berkeley, CA 94705, USA
e-mail: drjess@comcast.net

J. Broitman and J.M. Davis (eds.), *Treating NVLD in Children: Professional Collaborations for Positive Outcomes*, DOI 10.1007/978-1-4614-6179-1_16,

My mom let me express my feelings and frustrations, as much or as little I wanted. If something I had to do seemed difficult or unfair, she listened. When you have a different learning style many people will not understand how to be helpful. Having a space to freely express frustration helped me let off steam and it allowed me to feel heard. It helped me legitimize my experience to know that someone understood my perspective. Seeing my mom respect and understand me helped me learn to respect and understand myself. I learned to value my ability to face challenges that were more difficult for me than they were for the other kids.

It is hard to have difficulty with tasks that are generally considered to be enjoyable. It is isolating to not be able to connect with activities that peers love. Sometimes I needed to pretend to like things that were hard for me. I feared that not liking them meant I was inadequate. For example, I have never liked to read. It took me a long time to learn how to read and it is still tiring for me. I know that reading is a valuable skill. I enjoy discussing literature and I love the stories but the physical act of reading is not relaxing. I don't usually read on a warm summer day to pass the time. Yet, I don't like to admit this publicly. Saying that you don't like to read is like saying you don't vote or recycle; it makes you look like a jerk or an underachiever. The difficulty of having a learning disability is that you face challenges that people will not understand. You face the judgment of others and it is important to remember to go at your own pace and tackle the obstacles you think are worthwhile. It is okay to make the choice that something is not worthwhile; there are times when the effort required is not worth the potential result.

Having the courage and ability to discuss your learning disability with others is vital. It will help you deal with teachers and the occasional peer who may be troubled by some of the incoherencies you display. It is also important to know that you own the information, and that you get to choose who knows what about you. I sometimes need to be private in order to have the space to work through something without feeling pressured by the expectations of those around me. It is quite likely that I would have written off reading if I had not been given a safe environment where it was okay to not like it. In never having felt forced to like reading, I resolved my relationship with it at my own pace. I was not shamed for finding reading difficult and that helped me persevere. Eventually I respected my ability to face challenging obstacles, and I have utilized this respect to resolve other challenges in life.

Tough Love?

I don't like the concept of tough love. Some parents fear that if they don't lay down the law, they will let some lazy and malicious kid get the better of them. I believe that such a concern is misplaced when you have a child with NVLD. Whenever I discuss this issue with parents or peers, they talk about kids putting effort into a hobby that they don't appear to put into their schoolwork. It may seem look like the hobby is detracting from the student's academic potential. Instead I would argue that you should explore the hobby and try understanding the passion that the student has for it, and then build on this passion. This hobby may be the one thing from which the student can derive self-esteem when academics are a source of constant frustration. I found that being allowed to explore my interests has allowed me to be able to create goals for who I am as a person. My passions have helped me find the motivation to do well in school.

My parents never punished me when I had difficulties with a task. Some parents may fear that if they ease off on pressuring their child, their child will choose to do as little work as possible. I do not think this is true; in my experience most people want to learn and they want to succeed but they need the space to do it. Everyone learns that life is hard and unfair without their parents pushing them to do unfair and impossible tasks. I am not arguing that parents be negligent. There are of course times when a parent needs to make their child do something that they don't want to do. Not every child needs the same treatment; taking the time to learn about your child is very important. Thorough and comprehensive testing helps give some evidence-based guidance about how to approach a student's learning. These findings reveal what accommodations or modifications are actually needed. Listening does not mean always saying yes; it means trying to understand by creating a safe environment where the student can reveal what they need to you.

So, You Do Things Differently?

When you have a learning disability you experience the world differently than most people. Others make assumptions about your experience (what else can they do?) and those assumptions are often inaccurate. It is hard to remember that none of us are the baseline prototype for humanity, and it is hard to remember that others experience things differently than we do. I think this is probably a good thing for everyone to remember but it is particularly important and applicable to understanding the challenges of learning-disabled students.

Conversely, I had to learn about how most people saw me. I had to understand that my experience was not in sync with those around me; this was equally as important for me as it was for those dealing with me. I sometimes needed to be told to regulate my tone or react more keenly to a social cue; I had no other way of knowing how to adjust my behavior to fit in with my peers.

When I was first told I had a learning disability, I was shocked! I had worked with tutors for years but never received a conclusive diagnosis. I just had no idea. I always had known that my childhood was different than from everyone else's. I knew that my peers were not spending so much of their time meeting with eye doctors, occupational therapists (OT), neuropsychologists, math tutors, or English tutors. In the early half of elementary school I came to school a half hour late every Monday so I could work with an OT and work on my difficulties with body awareness. I would look at monkey bars and jump ropes and see everybody around me using them with ease and pleasure. For me, such activities were neither easy nor pleasurable. I would attempt them and my body would be unable to navigate them.

It was like trying to start a car with a dead battery—it feels like you are doing everything right only the car won't go. I moved bizarrely; I had a tendency to flail my arms and hit strangers accidentally on crowded streets.

I have not fully remediated all of these physical and social challenges but they have improved to the point that most people don't notice irregularities in my physical habits, and it would be almost impossible to connect them with my learning disability. My disability is practically invisible. I have put a lot of effort into being able to navigate my environment physically. I find crowded streets overwhelming and overstimulating (who doesn't?) but before my early teens, my brain was too distressed by the environment to make quick physical choices. I did not automatically respond to my environment. There is nothing worse than feeling like you are helpless, and I have found myself feeling that way about some pretty mundane tasks.

I experienced difficulty with an unbelievably large set of activities, but I had one where I excelled, and that was speaking. I could talk up a storm, and that ability set up a long-lasting confusion in my life—why did adults (who weren't my teachers) connect so easily to me, while kids didn't seem to like me at all? I know that this is probably something that a lot of kids have asked themselves, but my version of the question seemed very profound to me at the time; I felt like I was two different people. I did not make an active choice to act differently, but the difference in my experience with my peers versus my experience with my parents and their friends was so extreme that it felt like I was living in two different realities.

At school I felt lost and confused. I had no friends, and was either picked on or ignored. In class I was trying hard to keep my head down and get out as quickly as humanly possible. At home and around other adults I believe that my social ineptitudes were apparent, but I was not aware of this at the time. Some of this has to do with the fact that adults are often more outwardly understanding than children on a playground. Adults also have a greater appreciation for a child with an expansive vernacular. Around my parent's friends, I felt appreciated and accepted. I could talk freely and I could be funny, and they would respond to me in ways that people at school wouldn't. I am grateful for my ease with language; it has opened up more doors than it has closed but it has also created some unexpected challenges.

One major problem with my facility with speech was that I could articulate much bigger ideas than I could ever write down. I was inconsistent. Everyone was confused by the disparity between how I wrote and spoke. I had difficulty realizing how poorly I was doing in school because everything felt like hard work, and I have always associated work with success. It was a long time before I began to realize that the effort put in was far greater that the quality of products I produced.

This realization was very hard; more than anything I felt ashamed. I was horrified and angry that I could try so hard and accomplish so little. Even after I learned of my disability I couldn't forgive myself for being unable to produce work that was well received. It was difficult to accept that I had a learning disability. I made my mother promise not to tell anyone. If I found out that she did, I would throw a fit. I was so furious; it felt like the biggest betrayal to have that secret revealed.

In eighth grade I wrote an in-class essay and I felt really good about it! I loved the final sentence; it was witty and insightful. I received a high grade on it but when I actually got it back I saw that it was almost incomprehensible. It was riddled with spelling and grammatical errors. I am not sure what was more painful, seeing how unaware I was of the quality of work I had produced, or the realization that a good grade on that paper meant my teachers had either given up on me, or my standard of work was generally so low that I had actually made a major improvement. I bawled my eyes out because of this essay. When I turned the essay in I was not aware of the errors that I later noticed, because the process of writing the essay was so effortful that I was too fatigued to recognize the errors. I think I was just grateful to have finished.

I had gotten things back with lots of red ink on them before, but there was something about reading this particular paper and seeing the mistakes in it that made my deficits so clear to me. It was the first time that I saw my work the way my teachers did. It had taken me 4 years to begin to understand what my teachers were seeing. The knowledge of my learning disability that I had received in fourth grade was not enough.

People often misread external signs of my NVLD. Neurological problems were seen as psychological problems. People would suggest all sorts of ridiculous things about me. What other people saw as a psychological problem, like being too reserved and standoffish, is really an aspect of the way my brain processes information. I am pretty sure that the explanation for these "psychological issues" is in how my brain works. Some of my social behavior came from social anxieties that developed from years of being bullied. There are many rules to social interaction which most people take for granted. A lot of information is inferred through body language and tone. I didn't pick up on theses cues easily. For most neurotypical people when someone is not following these rules it is irksome. The sad thing is that it is not always apparent to people that the reason they are responding negatively to someone is because that person is simply having some difficulty navigating signals. That person, who is trying to make sense of the interaction but not succeeding, begins to look psychotic.

I remember being at a summer camp when I was 13 or 14 and a group of kids were being mean to me. I asked the counselor to intervene, and she did, but it was an intervention that ended in me being criticized by all parties involved. I ended up sitting through some dumb 16-year-old girl's explanation of the psychology of friendship, and how I had features that made me inherently unlikable. Even in that moment I knew that this was ridiculous, and that the counselor had subjected me to an even worse experience than I had been having before.

I cannot totally fault the people involved in this sadly painful experience. They didn't know what was going on with me, and were confused and freaked out by my atypical behavior. If they had understood what was actually going with me, I hope that they would have been a bit more sensitive. Like any disorder or handicap, there is nothing you can do about having NVLD other than try to work with it. In perfect world people would be more supportive of the truly good-natured attempts at connection made by the socially disadvantaged. As a disorder NVLD is not well understood, and people can be quick to draw unfair and inaccurate conclusions.

I was aware I had physical difficulties as far back as the monkey bars, but those were things that I could avoid. It took me a long time to realize that difficulty with monkey bars could relate to difficulties with other unavoidable activities, such as navigating how to use a public bus. My awareness of how my learning disability affected my whole being became clearer after age ten when I received the diagnosis. I have only recently been able to deal with my learning disability openly. In spite of having great support in my entire life, I have never been able to shake my desire to feel normal and to fit in. I have wanted to eradicate my learning disability and forget its existence. Hiding that you have a learning disability is rarely beneficial; the sooner that a student can speak openly about their learning disability the better. Academic life is full of evaluations from teachers; grades and report cards are meant to be a report of a student's performance but if a teacher is missing the full picture their evaluation is only based on their perception of your product. I have received painful report cards because a teacher misunderstood me. People who did not understand me have said things that were mean and inaccurate, but the truth is that these people were not always given information to help them contextualize my behavior.

The ability to self-advocate will make any student have a more successful relationship with the teachers and peers that they encounter. Those people will also be able to give better feedback in light of what they understand about you. That said, though external evaluations are useful and sometimes accurate, it is important to be able to see those evaluations as nothing more than someone else's opinion, take what is useful, and disregard the rest. I see external evaluations as good indicators of how I am being perceived but I rarely see them as more than that. Having this attitude is a double-edged sword—on the one hand it provides me with self-protection, but on the other hand it is very hard for me to accept the negative feedback. It is hard to allow yourself to openly fail in front of others. I spent so much time trying to sweep my difficulties under the rug. I learned that letting them sit out in the open is ultimately a better way of coping with them.

There are still individuals who cannot handle the responsibility of an LD student. But on the whole, openness with yourself and others is the best policy. I have rarely had someone reject me for telling them that I had a learning disability; I have gotten into way more trouble when I have tried to hide it. My understanding of my NVLD has evolved with my willingness to acknowledge its existence. I am now in a place where I can examine it. I have become more comfortable with my disability through time and through more positive social and academic experiences. As far as I am concerned there cannot be enough emphasis put on the importance of self-esteem. If you can avoid being ashamed of your NVLD you can accomplish amazing things; fear and self-loathing can really stunt your potential.

The School Day

School was embarrassing, and I did not want to be there. I didn't skip class physically, but my attempts to not stick out too much or admit to my difficulty meant I might as well have. I lived by a philosophy that I like to call "get through the day." So from the bus ride going to school, until the bus ride going home, I was focused on avoiding all possible conflicts or hiccups. This meant minimizing things as much as possible that made me feel terrible about myself, such as most of my more academic classes and P.E. I have always been a very quick thinker when it comes to speaking. If I was in gym class and we had to do cartwheels, I would come up with all sorts of reasons as to why I could not do cartwheels that day. I am sure that in retrospect many of those excuses were transparent, but even so they were compelling enough that teachers did not force the issue. I would say things like "going upside down gives me a headache," "I am sore," and "I am sick." I have faked sickness more times in my life than I would care to admit. I hated failing at things, and I would do or say anything to avoid the embarrassment.

I am fortunate that I went to schools with frequent parent–teacher conferences. The issues I was not willing to discuss with my teachers, my parents discussed for me. I did not always like knowing that my parents had talked to my teachers about my learning disability. But even when I got angry I always knew their talking to my teachers was in my best interest. The hardest part of my learning disability was acknowledging it, and having my parents address it directly for me ultimately felt like an act of kindness. Once my teachers knew about my learning disorder, they made an effort to be helpful. There were the rare few who didn't believe in learning disabilities, but they mostly joined the bandwagon, if only because they were given no other choice. One thing that worked in my favor is that I am generally a nice, well-behaved kid, and even when they were frustrated I think my teachers felt bad for me and tried to help.

The problem with my "get through the day" philosophy was that I was trying so hard to avoid embarrassment that I was not focused on making sure that I had everything I needed to be successful. I was trying to avoid admitting to being wrong or making mistakes. I said that I had forms I didn't have, and that I understood things I did not understand. The sad result of my "getting through the day" life meant that I wasn't honest at school; the only way that I survived was by having a really wonderful team of people who could help straighten out what had become so convoluted during the course of my day. School had one function: it was the place I went to be given homework. My team/parents had to figure out what completing that homework would require and relay it back to me. I went to school but most of my learning took place outside of it. I learned at home and then returned to school the next day acting as though I had in fact been getting the information like everyone else. I have clear memories of sitting in class and thinking "well, I have no idea what this guy's talking about, but I'll get that all sorted out later." So school was a time to sit, stare, nod, and be socially traumatized.

Frequently, a teacher would sit me down after class and suggest an alternative and creative version of a homework assignment, so as to even the playing field with the other kids. Understandably the teachers wanted a fuller understanding of what I did and didn't know. Many of these solutions were coming from good but uninformed places. I had a particularly uninspiring moment in a middle school science class where a teacher told me that I was getting a B on an assignment where I had really only earned a C. He said that in light of my difficulties he was going to boost my grade. This put me in an awkward and unfair situation. My teacher could have given me the C or he could have given me the B and not told me about it. He told me, and I felt both patronized and guilty for getting special treatment. I also felt bad for not doing well. I wanted to earn my successes, I struggled in that class and I worked hard to master the material, but the skills required of me were in some of my weakest areas. It is understandable that the teacher wanted to award my efforts but that was completely undermined when he told me I did not deserve the grade I received. Instead he only made me feel worse about my learning difficulties. I imagine that he felt guilty or uncomfortable with the choice he had made but he should have dealt with the issue differently. If he truly felt uncomfortable he could have talked one of his fellow teachers or my parents; telling me helped no one.

Modifying an assignment or shifting a standard might be necessary when dealing with an LD student. The goal of this should be to remove aspects of an assignment that are disproportionately difficult for an LD student and are not related to the core concept of the assignment. For example, if you are teaching a class about American history and you ask students to draw a map of the USA, you may wish to excuse the student with NVLD from this assignment. Many kids might find the map assignment fun and low stress, but the student with NVLD will struggle with the visual–spatial aspects of drawing and not learn a thing about geography. The artistic aspects of drawing a map might be one of the agents through which one was hoping to teach a lesson about the USA, but it is not the core concept. For a student with NVLD, the lesson about the geography of the USA would be obstructed by the difficult challenge of drawing. If the difficult aspect of an assignment is supposed to be difficult for everyone, then mastering this difficulty may be the point of the class and may not be avoidable (even if challenging). The ideal assignment modifications are the ones that remove the nonessential steps that are obstacles to obtaining critical conceptual understanding. These are steps that were never meant to be difficult. Allowing a student to use a laptop or having extended time on a test are examples of modifications that remove difficulties that the other kids don't experience.

Some classes are more difficult than others and there is not always an obvious way for an NVLD student to access the material. When most teachers suggested ways in which I could attempt to work to improve the product I was giving them, they often suggested generic LD aids like color coding and highlighting; these are things that don't happen to work for me. Once, a teacher noticed that I was talking under my breath while trying to solve a math problem and suggested that I actually record myself doing my homework so she could listen for what I was missing, or perhaps see that I understood more than I could put on the page. It was not right for me, but to her credit she was trying. I have to hand it to all my old teachers—for all the things I wish they never wrote or said about me, they were faced with a difficult task and many of them did try. There was a nightmarish moment in seventh grade when a teacher thought she was being inspirational or doing what no one else dared do, and she yelled at me telling me that I was lazy and that she saw through my "act." This woman really has no business being an educator and I hope that she has since changed careers, but the point is that even she was trying her best. Even though it could feel like a battle, everyone wanted to see me succeed.

The Team

I attended a very nice private middle school and for most kids I think it was ideal. They nurtured the "whole child." My mother did a lot to help educate the staff about NVLD and learning disabilities in general. They had their hearts in the right place, but to be truthful I hated almost every second of my time there. As toxic as school may have been, the places I went afterward were always supportive. I truly discovered how I learn with my team. There were times when we were all stumped about how I was going to learn something but it didn't stop us; instead we just dove in together.

The team was successful because the team tailored my education to my specific needs. Most large middle schools and high schools are unable to do that. The general assumption of a lot of educators is that they need to do something to get kids to learn. My team approached me from a different angle—they assumed that my heart was in the right place and that I wanted to learn. They worked to figure out how I could learn best. They were my allies and I felt very comfortable around them; I was able to honestly tell them what I was struggling with. I could say things that I was unable to say to anyone else, and the best part is that they believed in my potential and never thought I was a lost cause. They made me feel like my achievements were legitimate achievements as opposed to making me feel like I was constantly playing catch up.

Anxiety was detrimental to my success. The team helped me lower and/or contain my anxiety. If something went wrong at school, I began to learn how to tolerate it and deal with it later. I enjoyed working with my team; they taught me that I actually liked to learn. Since school was often nothing more than a physical location I visited between 8:30 am and 3:30 pm, you may wonder why I didn't just switch schools or become homeschooled; the answer is complicated. I really didn't want to change schools because I was scared of the changes I might face, and I actually begged my parents to let me stay. There was a part of me that felt like I would be giving up if I didn't tough it out. I didn't want to feel like my school "beat me." Should I have left? Homeschooling would not have worked. I had trouble making friends but I desperately wanted friends and needed to be around people. It is a weird truth of NVLD—connections are craved yet very difficult to make. I didn't want extended family and members of the outside world to see how affected I was.

A lot of it was about my ego, and again I can't say what the "right" choice would be. It is very personal. I can't even say if I regret staying there or not.

My team has been both large and small depending on my developmental needs. In the beginning I saw someone almost every day, and by the end I was basically just seeing a single neuropsychologist. By the end of my time with this man I was prepared to teach myself. The thing that he got more than anyone else was the importance of breaking down an assignment into individualized steps. My learning specialist realized that the more crowded a page was, the harder it was for me to see essential information. We spent a lot of time breaking down an assignment into chunks of essential information and tackling them one by one. Because NVLD has an organizational deficit, it was important for me to have someone teach me how to break down tasks into manageable chunks. He would literally go over each and every step of something repeatedly till I knew how to replicate it. The best way I can describe what he did is say that he made space for me to learn. He took what was too convoluted and congested for me and helped give it breathing room so I could digest it. He called it "reducing cognitive overload." I wish I could be more descriptive about his process but as the recipient of his wisdom I didn't know his thought process when he made the choices he made. I do know that working with him helped me immensely. His goal was to understand me; he spent a lot of time listening to me and trying to see all the factors that contributed to my struggles. My neuropsychologist's office felt like a sanctuary, where I felt the most free to honestly express my difficulties. I am enormously grateful and could never thank him enough for what he did for me. I only hope that others in my position are so lucky.

A Safe Environment for Academic and Social Growth

A huge mistake people can make is to find themselves in a teacher/parent/student battle. As soon as that relationship becomes adversarial it becomes impossible. Everyone needs to work from the perspective that the student wants to be successful, and that any sense of dishonesty or laziness is probably coming from the student feeling discouraged, scared, and ashamed of difficulties. There are a myriad of reasons why someone may be averse to certain tasks and the most important thing is to create an optimal working environment.

I have learned that most things can be accomplished with patience and perseverance. The biggest hindrance to my success has been the fear I had of expressing when things were hard for me. It would allow me to sit in a class for weeks and not know what was going on. No one would be the wiser until a test came around and it was clear I had learned nothing. The most valuable lesson I have learned so far is to be okay with failing—this is different from accepting failure. What I mean is learning how to say "okay, that didn't work, so it is time to go back to the drawing board and try something different." I don't think that self-laceration does much for anyone.

One problem is that I had been at the same school from kindergarten through eighth grade. Going to the same school for 9 years makes it difficult to reinvent yourself or the way people see you. You may change, but it can be hard for others to see that change. When I left middle school my life changed drastically. Kids are mean, and that is just a fact. The other fact is that I was weird, and although there may be no such thing as "normal" it is really important to acknowledge that while we are all unique snowflakes, some snowflakes are just a tad more unique than others. I was a great target for bullying, which sadly denied me the social world I so desperately wanted to be a part of. This social world was infinitely more important to me than my academic advancement. My hatred of school was more linked to these social issues than to my actual struggles with academics. My fear of the social ramifications and potential problems caused me to hide my learning disability, and it meant that I sabotaged my academic success because of social anxiety.

Life at that school was very unpleasant, and I can't stress enough how important it is to deal with the social element. When I was socially prosperous, I felt emotionally confident enough to manage other things. When I was insecure and depressed, I became unmotivated. When I was more excited to go to school and not actively afraid of being bullied or teased, I performed better academically.

When looking into high schools, one option that I considered was a large public school. I had to get an IEP done in order to see what accommodations I would need. I remember meeting with a counselor from that school who told me that I would be put into special ed for a few of my classes. She asked me how I would feel about being a "special ed kid" and in the moment I said I could handle it, but from that moment on I realized that I had no intention of ever going there. I hate to say it but my ego would not allow me to accept that label I was not willing to call myself a "special ed kid"; it felt wrong. I just didn't need another school where I would be isolated, teased, or bullied.

I left the school that I attended for the first 9 years with specific goals. I was determined to have friends and feel normal. In my new high school, I initially tried to make myself as small as possible and not offend anyone; it became the art of becoming invisible. I pretended that my NVLD was over and that I could move on. I was forced to meet with the school's learning specialist, and though initially reluctant, I learned she was a resource.

My high school experience was infinitely better than my previous 9 years of education had been. I ended up choosing a small school tailored to kids who had not been successful in their previous learning environment. Many had some kind of learning disability, but there were a variety of reasons why students ended up there. My freshman year math teacher was dedicated and gave me as much help as necessary for me to succeed in his class. I did not get an A but I did learn, and I gave my best effort. The teacher paid enough attention to me to understand how it was difficult for me; even if I did not become the best student in his class, he recognized my hard work and progress. Being seen honestly is a big deal.

My social life evolved enormously during high school. The small size of my high school allowed me to not become overwhelmed; I could navigate my world with ease. My high school attracted kids with a variety of backgrounds, but the thing that we all had in common was that we had some kind of difficulty that kept us from thriving at a more traditional school. This meant that the students shared a common need to fit in and succeed although we were also very different from one another. In learning to get along with a variety of people in a safe environment I become more confident and ultimately able to interact with people anywhere. By the end of my time there, I barely needed my school anymore. I outgrew it. I don't think that my school had a particularly strong pedagogy, but most of my teachers were at least adequate. The school catered to a less academically rigorous track of students than the school that I previously attended and that meant my freshman year of high school was basically a repeat of what I learned in eighth grade. Learning something twice has proven to work very well for me. I was academically a big fish at this school and that was refreshing. It helped me feel better about myself; it's nice to feel like you are good at things.

Developing a Social Life

At this point I need to talk about something that I have very mixed feelings about. This idea of learning how to be socially successful is complicated; I can't quite tell you what did it for me. I watched a lot of situational comedies, which I think were useful because of their exaggerated quality—they made certain dynamics clearer than they might have been in real life.

Another learning technique for me was trial and error; I learned a lot from watching other people. Once I learned that everyone was scared to meet new people I realized that I could take more risks to render myself more socially vulnerable. Nervousness had hindered me, and I was defensive when it wasn't called for. There is an unwritten rulebook that you need to study in terms of how far to stand away from people and when to make eye contact, and I learned that the rules were less concrete than I thought. I learned that if you watch and listen to other people they will show you how they want to be interacted with. Everyone learns how to interact from their environment; it just took me longer.

Here is the part that I have reservations about. I read a book on NVLD that suggested one should learn to fake certain kinds of interactions and join clubs, learn how to throw parties, etc. for the sake of guaranteeing contact with others, but it did not say anything about learning how to preserve your sense of a true self. I spent a lot of energy in my early teen years becoming friends with people I didn't even like just because they were willing to talk to me. I had a lot of superficial interactions, and even though I think that some of this behavior comes with the age, I believe I did it more than most. I put a lot of effort into managing a façade in order to just have any kind of social life. It took me a long time to be able to choose who I actually wanted to be friends with and to understand that I didn't have to fake social interactions. I could be true to who I was and do the things I wanted to do.

I don't want people with NVLD to think that all of their natural behaviors and inclinations need to be stamped out in order to be successful. I think you need to be very kind and forgiving to yourself and willing to get to know yourself in such a way that you can be your own guide. No one else is going to quite get what's going on in there so you need to be okay with it and work through your deficits in a way that still allows you to enjoy your life. So much of my life has been strained and effortful; there are times when it is too much. It's important to be able to find time to relax and accept yourself.

Picking a College

Applying to college was another hurdle. My GPA was a 4.0, but my SAT scores would put me at a disadvantage. My math score alone would eliminate colleges that would otherwise be a good fit. I realized that I was no longer interested in struggling; I wanted college to be a time where I studied what interested me in environments where I could do well. And so I chose not to take the SAT. I only applied to schools that did not require it, and furthermore, I was only interested in schools that had minimal general education requirements. All of these choices could look lazy to the outside world, but they were made because I was ready to attend a school that allowed me to custom design my education. I'd been thinking about my learning process for many years. My choice of a college was about finding an environment that not only tolerated but respected approaches to learning that suited my strengths and skills. The school I chose proven to be an excellent learning environment for me.

So, What Do You Do with All of This Information?

I have learned that trial and error combined with perseverance eventually yields growth. The one thing I hope that others take away from what I have written is that it is essential to set clear personal goals based on who a student is as a unique individual. Sometimes the goals you want to achieve are not realistic for where you are at a given point in your development, but it is the very act of establishing and examining goals that ultimately prepares someone to take control of their own development. If you have NVLD never cease to challenge yourself but always allow yourself the space to step away from a problematic situation and examine what you want to get out of it. The biggest reason the team is important is that they are independent consultants who are devoted to YOUR education. If having a team is not financially feasible, it is still important to think about what you want, separate from what a school or teacher asks you to want. This does not mean never cooperating with teachers; it just means that you must be protective of your own needs while you work with them.

Once you accept your learning disability as a lifelong process, you can focus more specifically on achieving goals that will lead to a happy life. I have said it a few times but I'll say it again: my parents were my key. They were supportive, and without that support I could not have achieved what I have achieved. It is so important for parents to be active. I felt like they would have stayed up all night with me if that was needed for me to learn something. I wish that I had grown up in an environment where a learning disability was not something to be ashamed of. I hope it becomes something that kids can communicate clearly and honestly about.

Dealing with NVLD: A Family's Perspective

Brett Mill's Father

As Brett's father I write with something of an "outsider's" perspective, since I had very little knowledge or experience with learning disabilities before Brett came into our lives. I understood the perspective of Brett's teachers: the incomprehension, the feeling that it was somehow Brett's fault for not paying sufficient attention, and the frustration of having what had worked before suddenly not work when trying to teach him about school subjects or about social interactions. I am an engineer, a linear thinker, someone for whom long chains of logic are both pleasurable and the way to approach problems or learning.

Brett and I both owe a great debt to his mother. I'm sure that without her knowledge and perspective things would not have gone nearly as well. I'm not sure I would have identified on my own what was making Brett so unique, and it is far from clear that the schools would have either. One thing I will take credit for is the early resolution not to try to force Brett into my own ideas about what would be fun to do or study, or to try to get him to be like me. I was agnostic about whether he should like science, or sports, or hiking, or watching educational television, or reading (even though I really like those things and had initial hopes of sharing them with my son). I do strongly believe (along with my wife) that each person should figure out their passions and then pursue them, and I think we left room for Brett to aim his life in the direction that appealed to him.

It didn't take very long to notice that Brett was different than I expected. He had a series of obsessions as a toddler (spray bottles, vacuum cleaners, car keys) that he was very single-minded about. He became quite an expert in each, and was unhappy if not able to return to the favored type of object with high frequency. The car key thing got to be a great source of entertainment; he could identify keys of a great many models and years with no brand identification, to the amazement of our friends. On the other hand, the simplest of puzzles was beyond him. I also became aware that at about 3 years of age, while he knew numbers (in several languages), he couldn't count. The ordered one-to-one connection between the number words and a small collection of marbles was opaque to him.

Our greatest source of pride at these early ages was Brett's amazing articulateness. He picked up adult words easily, and used them correctly in complex sentences. He was always far more comfortable among adults, who were generally impressed with how smart he was. This was in great contrast to being with his fellow toddlers, where his interests had little intersection with theirs. They were far more into physical play than he was; he preferred to engage teachers or babysitters in a discussion beyond his years. Kids seemed to pick up that he wasn't like them, and didn't treat him well. He was averse to our attempts to bring him to "kid events," be they birthday parties, play dates, gym classes, or the like.

Our choices of day care, then schools, were first informed by what we thought would be best for him (with a model of ourselves in mind). His preschool was creative and free-form, but he clearly did not take advantage of that. He tended to stick closely to his teacher and only enjoy highly structured activities. The social difficulties were apparent fairly quickly, and became more obvious over time. He really hated to go to school; by the time we were carpooling to elementary school it was often quite a drama to go to the car or to say goodbye. His great verbal adeptness contrasted more and more with deficits in other areas. One of my favorite examples is when he was "interviewing" for kindergarten at a snooty private school. They asked kids to sign in at the door, but Brett was not capable of writing his name at that time. I think he sensed it was a test, but in any case he informed the teacher that he preferred to check the school out first before deciding whether to leave his name. This seemed to be a novel response that they enjoyed; they warmly let him go on in (but didn't admit him).

I was inclined to view Brett's characteristics as quirky, but didn't think much about whether anything more serious was in play. My wife was much more tuned into Brett's oddities, partly because she understood child development much more deeply. She kept insisting on tests, and then treatments. I was skeptical, but went along. As we proceeded into the early grades, however, it became increasingly clear that she was right. We didn't have a name to put to it until the diagnosis of NVLD. Upon hearing the description of this rather poorly known (at the time) LD, we immediately saw how well it fit. Brett's various physical, academic, and social struggles suddenly fell into place. This caused me to change how I basically thought about Brett, but it didn't solve for me the problem of how to teach him. I'm sorry to say that both he and his mom had to argue with me on many occasions about how things were going at school, and what could be done about it. After a while I felt it was better to defer to him and the experts; I was clearly out of my known territory.

I was one of the "team," and one of my main ongoing tasks was to provide homework help. This was part of what Brett has described as repeating in a safer environment what the school thought it was accomplishing. I'm afraid that I wasn't really in any better shape than his teachers to understand what would work in teaching him, though of course I was very sympathetic to the idea that something new needed to be found. I would engage in long patient explanations, going over material again and again if he didn't seem to get it, but still employing my linear logical way of seeing things. At first I was a believer in "tough love," but after a while it was clear that I needed to get on Brett's side, because he was a motivated and disciplined kid and when things didn't work it had nothing to do with a lack of motivation on his part. It was many years before I understood that part of what Brett had to do differently was in organizing these logical chains; he couldn't really keep track of the whole thing at once. Tasks had to be broken down into subtasks that he could master.

There were frankly things in his high school science and math classes that he simply couldn't master; the things that relied on getting a whole long chain of things right and in the right order. I gained a new appreciation of "math phobia," and a new sympathy for the idea that the population is not homogeneous on the basic thought structures that take place in disparate areas like math, art, writing, etc. This has helped me as I do trainings for people in my own work. I came to appreciate as well that it was not important that he master some of these things. He was much better than I in other areas and his interests were aligned with his abilities.

One arena where Brett made steady progress was in writing. His verbal output had always shown that he was a deep and sophisticated thinker. The physical act of handwriting was difficult for him, and used up too much of his cognitive bandwidth. This meant that his early essays had poor handwriting, a lot of syntactical and grammatical problems, and organizational problems. He would repeat himself, and had little concept of paragraphs. Needless to say, teachers had trouble judging such work, even if it actually contained a unique and sophisticated thought at the core of it. You could talk to him about the subject of the essay and easily find that he brought a high level of analysis to it. More importantly, he often also brought a perspective that nobody else had thought of, yet was very interesting or compelling.

I (and some of his English teachers) saw that with enough practice and instruction there was real hope that he would become a fine writer. I did not, therefore, feel any regret about letting him dictate essays to me when possible, and correcting mechanical errors in them (while we slowly worked on what those were, along with the organizational problems). He finally developed the ability to keyboard, which removed the appearance of sloppiness that his handwriting conveyed. By the time he finished high school he was an accomplished writer, and he successfully went to college.

On the social side of things, it was easier for me to sympathize with Brett. Having been a "nerd" myself, I could understand how other kids respond to behaviors outside their norms. I also understood that Brett didn't have the advantages I had in dealing with it; I was understood to be the "smart kid," and was also athletically adept. It was very painful to see how much Brett wanted to be social, and how hard it was for him before high school. My own defense mechanism had been to work very hard not to care what others thought or need their company; I developed a number of solitary activities that I greatly enjoyed. I tried to impart this strategy to Brett, but it clearly did not fit his personality. At the end of the day, this was something that Brett had to figure out for himself. It was clearly tied to his level of self-esteem, and when that got high enough (as he understood himself better), he began to find more social success.

Speaking of self-esteem, this was another area that his mother worked incessantly on, always validating what he was doing and expressing love at every opportunity. At first I thought she was being excessive (being more a fan of tough love myself, as my parents had been). This led to increasing strains in our marriage, as I felt undermined in what I viewed as an important component of childrearing.

It was a source of conflict, and probably confusing for Brett as we battled about whether he was being coddled about something, or should be made to take more energy to figure something out. As my understanding of the true situation grew and the depth of Brett's learning disability became apparent, I was able to stand down from my tough love philosophy. It became clear that the world was providing a much clearer picture of all its hazards than any lessons I might concoct. I realized that there was no question that Brett had a strong work ethic, and he was putting much more effort into difficult tasks than the output made obvious. Indeed, being supportive loving parents became obviously essential to our child's health. I wish I had grasped this from the beginning, but fortunately (for both Brett and our marriage) I was able to adjust in time. There was a time when we despaired whether Brett would ever be able to function independently in the world. Through his own perseverance and strength and our support, he has put those fears to rest permanently. He is well launched, and is his own man successfully navigating his own path. We are very proud of him.

Dealing with NVLD: A Family's Perspective

Brett Mill's Mother

As Brett Mills' mother I have been asked to describe our process of developing and working with a team of professionals in order to help our son figure out how he learns. What follows is his history. By no means am I suggesting that this is the only way or even best way to work with a child with NVLD, it's just what we did. Each child with NVLD is unique; each family must sort out how to best allocate their resources. Our family was in the fortunate position of having only one child and sufficient financial resources, and a parent (me) who could devote herself full time to managing his care.

We first noticed that Brett had issues when at 8 months old he was talking in full sentences but hardly crawling. Although he did walk at one he wasn't very physical, hated all the typical baby gym activities like Gymboree, and seemed overstimulated and overly anxious when separations occurred. Brett was visibly agitated and uncomfortable at birthday parties, or in large groups. Although it alarmed his father and me we developed a wait-and-see attitude.

By the time he was 4 years of age he still initiated little physical exploration or manipulation of his environment. Our entire baby-proofing efforts were wasted! His fine motor skills seemed delayed. For example he couldn't manipulate scissors. His drawings seemed immature, with no awareness of line. By kindergarten he still had no ability to form or recognize letters, even his own name. He could count with a perfect accent in five languages but had no letter or number recognition until first grade. There were clearly unexplainable gaps in his abilities.

In kindergarten Brett had his first assessment by the learning specialist at his school. The findings were positive for a visual/perceptual disability and a motor coordination problem. This was the beginning of both the ever-changing diagnoses and creating our team. Brett was referred for a physical therapy (PT) evaluation, which was positive for sensory motor difficulties. We were told he had "dyspraxia," which we described to him saying "your muscles are having trouble understanding/hearing what your brain wants you to do. We are going to train your muscles to get the messages better so you can have more fun and control."

Brett began occupational therapy twice a week. In addition he was referred to an educational specialist for reading/handwriting assistance. Brett began educational therapy twice a week and weekly psychotherapy. In addition we were referred an optometry clinic for eye tracking training. There he began what would be 6 months of daily eye exercises that would need to be repeated again at age 14. His team now consisted of four professionals: an occupational therapist (OT), a physical therapist (PT), a learning specialist, and a cognitive behavioral therapist.

By the time Brett entered fourth grade it was apparent that his "problem" was more than simple dyspraxia, evidenced by the fact that his math skills were still significantly below grade level and his thinking appeared "unique." Social problems had continued and he was often found isolated without friends, wandering around talking to himself in the school yard.

At this time a referral was made for a comprehensive neuropsychological evaluation, which found a 40 standard score point discrepancy between his very high verbal IQ and his performance IQ, significant visual–spatial, organizational difficulties, and motor difficulties. His diagnosis was atypical NVLD. I had never heard of this disability and my catch up intensive learning process began. We told him we had learned that "You see things differently than most people and have your own unique way of understanding things … that you had been aware of this and devised your own ways of coping but some of the mechanisms took great effort and interfered with learning things … and some of these things get you into trouble and teased by kids at school (like talking to yourself to decompress). We will sort it out together and figure out how to help you."

We made a lot of apologies for failing to understand how difficult things were for him and not recognizing how hard he had been trying. We were confused and hadn't known if the problem was that he wasn't trying hard enough or if he was being oppositional. We adjusted the team—adding twice-weekly learning therapy with a neuropsychologist. This continued until the end of high school. These sessions helped Brett figure out how he learned best, by focusing on his executive functions and math skills and reducing his cognitive overload. During the next 8 years Brett also had a variety of team members who came and went. We generally used his interests and passions to guide us.

We were able to arrange the following accommodations with his middle school:

1. *Registration and teacher choice*: Preferential registration to classes with teachers sensitive to LD issues. We looked for teachers who were known to be clear about their expectations and assignments, who were willing to modify assignments that emphasized visual–spatial issues or sequential multistep processes in order to allow him alternative ways of showing his mastery, who did not penalize him

unduly for spelling errors or reversals, and who supported his thinking and creativity. We helped them understand why materials might not get to or from school in a timely manner.

2. *Test taking*: We were able to arrange longer test time in a distraction-free environment, a recorder for bubble tests, and a revised spacing on tests when needed.
3. *Homework*: We arranged for his homework assignments to be listed on the web, faxed, or emailed home, explaining that verbal instructions or handouts were easily lost in the transitions. Brett was also given permission to dictate or verbally record long homework assignments.
4. *Gym*: We had Brett's P.E. reassigned to appropriate activities as needed.
5. *Class notes*: We arranged for copies of class notes to be made available directly to us and all of the team members.
6. *Math accommodations*: The school also agreed to make modifications of assignments involving visual–spatial skills such as graphs and or charts. Brett was permitted the use of a laptop and a calculator in math and eventually was allowed to do math as an independent study.

You might ask why we didn't homeschool Brett or find a better K-8 school for him? For one thing, we didn't want to isolate him at home since we knew his future success depended on his capacity to make friends and form connections. By the time Brett was diagnosed in fourth grade he seemed to have a few friends he didn't want to lose by moving to a new school. Also, there just weren't any better options in our area. There wasn't a school that could encourage his curiosity, support his superb verbal skills, and work with his math and visual–spatial deficits. We worked very closely with Brett's team to continually assess what made the most sense at each stage of his development. At various points his team consisted of OT, a learning specialist, neuropsychologist, physical trainer, and a music teacher. To this day I can't decide if leaving him in the same school until high school was the correct decision or not.

Remaining in such a difficult environment for 9 years deeply affected Brett emotionally, but he claims he gained a lot from making it through those unpleasant years. Was the cost was too high? I don't know. The decision was partially impacted by how hard I had worked with his school to arrange for him to receive the accommodations that he needed. In-service trainings were arranged and created for the entire school to educate them about working with learning disorder and NVLD in particular. They were open to, and excited about, better serving this population. I feared that no matter which school he was enrolled in, he would need the same learning aids. That is because they weren't as related to how hard or fast paced the curriculum was so much as to how the information was presented or how much material he was required to produce.

Luckily, Brett's high school suited him exceptionally well. By then we knew what worked best for Brett. The high school was small, very structured (almost rigid), and had rules and consequences for everything. It specialized in all sorts of different learners and was open to individualized programs. It had a good history and English faculty and an excellent arts program. The school allowed Brett to take advanced math and chemistry through an independent study program set up as a one-on-one tutorial. He worked very hard during extremely long days (including homework), but learned a tremendous amount, graduating with a 4.00 GPA. He made friends and seemed happier, though his chapter suggests this period was still fraught with difficulty. He learned that he liked to write and was good at it.

Brett was accepted early decision at his first choice college. As he stated, he wanted a place where he could individualize his education and not be forced to learn in ways that were a struggle for him. True to his nature, he took several advanced level classes in his first term and once again repeated his pattern of working like crazy to prove to himself that he could succeed. And indeed he did—at a prestigious college! Thankfully he appears to have moved on from that need, and now has fun learning things he enjoys in a manner that suits his learning style.

When I look at his current success, I have great awe and admiration for his perseverance and strength. Brett is an independent, professional young man with clear goals and a realistic plan for obtaining them. He has talent, passion, and healthy close relationships. He knows how to use his unique and creative mind. Life truly got better for Brett once he was out of middle school! One of the secrets to his success was that we were able to pull together and thoroughly use a superb team of professionals. They made it their mission and business to figure out what Brett needed to successfully learn. My model was that if he didn't understand me, it was my error and I needed to learn how to explain it better so that he could understand.

I'm very sorry that public resources are extremely limited for children with NVLD. Brett is fortunate in that we were able to provide all the services he needed and one can see that he required a lot of services. Each member of the team provided crucial training and guidance. Professionals such as these can help families to create their own team based on the unique needs of their child with NVLD. Our journey had no road maps or suggestions to guide us. I'm guessing and hoping that it will be easier for those who walk this path after Brett.

Chapter 17
Conclusion

Jessica Broitman and John M. Davis

We now summarize some of the key points in each chapter, and end with some final thoughts. Chapter 2 provides a history of NVLD. We survey the etiology and symptoms of the disorder. It is estimated that 10–15% of all learning disabled students have NVLD (Ozols & Rourke, 1988)). The most current model of understanding NVLD is from a neurological perspective and commonly called the "white matter model." We offer a developmental picture of how the child with NVLD might appear throughout his/her lifespan. We identify five major categories of deficits and dysfunction: motor, visual–spatial, organizational, social, and sensory. Motor deficits include poor coordination, severe balance problems, and difficulties with graphomotor skills. Visual–spatial/organizational deficits reflect a lack of image formation, poor visual recall, faulty spatial perceptions, and difficulties with executive functions. These executive functioning difficulties include decision making, planning, initiative, assigning priority, sequencing, motor control, emotional regulation, problem-solving, planning, impulse control, establishing goals, monitoring results of action, self-correcting, and problems with spatial relations. Social deficits include difficulties comprehending nonverbal communication, adjusting to transitions and novel situations, along with deficits in social judgment and social interaction. The last category refers to sensitivity in any of the sensory modes: visual, auditory, tactile, taste, or olfactory.

In addition we offer a four-subtype model and the research which supports our model. It is our contention that all children who present with NVLD have visual–spatial and executive function difficulties relative to their non-impacted peers.

J. Broitman, Ph.D. (✉)
San Francisco Psychotherapy Research Group, 9 Funston Street,
San Francisco, CA 94129, USA
e-mail: drjess@comcast.net

J.M. Davis, Ph.D.
California State University, East Bay, 25800 Carlos Bee Blvd,
Hayward, CA 94542-3095, USA
e-mail: jack.davis@csueastbay.edu

J. Broitman and J.M. Davis (eds.), *Treating NVLD in Children: Professional Collaborations for Positive Outcomes*, DOI 10.1007/978-1-4614-6179-1_17,

Therefore we consider these deficits to be the primary components of NVLD, constituting our first and core subtype. Our second subtype includes children with visual–spatial and executive function difficulties that significantly impact their social functioning. The third subtype is characterized by children with significant visual–spatial and executive function difficulties which are functionally impacting their academic work. The fourth and final subtype is characterized by children with visual–spatial, executive function, social difficulties, and academic deficits, wherein all areas are functionally impaired.

In Chap. 3 Occupational Therapist Rebecca Schatz provides an overview of assessment in the OT field. She covers how the information would go into a report, be presented to parents and educators, and would serve to develop an OT treatment plan. When assessing children with NVLD, there are a number of different areas that require evaluation before an appropriate treatment plan can be determined. As part of the assessment process, an occupational therapist utilizes motor skills assessments, handwriting and visual motor evaluations, sensory processing, visual processing, and clinical observations (Bowyer & Cahill, 2009). She introduces many of the assessment tools that may be included in the evaluation process and emphasizes the most important areas to include in the report: test results, interpretation, intervention plan consisting of goals for home and school, classroom accommodations, and reevaluation. Finally she discusses treatment intervention for the following areas: gross motor skills development, fine motor skills development, handwriting, sensory processing, and social skills development, especially as they pertained to any evidence-based interventions that were included.

In Chap. 4 Speech and Language Therapist Joanne Volden, Ph.D., explores the communicative characteristics associated with NVLD specifically language form: phonology, morphology, syntax, semantics, and pragmatics. Dr. Volden examines areas of overlap with other diagnostic categories, in particular Asperger's disorder (ASD), and suggests that guidance in terms of assessment and potentially effective intervention may cautiously be taken from the research evidence that has amassed around ASD. She also emphasizes how the pragmatics area is most often impacted for children with NVLD, and recommends the use of the CCC-2 as a useful assessment instrument to document the presence of pragmatic communication disorder.

In Chap. 5 Psychologists John M. Davis, Ph.D., and Jessica Broitman, Ph.D., (coeditors) address the role of a comprehensive psychoeducational and/or neuropsychological assessment in the identification of the issues that need to be better understood and addressed for students with NVLD. We provide a model for approaching this assessment as well as a table of tools that can be utilized. We explain how our subtyping model can help drive the assessment process and aid in understanding the student's difficulties. Finally a brief case is presented to illustrate some of the difficulties inherent in diagnosing this disorder.

In Chap. 6 Pediatric Neurologist Meryl Lipton, M.D., covers the role of medical personnel who deal with developmental disorders, and how these professionals may encounter and work with children with NVLD and their parents. She uses this chapter to address the following questions she believes are pertinent to the medical profession:

1. What are the NVLD characteristics that prompt a referral to a physician?
2. What are the developmental NVLD milestones families and professionals should know about?
3. What types of physicians are most likely to be skilled in caring for patients with NVLD?
4. Why aren't some doctors able to provide what these children need?
5. How can parents and professionals partner with their physicians to create the best outcomes?
6. What medications might be useful for which symptoms?
7. What is a clinical model of physician as case manager and what are some case histories that can highlight important issues including the role of medication in treatment?

The topic of whether any medications may be useful for the client and how the developmental pediatrician goes about thinking about the issues to help make those decisions is explored through case studies.

In Chap. 7 Dr. Catherine Brown and Bridget Leary discussed the role of the coach, and what services parents, teachers, and professionals working with a child with NVLD in pre-K-12 may need to consider for future academic and social success. We believe this to be a particularly important chapter, as "coaching" is becoming a more accepted approach to working with students with NVLD.

They begin by pointing out that the primary focus for many school evaluations is to determine eligibility for special education. That being determined, school-based professionals often include recommendations for treatment or accommodations like waivers for or time extensions for testing, course substitutions, modifications to course content, and para-educator assistance in the classroom should the student meet criteria for special education. Other recommendations may also include transportation, counseling, and physical, occupational, and speech therapy (see Chap. 5 for more types of interventions). Often, other psychosocial issues and executive functioning issues are associated with students with NVLD. These issues most often include comorbid diagnoses and delayed development of social and independent living skills. We suggest that additional non-mandated social supports outside of the school setting such as the use of "coaches" or tutors might better prepare children with NVLD for positive psychosocial outcomes in various environments.

In Chap. 8 Marion Marshall, M.S., BCET, FAET, discusses the role of the educational therapist and presents academic interventions for reading and writing for students with NVLD. Her chapter has three main foci: first is an introduction and overview of what an educational therapist does, the second includes specific recommendations for treatment of reading comprehension disorders, and finally there are recommendations for treatment of written expression disorders. The recommendations cited are evidence-based whenever possible. Teaching essential skills, such as summarization and notetaking, is discussed in detail in this chapter. Ms. Marshall warns that multisensory methodologies may not be best practice, as they may cognitively overload some students with NVLD. She emphasizes that one should reduce, eliminate, or *narrate* visual elements, much as if you had to modify a learning task for a student with low vision. She also suggests that techniques that support reading comprehension also improve writing; hence *cross training* can be highly effective. She concludes with the notion that an educational therapist can be an effective educator for the student with NVLD.

In Chap. 9 Dianne Matthaei, M. Ed., Educational Therapist, specifically addresses how to teach and how to remediate math difficulties with the children who have NVLD. She explains how the characteristics of a child with NVLD can interfere with learning math, offering principles for mathematics instruction for students with NVLD. She describes the importance of learning the *vocabulary* of mathematics, the *procedures* of mathematics, and the *major concepts* of mathematics. Ms. Matthaei offered three main principles of effective instruction:

- Instruction must involve several important components including number sense, counting skills, math vocabulary, procedural skills, conceptual skills, fluency with number combinations (math facts), and skills for solving word problems.
- Instruction needs to follow the progression of learning by first starting at the three-dimensional, concrete level before moving on the two-dimensional level with pictures, diagrams, workbooks, and textbooks.
- Instruction must be specifically matched to the learning strengths as well as core deficits inherent to the profile of the individual with NVLD.

She shows how with support students with NVLD can become more competent at mathematics and achieve their learning goals.

In Chap. 10 Psychologist and Social Skills Specialist Bernadette Evans, Ph.D., provides an overview of the socio-emotional learning needs of children with NVLD from two complementary theoretical perspectives, neurodevelopmental behavioral (Lipton & Evans-Smith, 2006; Lipton & Nowicki, 2009; Siegel, 1999; Stern, 2000) and interpersonal neurobiology (Palombo, Bendicsen, & Koch, 2011; Schore, 2003, 2005; Siegel, 1999). Primary psychotherapeutic approaches that address these socio-emotional needs are described along with a way to conceptualize their integration in therapy. These approaches include cognitive–behavioral therapy (CBT), dialectical behavior therapy (DBT), control mastery theory (CMT), mindfulness, relaxation, relational, and systemic interventions. Studies assessing peer group interventions in particular are also reviewed, with a special emphasis on the Intervention-Social Emotional Learning Framework (I-SELF). A pilot study based on the I-SELF model's theoretical framework for assessing and treating children with socio-emotional learning challenges such as those with NVLD is presented in detail.

In Chap. 11 Licensed Educational Psychologist Jane McClure MA/LEP writes about the role of a college counselor, and the process of helping young adults with NVLD find their best fit for college. She explores the variety of challenges facing the college-bound student with NVLD and his or her family. This includes the typical academic and social issues of students with NVLD, and academic and social interventions and accommodations for college-bound and college-transitioning students with NVLD. In addition she offers an overview of relevant laws, and describes a model for how to think about the differing levels of support provided by colleges for students with NVLD. She identifies the crucial issues to be considered and discusses the application process including considerations regarding disclosure. Ms. McClure also discusses the role of a counselor in K-12 placement decisions including private school versus public schools and homeschooling. Lastly, Ms. McClure presents a case study illustrating this kind of work with a student with NVLD and her family.

In Chap. 12 Psychologist Catherine Brown and Bridget Leary address the issues that children with NVLD face as they transition from high school to college. Students with NVLD that qualify under ADA will receive mandated accommodations from a case counselor (usually associated with a disability resource center) who is designated to review documentation of students with NVLD and other disabilities. The counselor's primary focus is to determine academic accommodations needed to provide the student with equal access to the curriculum as mandated by law, such as extra time on tests, note takers in the classroom, etc. However, these counselors must also be aware of other psychosocial issues associated with students with NVLD. These issues most often include comorbid diagnoses, delayed development of social and independent living skills, and significant deficits in executive functioning. Therefore, some students with specific types of NVLD are forced to use non-mandated supports in college to address these psychosocial issues.

In Chap. 13 Psychologist and Vocational Specialist Lynn C. Koch, Ph.D., reviews post-high school vocational services for those students with NVLD who are not college bound. She outlines an overview of the kinds of services a vocational rehabilitation counselor and workforce specialist can provide. Dr. Koch informs how the state/federal vocational rehabilitation (VR) program can be a resource for individuals with NVLD who qualify for assistance by helping to overcome the many barriers to meaningful employment that she discusses. Dr. Koch also describes the vocational implications of NVLD, provides an overview of the federal–state vocational rehabilitation (VR) programs, and examines the VR process and specific VR services that could benefit individuals with NVLD in terms of maximizing their vocational potential and achieving their self-determined employment goals.

In Chap. 14 Neuropsychologist Margaret Semrud-Clikeman, Ph.D., and Dr. Jennifer Wheeler Maedgen cover the role of the pediatric neuropsychologist as an advocate in the treatment of NVLD. Dr. Semrud-Clikeman familiarizes neuropsychologists with the four major pieces of legislation which directly affect the provision of services to people with physical, cognitive, and mental health disabilities laws and affect the provision of accommodations in the secondary and postsecondary settings. She discusses their scope and purposes, and how related legislation has been interpreted by the courts and educational institutions. She reviews issues related to the transition from high school to college, and how these affect neuropsychologists who are working with incoming college students. She offers practical strategies relating to how clinicians can best work with school personnel and clients in secondary and postsecondary settings, and how to best utilize the framework of

IDEA, Section 504, and the ADA/ADAAA to obtain appropriate services. However, the laws governing accommodations in higher education are continually changing and one must consult the university in which you are interested for the latest rules and regulations and/or how that specific university is implementing them. See for example: the Association of Higher Education and Disability site 2011 paper on Supporting Accommodation Requests: Guidance on Documentation Practices (http:/www.ahead.org/resources/documentation_guidance). Lastly Dr. Semrud-Clikeman discusses why neuropsychologists, by virtue of their training, may be especially well suited to perform disability and education-related evaluations.

In Chap. 15 Research Psychologist Jodene Fine, Ph.D., offers an update on the ongoing research on children, adolescents, and adults with NVLD. She describes how NVLD research tends to be divided between neurological/medical explorations into the white matter model and research addressing the learning and psychosocial characteristics of children with nonverbal learning problems. Dr. Fine writes about how the literature as a whole evolved, explaining that NVLD has been conceptualized from many different perspectives: clinical, medical, and academic. She then provides some guidelines about how one might assess the utility of available research articles. She notes that the body of research has ranged widely in terms of how study samples have been defined, as well as the instruments used to measure the characteristics of this population. Because of this, Fine cautions that clinicians are wise to give thought as to how our conceptions about NVLD have evolved. When looking to the literature, she suggests careful consideration about how an NVLD group was defined for a study, and whether the findings can be reasonably applied to the population with which you are working. Finally, Fine offers some of the more reliable findings in the literature, and raises some still unresolved questions.

In Chap. 16 Brett Mills offers his personal account of growing up with NVLD (he was previously heard from in the afterword in our last book). This chapter includes some of the most important things parents/educators must know about dealing with a child with NVLD from the perceptive of a young adult with NVLD and his family. His parents offer their insights as well.

We close this chapter with questions regarding the future of how NVLD will be conceptualized and researched. There remains a considerable controversy regarding the relationship, or lack thereof, between NVLD and Asperger's disorder (AS). Some, for example, postulate that they are virtually the same disorder assessed by two different systems, psychiatric evaluations and neuropsychological evaluations, respectively (Klin, Volkmar, Sparrow, Cicchetti, & Rourke, 1995; Volkmar & Klin, 1998). However, other researchers believe that AS should be identified as a high-functioning autism (Lord & Spence, 2006; Schopler, 1996), as part of the pervasive developmental disorder spectrum (Szatmari, 1998), or as schizoid–schizotypal disorders (Wolff, 1995). In addition there is considerable symptom overlap between NVLD and attention deficit hyperactivity disorder (ADHD).

In our first book (Davis & Broitman, 2011) we reviewed both the research and clinical data, looking at the evidence and arguments about whether AS and NVLD are actually the same disorder from two differing perspectives: psychiatric and neuropsychological. We found that one of the major problems with the research in this area is the lack of consistent inclusion criteria for selection for the clinical groups (see for instance Fine, Semrud-Clikeman, Bledsoe, & Hasson's meta-analysis of NVLD research, 2010). It seems clear that the question of the relation between children with NVLD and children with AS needs additional research. Future studies that attempt to understand any similarities or differences between AS and NVLD might investigate a variety of cognitive, affective, behavioral, and social differences. Centers currently working on this include the University of Padua in Italy, Rush Neurobehavioral Center in Chicago, the Center for Neurodevelopment Studies at Michigan State University, and the Pediatric Behavioral Neuroscience Center at the University of Minnesota Medical School. We believe these diagnostic concerns are important not just for the sake of diagnosis, but because they may help us understand how to develop the most appropriate interventions.

We currently believe that it is necessary to view NVLD from two different vantage points—the clinical vantage point, which is addressed by our subtype model, and the research vantage point, which Dr. Fine writes about in Chap. 15. The clinical model functions as a heuristic tool that enables the clinician to assess, investigate, and understand the processes most often impacted for children with NVLD. As pointed out by Dr. Fine, the clinician needs to be guided as best as they can by the available research data on NVLD. We have tried to follow this advice.

Unfortunately clinical models are currently too complex for research purposes. As Dr. Fine and others have pointed out, most studies on children and adolescents with NVLD have very few subjects. NVLD is a relatively low-incidence disorder, so gathering enough subjects is a daunting task. For that reason, most researchers in this area agree that at some point in time a multisite study, much like the NIMH Multimodal Treatment of ADHD Jensen et al. (2001), will be needed to provide the number of subjects necessary for more generalizable research. Gaining agreement on the selection criteria for these studies may prove difficult, but it is essential for progress to be made.

To conclude, this book concentrates on two primary points. The first is to emphasize that a team approach is needed for the treatment of NVLD. The team functions best when there is a designated team leader who can manage the advocacy and treatment plans needed for the child. This leader can be the child's parent or any of the participating professionals. The leader is likely to change over the course of the child's or even adult's lifetime. The crucial concern is not who serves as team leader, but rather that the leader is a person who the family can trust, work and communicate well with, and who can establish a similar relationship with the other professionals on the team. Secondly, we provide information to all professionals about how colleagues from different trainings and perspectives understand NVLD, and what types of interventions they can provide for the child and family. We hope that this book provides a guide to, and overview of, the understanding and work needed to best serve children with NVLD.

References

Association of Higher Education and Disability. (2011). Supporting Accommodation Requests: Guidance on Documentation Practices. Retrieved April 2012 from http:/www.ahead.org/resources/documentation_guidance.

Bowyer, P., & Cahill, S. (2009). *Pediatric occupational therapy handbook*. St. Louis, MO: Mosby.

Davis, J. M., & Broitman, J. (2011). *Nonverbal learning disability in children: Bridging the gap between science and practice*. New York: Springer.

Fine, J. G., Semrud-Clikeman, M., Bledsoe, J., & Hasson, R. (2010). *Meta-analysis of the NVLD empirical literature: Scientific rigor of extant research*. San Diego, CA: American Psychological Association Annual Meeting.

Jensen, P. S., Hinshaw, S. P., Swanson, J. M., Greenhill, L. L., Conners, C. K., Arnold, L. E., et al. (2001). Findings from the NIMH multimodal treatment study of ADHD (MTA): Implications and applications for primary care providers. *Developmental and Behavioral Pediatrics., 22*(1), 60–73.

Klin, A., Sparrow, S. S., Volkmar, F., Cicchetti, D. V., & Rourke, B. P. (1995). Asperger syndrome. In B. P. Rourke (Ed.), *Syndrome of nonverbal learning disabilities: Neurodevelopmental manifestations* (pp. 93–118). New York: Guilford Press.

Lipton, M., & Evans-Smith, B. (2006, August). *Social emotional learning framework (SELF): Conceptual, clinical, and research aspects*. Davis, CA: The summer institute on neurodevelopmental disorders, MIND Institute, University of California.

Lipton, M., & Nowicki, S. (2009). The social emotional learning framework (SELF): A guide for understanding brain-based social emotional learning impairments. Journal of Developmental Processes, 4(2), 99–115.

Lord, C., & Spence, S. J. (2006). Autism spectrum disorders: Phenotype and diagnosis. In S. O. Moldin & J. L. R. Rubenstein (Eds.), *Understanding autism: From basic neuroscience to treatment* (pp. 1–23). Boca Raton, FL: CRC Press.

Ozols, E. J., & Rourke, B. P. (1988). Characteristics of young learning-disabled children classified according to patterns of academic achievement: Auditory-perceptual and visual-perceptual abilities. *Journal of Clinical Child Psychology, 17*, 44–52.

Palombo, J., Bendicsen, H., & Koch, B. (2011). *Guide to psychoanalytic developmental theories*. USA: Springer.

Schopler, E. (1996). Are autism and Asperger syndrome different labels or different disabilities? *Journal of Autism and Developmental Disorders, 26*, 109–110.

Schore, A. (2003). *Affect dysregulation and disorders of the self*. NY: Norton.

Schore, A. (2005). Attachment, affect regulation, and the developing right brain: Linking developmental neuroscience to pediatrics. *Pediatrics in Review, 26*(6), 204–217.

Segal, Z., Williams, J., & Teasdale, J. (2002). *Mindfulness-based cognitive therapy for depression: A new approach to preventing relapse*. NY: Guilford.

Siegel, D. (1999). The developing mind: How relationships and the brain interact to shape who we are. NY: Guilford.

Stern, D. (2000). *The interpersonal world of the infant: A view from psychoanalysis and developmental psychology*. New York: Basic Books.

Szatmari, P. (1998). Differential diagnosis of Asperger disorder. In E. Schopler, G. B. Mesibov, & L. J. Kunce (Eds.), *Asperger syndrome or high-functioning autism?* (pp. 61–76). New York: Plenum.

Volkmar, F. R., & Klin, A. (1998). Asperger syndrome and nonverbal learning disabilities. In E. Schopler, G. B. Mesibov, & L. J. Kunce (Eds.), *Asperger syndrome or high-functioning autism? Current issues in autism* (pp. 107–121). New York: Plenum.

Wolff, S. (1995). *Loners: The life path of unusual children*. London: Routledge.

Appendix

The following is a list of potentially useful Web sites. *The authors do not endorse or recommend any of them but offer the list as a resource.*

504 PLAN INFORMATION	http://www.burltwpsch.org/
ADVOCACY	http://www.conductdisorders.com
American Hyperlexia Association	http://www.hyperlexia.org
American Speech-Language-Hearing Association (ASHA)	http://www.asha.org
Anxiety Disorders Association of America (ADAA)	http://www.asha.org
ANXIETY	http://www.nimh.nih.gov/anxiety
ASPEN	http://www.AspenNJ.org
Asperger's	http://www.asperger.org/
Assistive Technology and LD	http://www.ldresources.com
ASSISTIVE TECHNOLOGY	http://www.assistivetech.com
Association on Higher Education and Disability (AHEAD)	http://www.ahead.org
Association on Higher Education and Disability (AHEAD)	http://www.ahead.org/resources/documentation_guidance
BOOKS ON TAPE TALKING BOOK LIBRARY—California	http://www.library.ca.gov/html/pubser05.html
BOOKS ON TAPE: RECORDING FOR THE BLIND AND DYSLEXIC	http://www.rfbd.org/
Brain Connection	http://www.brainconnection.com
Center for Speech and Language Disorders	http://www.csld.org
Central Auditory Processing Disorder CAPD	http://kidshealth.org/parent/healthy/central_auditory.html
Children and Adults with Attention Deficit/Hyperactivity Disorder (CHADD)	http://www.chadd.org
CHILDREN WITH SPINA BIFIDA, A RESOURCE PAGE FOR PARENTS	http://www.waisman.wisc.edu/~rowley/sb-kids/
CONDUCT DISORDERS	http://www.conductdisorders.com/

(continued)

J. Broitman and J.M. Davis (eds.), *Treating NVLD in Children: Professional Collaborations for Positive Outcomes*, DOI 10.1007/978-1-4614-6179-1,

CONSORTIUM FOR CITIZENS WITH DISABILITIES	http://www.c-c-d.org/
Council for Learning Disabilities	http://www.cldinternational.org
Council of Parent Attorneys and Advocates	http://www.copaa.net
DUTCH NLD SITE	http://www.geocities.com/Athens/Academy/1644/
DYSPRAXIA ARTICLE	http://www.allhealth.com/childrens/qa/0,4801,1620_121375,00.html
DYSPRAXIA FOUNDATION	http://www.emmbrook.demon.co.uk/dysprax/homepage.htm
Educational Resources Information Center (ERIC)	http://www.eric.ed.gov
Educational Therapy's Web site	http://www.edtherapy.com/students/htm
EXCELLENT LITERATURE, HOMEWORK INFORMATION	http://www.embracingthechild.com (*look in the tutor section for literature*)
FACTS FOR FAMILIES…ABOUT PSYCHIATRIC DISORDERS AFFECTING CHILDREN AND ADULTS	http://www.aacap.org/web/aacap/factsFam/
Free Advocacy for Parents	http://www.amicusforchildren.org
Gifted and LD	http://www.uniquelygifted.org
Gifted and LD	http://www.uniquelygifted.org
Good Basic Information + Self Advocacy info	http://www.LDinfo.com
HANDWRITING	http://www.BFHhandwriting.com
HOAGIES' GIFTED EDUCATION PAGE	http://www.hoagiesgifted.org/
HYPERLEXIA	http://www.hyperlexia.org/
IDEA Information	http://www.ideapractices.org/docs/ideadepot/userguide.htm#guidepurpose
IEP Information	http://www.cesa7.k12.wi.us/sped/
IEP Information	http://www.awesomelibrary.org/Library/Special_Education/Individualized_Education_Plans/Individualized_Education_Plans.html
IEP/advocacy INFORMATION	http://www.wrightslaw.com
Interactive Metronome	http://www.interactivemetronome.com/
ISER—internet special education resources	http://www.iser.com
LD On Line	http://www.ldonline.org/
LD ON LINE SOCIAL SKILLS WITH RICK LAVOIE	http://ldonline.org/ld_indepth/social_skills/lavoie_quest.html
LD Online	http://www.ldonline.org
LD PRIDE ONLINE	http://www.ldpride.net
LEARNING DISABILITIES ASSOCIATION OF AMERICA	http://www.ldanatl.org
LEARNING DISABILITIES ASSOCIATION OF AMERICA, CALIFORNIA	http://www.ldaca.org
Lisa Marti's Nonverbal Learning Disability Cyber Advocacy and Support Group	http://www.geocities.com/Athens/Pantheon/3433
LITERATURE, HOMEWORK INFORMATION	http://www.embracingthechild.com (*look in the tutor section for literature*)
Margaret Kay, Ph.D.	http://www.margaretkay.com
MATRIX	http://www.matrixparents.org/faq.html

(continued)

MIND STEPS CAREER SOFTWARE	http://www.mind-steps.com
Misunderstood Minds	http://www.pbs.org/misunderstoodminds
NATIONAL CENTER FOR LEARNING DISABILITIES	http://www.ncld.org
NATIONAL INFORMATION CENTER FOR CHILDREN/YOUTH WITH DISABILITIES	http://www.nichcy.org/
NATIONAL INSTITUTE OF NEUROLOGICAL DISORDERS & STROKE	http://www.ninds.nih.gov/
Nerd World	http://www.nerdworld.com
NLD ARTICLES	http://www.laran.waisman.wisc.edu/fv/www/lib_nvld.html#Articles
NLD On the Web	http://www.nldontheweb.org/
NLDA	http://www.nlda.org
NLDA, Nonverbal Learning Disorders Association	NLDResources@aol.com, http://www.nlda.org/
NLDline	http://www.nlda.org/
NLDontheweb.org	http://www.NLDontheweb.org/
Nonverbal Dictionary (Center for Nonverbal Studies)	http://members.aol.com/nonverbal2/index.htm
NOONAN SYNDROME	http://noonansyndrome.org
OASIS	http://www.udel.edu/bkirby/asperger/
Obsessive Compulsive Disorder (OCD)	http://www.ocdawareness.com/
Online Asperger Syndrome Information and Support (O.A.S.I.S.)	http://www.udel.edu/bkirby/asperger
OUT-OF-SYNC CHILD WEBPAGE	http://www.comeunity.com/disability/sensory_integration/bksync.html
PARENT TO PARENT SUPPORT	http://www.NPPSIS.org
PARENTS AND EDUCATORS RESOURCE CENTER	http://www.perc-schwabfdn.org
Parents of Gifted/Learning Disabled Children	http://www.geocities.com/Athens/1105/gtld.html
Pathways to Technology	http://pathwaystotechnology.org
Recording for the Blind & Dyslexic (RFB&D)	http://www.rfbd.org
Rondalyn Whitney's Web site	http://www.thelighthouseproject.com
Rush Neurobehavioral Center	http://www.rush.edu/rnbc
SENSORY INTEGRATION RESOURCE NETWORK	http://www.sinetwork.org/
SOS-Executive Function	http://www.sos4students.com
Special Ed Advocacy	http://www.reedmartin.com/
Special Ed Links	http://alpha.fdu.edu/~dumont/extended_links.htm
Special Ed News (updated weekly)	http://www.specialednews.com/
Special Needs online Newsletter	Subscribe: special-needs-books-subscribe@onelist.com, http://home.freeuk.net/theadhdgazette
SPEECH AND LANGUAGE SOFTWARE	http://www.locutour.com/
Spirited Kids Family Resource Center	http://www.network54.com/Realm/Spirited_Kids
Stern Center for Language and Learning	http://www.sterncenter.org

(continued)

STERN CENTER, WILLISTON, VERMONT	http://www.sterncenter.org
Struggling Teens	http://www.strugglingteens.com/
TAWK	http://www.nldsupport.org.
TERA KIRK: (an NLD teenager's great Web site)	http://www.geocities.com/HotSprings/Spa/7262
TONY ATTWOOD	http://www.tonyattwood.com
Web site for Learning Disabilities	http://www.abilityhub.com
Wrightslaw	http://www.wrightslaw.com
Yale Study	http://www.info.med.yale.edu/chldstdy/research.htm

Alternative Methods / Interventions / Programs

(*not tested or recommended by authors!!*)

http://icdl.com/forparentsbyparents/sensoryprocessing/sensorycontent.htm

Dalcroze Eurhythmics (http://www.dalcrozeusa.org/) uses movement and music, rhythmic responses, and social integration.

NeuroNet (http://www.neuronetonline.com/pro.php) a lot of balancing, following a rhythm (we use metronome), throwing, catching, counting, naming, visual tracing, controlling body movements—and integrating of all of the above.

The Alexander Technique (www.alexandertechnique.com)

Yoga and a class at the local gym called Neuro-muscular Integrative Action (NIA; http://www.nia-nia.com/) which is a form of low impact aerobics, dance and martial arts balance exercises.

Improv workshops

EMDR (Eye Movement Desensitization and Reprocessing; http://www.emdr.com/) and BIOLATERAL TAPES (http://www.biolateral.com/products.htm)

Balametrics (http://www.balametrics.com/)

Interactive Metronome (http://www.interactivemetronome.com/home/index.asp)

Juggling (http://news.bbc.co.uk/1/hi/health/3417045.stm)

Brain Gym (http://www.braingym.org/)

Sensory Learning (http://www.sensorylearning.com/)—Bolles Method The treatment retrains the brain to coordinate and send information from mind to body.

http://www.neuroacoustics.com/

http://www.mentalskills.com

Neurobiofeedback (http://www.nldline.com/neurobiofeedback.htm)

Index

J. Broitman and J.M. Davis (eds.), *Treating NVLD in Children: Professional Collaborations for Positive Outcomes*, DOI 10.1007/978-1-4614-6179-1,

F

G

H

I

J

L